RN

Expert
Guides

Respiratory
Care

Wolters Kluwer | Lippincott Williams & Wilkins
Health

Philadelphia · Baltimore · New York · London
Buenos Aires · Hong Kong · Sydney · Tokyo

STAFF

EXECUTIVE PUBLISHER
Judith A. Schilling McCann, RN, MSN

EDITORIAL DIRECTOR
H. Nancy Holmes

CLINICAL DIRECTOR
Joan M. Robinson, RN, MSN

ART DIRECTOR
Elaine Kasmer

EDITORIAL PROJECT MANAGER
Ann E. Houska

CLINICAL PROJECT MANAGER
Beverly Ann Tscheschlog, RN, BS

EDITORS
Rita Doyle,
Jennifer Dellarossa Kowalak

COPY EDITORS
Kimberly Bilotta (supervisor),
Tom DeZego, Amy Furman,
Liz Mooney, Dorothy P. Terry,
Pamela Wingrod

DESIGNERS
Debra Moloshok

DIGITAL COMPOSITION SERVICES
Diane Paluba (manager),
Joyce Rossi Biletz, Donna S. Morris

ASSOCIATE MANUFACTURING MANAGER
Beth J. Welsh

EDITORIAL ASSISTANTS
Karen J. Kirk, Jeri O'Shea,
Linda K. Ruhf

INDEXER
Barbara Hodgson

The clinical treatments described and recommended in this publication are based on research and consultation with nursing, medical, and legal authorities. To the best of our knowledge, these procedures reflect currently accepted practice. Nevertheless, they can't be considered absolute and universal recommendations. For individual applications, all recommendations must be considered in light of the patient's clinical condition and, before administration of new or infrequently used drugs, in light of the latest package-insert information. The authors and publisher disclaim any responsibility for any adverse effects resulting from the suggested procedures, from any undetected errors, or from the reader's misunderstanding of the text.

RNERESP010707

**Library of Congress
Cataloging-in-Publication Data**

RN expert guides. Respiratory care.
   p. ; cm.
  Includes bibliographical references and index.
  1. Respiratory organs—Diseases—Nursing—Handbooks, manuals, etc. I. Lippincott Williams & Wilkins. II. Title: Respiratory care.
  [DNLM: 1. Respiratory Tract Diseases—nursing. 2. Nursing Care—methods. WY 163 R627 2008]
   RC735.5.R62 2008
   616.2'004231—dc22
ISBN-13: 978-1-58255-707-6 (alk. paper)
ISBN-10: 1-58255-707-1 (alk. paper)
             2007012522

Contents

Contributors and consultants

Ruth A. Chaplen, RN, MSN, APRN-BC, AOCN
Clinical Instructor
Wayne State University College of Nursing
Nurse Practitioner
Karmanos Cancer Institute
Detroit

Karen Demzien-Connors, RN, MSN
Faculty
Central New Mexico Community College
Albuquerque

Shelba Durston, RN, MSN, CCRN
Nursing Instructor
San Joaquin Delta College
Stockton, Calif.

JoAnn C. Green, RN, MSN, CCRN
Consultant
Riverview, Fla.

Kenneth Hazell, PhD[C], MSN, ARNP
Nursing Program Director
Keiser University
Ft. Lauderdale

Jennifer M. Lee, MSN, FNP-C, CCRN
Nurse Practitioner
Greenville (S.C.) Hospital System–Pulmonary Disease Associates

Lynda A. Mackin, PhD [C], APRN,BC, CNS, ANP
Associate Clinical Professor
University of California, San Francisco, School of Nursing

Cecilia Jane Maier, RN, MS, CCRN
Assistant Professor
Mount Carmel College of Nursing
Columbus, Ohio

Dana Reeves, RN, MSN
Assistant Professor
University of Arkansas
Fort Smith

Anatomy and physiology

The respiratory system includes the airways, lungs, bony thorax, and respiratory muscles. These structures and the central nervous system work together to deliver oxygen to the bloodstream and remove excess carbon dioxide from the body.

RESPIRATORY ANATOMY

Knowing the basic anatomy of the respiratory system will help you perform a comprehensive respiratory assessment and recognize any abnormalities. (See *Structures of the respiratory system,* page 2.)

Airways and lungs

The airways are divided into the upper and lower airways. The upper airways include the nasopharynx (nose), oropharynx (mouth), laryngopharynx, and larynx. Their purpose is to warm, filter, and humidify inhaled air. They also help to make sound and send air to the lower airways.

The epiglottis is a flap of tissue that closes over the top of the larynx when the patient swallows. It protects the patient from aspirating food or fluid into the lower airways. The larynx is located at the top of the trachea and houses the vocal cords. It's the transition point between the upper and lower airways.

The lower airways begin with the trachea, which then divides into the right and left mainstem bronchial tubes. The bronchial tubes divide into bronchi, which are lined with mucus-producing ciliated epithelium, one of the lungs' major defense systems.

STRUCTURES OF THE RESPIRATORY SYSTEM

The major structures of the upper and lower airways are illustrated below.

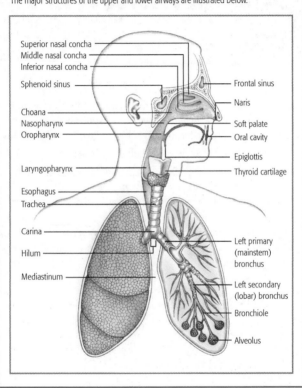

The bronchi then divide into secondary bronchi, tertiary bronchi, terminal bronchioles, respiratory bronchioles, alveolar ducts and, finally, alveoli, the gas-exchange units of the lungs. The lungs in an adult typically contain about 300 million alveoli.

Each lung is wrapped in a lining called the *visceral pleura*. The right lung is larger and has three lobes: upper, middle, and lower. The left lung is smaller and has only an upper and a lower lobe. The lungs share space in the thoracic cavity with the heart and great vessels, the trachea, the esophagus, and the bronchi. All areas of the thoracic cavity that come in contact with the lungs are lined with *parietal pleura*.

A small amount of fluid fills the area between the two layers of the pleura. That fluid, called *pleural fluid,* allows the layers of the pleura to slide smoothly over one another as the chest expands and contracts. The parietal pleura also contains nerve endings that emit pain signals when inflammation occurs.

Thorax

Composed of bone and cartilage, the thoracic cage supports and protects the lungs. The vertebral column and 12 pairs of ribs form the posterior portion of the thoracic cage. The ribs, the major portion of the thoracic cage, extend from the thoracic vertebrae toward the anterior thorax. Along with the vertebrae, they support and protect the thorax, permitting the lungs to expand and contract. The vertebrae and ribs are numbered from top to bottom. Posteriorly, certain landmarks are used to help identify specific vertebrae. In 90% of people, the seventh cervical vertebra (C7) is the most prominent vertebra on a flexed neck; for the remaining 10%, it's the first thoracic vertebra (T1). Thus, to locate a specific vertebra, count along the vertebrae from C7 or T1. (See *Respiratory assessment landmarks*, page 4.)

The manubrium, sternum, xiphoid process, and ribs form the anterior thoracic cage, which has the additional duty of protecting the mediastinal organs that lie between the right and left pleural cavities. Ribs 1 through 7 attach directly to the sternum; ribs 8 through 10 attach to the cartilage of the preceding rib. The other two pairs of ribs are "free floating"; they don't attach to any part of the anterior thoracic cage. Rib 11 ends anterolaterally and rib 12 ends laterally. The lower parts of the rib cage (the costal margins) near the xiphoid process form the borders of the costal angle—an angle of about 90 degrees normally.

Above the anterior thorax is a depression called the *suprasternal notch*. Because this notch isn't covered by the rib cage like the rest of the thorax, it allows you to palpate the trachea and check aortic pulsation.

RESPIRATORY ASSESSMENT LANDMARKS

The common landmarks used in respiratory assessment are illustrated below.

ANTERIOR VIEW

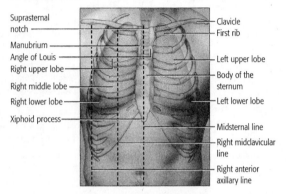

- Suprasternal notch
- Manubrium
- Angle of Louis
- Right upper lobe
- Right middle lobe
- Right lower lobe
- Xiphoid process
- Clavicle
- First rib
- Left upper lobe
- Body of the sternum
- Left lower lobe
- Midsternal line
- Right midclavicular line
- Right anterior axillary line

POSTERIOR VIEW

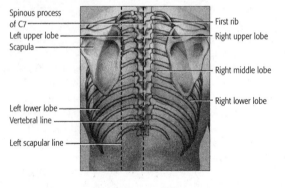

- Spinous process of C7
- Left upper lobe
- Scapula
- Left lower lobe
- Vertebral line
- Left scapular line
- First rib
- Right upper lobe
- Right middle lobe
- Right lower lobe

THE MECHANICS OF BREATHING

These illustrations show how mechanical forces, such as the movement of the diaphragm and intercostal muscles, produce a breath. A plus sign (+) indicates positive pressure, and a minus sign (–) indicates negative pressure.

AT REST

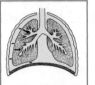

- Inspiratory muscles relax.
- Atmospheric pressure is maintained in the tracheobronchial tree.
- No air movement occurs.

INSPIRATION

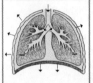

- Inspiratory muscles contract.
- The diaphragm descends.
- Negative alveolar pressure is maintained.
- Air moves into the lungs.

EXPIRATION

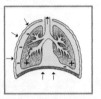

- Inspiratory muscles relax, causing lungs to recoil to their resting size and position.
- The diaphragm ascends.
- Positive alveolar pressure is maintained.
- Air moves out of the lungs.

Respiratory muscles

The diaphragm and the external intercostal muscles are the primary muscles used in breathing. They contract when the patient inhales and relax when the patient exhales.

The respiratory center in the medulla initiates each breath by sending messages to the primary respiratory muscles over the phrenic nerve. Impulses from the phrenic nerve adjust the rate and depth of breathing, depending on the carbon dioxide and pH levels in the cerebrospinal fluid. (See *The mechanics of breathing.*)

Accessory inspiratory muscles, which also assist in breathing, include the trapezius, the sternocleidomastoid, and the scalenes, which combine to elevate the scapula, clavicle, sternum, and upper ribs. That elevation expands the front-to-back diameter of the chest when the diaphragm and intercostal muscles aren't effective.

Expiration occurs when the diaphragm and external intercostal muscles relax. If the patient has an airway obstruction, he may also use the abdominal muscles and internal intercostal muscles to exhale.

RESPIRATORY PHYSIOLOGY

The primary function of the respiratory system is gas exchange, which involves pulmonary circulation, respiration, ventilation, pulmonary perfusion, diffusion, and acid-base balance.

Pulmonary circulation
Oxygen-depleted blood enters the lungs from the pulmonary artery of the right ventricle. It then flows through the main pulmonary arteries into the pleural cavities and the main bronchi, where it continues to flow through progressively smaller vessels until it reaches the single-celled endothelial capillaries serving the alveoli. Here, oxygen and carbon dioxide diffusion takes place. After passing through the pulmonary capillaries, blood flows through progressively larger vessels, enters the main pulmonary veins, and finally flows into the left atrium.

Respiration
Effective respiration requires gas exchange in the lungs through external respiration and in the tissues through internal respiration. Three processes contribute to external respiration:
- ventilation—gas distribution into and out of the pulmonary airways
- pulmonary perfusion—blood flow from the right side of the heart, through the pulmonary circulation, and into the left side of the heart
- diffusion—gas movement from an area of greater to lesser concentration through a semipermeable membrane.

Internal respiration occurs only through diffusion. These processes are vital to maintain adequate oxygenation and acid-base balance.

Ventilation

Adequate ventilation depends on the nervous, musculoskeletal, and pulmonary systems for the requisite lung pressure changes. Dysfunction in any of these systems increases the work of breathing, diminishing its effectiveness.

NERVOUS SYSTEM EFFECTS

Although ventilation is largely involuntary, individuals can control its rate and depth. Involuntary breathing results from neurogenic stimulation of the respiratory center in the medulla and the pons of the brain stem. The medulla controls the rate and depth of respiration; the pons moderates the rhythm of the switch from inspiration to expiration. Specialized neurovascular tissue alters these phases of the breathing process automatically and instantaneously.

When carbon dioxide in the blood diffuses into the cerebrospinal fluid, the respiratory center of the brain stem responds. At the same time, peripheral chemoreceptors in the aortic arch and the bifurcation of the carotid arteries respond to reduced oxygen levels in the blood. Noticeable increases in the carbon dioxide level or declines in the oxygen level trigger the respiratory center of the medulla to start respiration.

MUSCULOSKELETAL EFFECTS

The adult thorax is a flexible structure—its shape can be altered by contracting the chest muscles. The medulla controls ventilation primarily by stimulating contraction of the diaphragm and the external intercostals, the major muscles of breathing. The diaphragm descends to expand the length of the chest cavity, while the external intercostals contract to expand the anteroposterior and lateral chest diameter. These musculoskeletal actions produce changes in intrapulmonary pressure that cause inspiration.

PULMONARY EFFECTS

During inspiration, air flows through the right and left mainstem bronchi into increasingly smaller bronchi; then into bronchioles, alveolar ducts, and alveolar sacs; and finally into the alveolar membrane. Pulmonary effects that can alter airflow distribution include airflow pattern, volume and location of the functional reserve capacity (air retained in the alveoli that prevents their collapse during respiration), amount of intrapulmonary resistance, and presence of lung disease. If disrupted, airflow distribution will follow the path of least resistance. For example, an intrapulmonary obstruction or forced inspiration will cause an uneven distribution of air.

Normal breathing requires active inspiration and passive expiration. Forced breathing, as in patients with emphysema, demands active inspiration and expiration. It activates accessory muscles of respiration, which requires additional oxygen to work, resulting in less efficient ventilation with an increased workload.

Other alterations in airflow, such as changes in compliance (distensibility of the lungs and thorax) and resistance (interference with airflow in the tracheobronchial tree), can also increase oxygen and energy demands and lead to respiratory muscle fatigue.

Pulmonary perfusion

Optimal pulmonary perfusion aids external respiration and promotes efficient alveolar gas exchange. However, factors that reduce blood flow, such as a cardiac output that's less than average (5 L/minute) and elevated pulmonary and systemic vascular resistance, can interfere with gas transport to the alveoli. Also, abnormal or insufficient hemoglobin picks up less oxygen than is needed for efficient gas exchange. (See *Exchanging gases.*)

Gravity can affect oxygen and carbon dioxide transport by influencing pulmonary circulation. Gravity pulls more unoxygenated blood to the lower and middle lung lobes than to the upper lobes, where most of the tidal volume also flows. As a result, neither ventilation nor perfusion is uniform throughout the lungs. Areas of the lung where perfusion and ventilation are similar have good ventilation-perfusion matching. In such areas, gas exchange is most efficient. Areas of the lung that demonstrate ventilation-perfusion inequality result in less-efficient gas exchange. (See *What happens in ventilation-perfusion mismatch*, pages 10 and 11.)

Diffusion

In diffusion, molecules of oxygen and carbon dioxide move between the alveoli and the capillaries. Partial pressure—the pressure exerted by one gas in a mixture of gases—dictates the direction of movement, which is always from an area of greater concentration to one of lesser concentration. During diffusion, oxygen moves across the alveolar and capillary membranes, then dissolves in the plasma and passes through the red blood cell (RBC) membrane. Carbon dioxide moves in the opposite direction.

Successful diffusion requires an intact alveolocapillary membrane. Both the alveolar epithelium and the capillary endotheli-

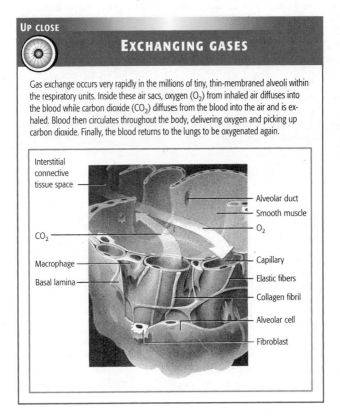

UP CLOSE

EXCHANGING GASES

Gas exchange occurs very rapidly in the millions of tiny, thin-membraned alveoli within the respiratory units. Inside these air sacs, oxygen (O_2) from inhaled air diffuses into the blood while carbon dioxide (CO_2) diffuses from the blood into the air and is exhaled. Blood then circulates throughout the body, delivering oxygen and picking up carbon dioxide. Finally, the blood returns to the lungs to be oxygenated again.

Interstitial connective tissue space

Alveolar duct

Smooth muscle

O_2

CO_2

Capillary

Macrophage

Elastic fibers

Basal lamina

Collagen fibril

Alveolar cell

Fibroblast

WHAT HAPPENS IN VENTILATION-PERFUSION MISMATCH

Effective gas exchange depends on the ventilation and perfusion ($\dot{V}/\dot{Q}$) ratio. The diagrams shown here demonstrate what happens when the $\dot{V}/\dot{Q}$ ratio is normal and abnormal.

Normal ventilation and perfusion

When $\dot{V}/\dot{Q}$ are matched, unoxygenated blood from the venous system returns to the right ventricle through the pulmonary artery to the lungs, carrying carbon dioxide (CO_2). The arteries branch into the alveolar capillaries. Gas exchange takes place in the alveolar capillaries.

Inadequate perfusion (dead-space ventilation)

When the $\dot{V}/\dot{Q}$ ratio is high, as shown here, ventilation is normal, but alveolar perfusion is reduced or absent. Note the narrowed capillary, indicating poor perfusion. This typically results from a perfusion defect, such as pulmonary embolism or a disorder that decreases cardiac output.

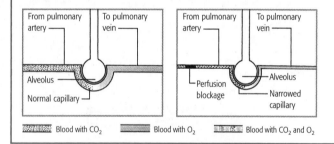

um are composed of a single layer of cells. Between these layers are minute interstitial spaces filled with elastin and collagen. Normally, oxygen and carbon dioxide move easily through all of these layers. Oxygen moves from the alveoli into the bloodstream, where it's taken up by hemoglobin in the RBCs. Once there, it displaces carbon dioxide (the by-product of metabolism), which diffuses from the RBCs into the blood; then it moves to the alveoli. Most transported oxygen binds with hemoglobin to form oxyhemoglobin, whereas a small portion dissolves in the plasma (measurable as the partial pressure of arterial oxygen).

After oxygen binds to hemoglobin, the RBCs travel to the tissues. At this point, the blood cells contain more oxygen, and

Inadequate ventilation (shunt)

When the $\dot{V}/\dot{Q}$ ratio is low, pulmonary circulation is adequate, but not enough oxygen (O_2) is available to the alveoli for normal diffusion. A portion of the blood flowing through the pulmonary vessels doesn't become oxygenated.

Inadequate ventilation and perfusion (silent unit)

The silent unit indicates an absence of ventilation and perfusion to the lung area. The silent unit may help compensate for a $\dot{V}/\dot{Q}$ imbalance by delivering blood flow to better-ventilated areas.

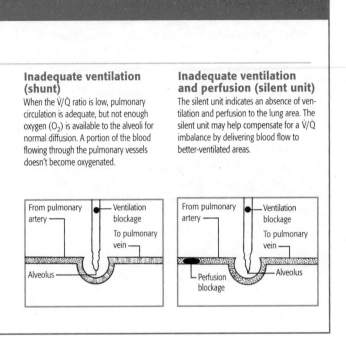

the tissue cells contain more carbon dioxide. Internal respiration occurs during cellular diffusion, as RBCs release oxygen and absorb carbon dioxide. The RBCs then transport carbon dioxide back to the lungs for removal during expiration.

Acid-base balance

The lungs help maintain acid-base balance in the body by maintaining external and internal respiration. Oxygen collected in the lungs is transported to the tissues by the circulatory system, which exchanges it for the carbon dioxide produced by cellular metabolism. Because carbon dioxide is 20 times more soluble than oxygen, it dissolves in the blood, where most of it forms bicarbonate (base) and smaller amounts form carbonic acid (acid).

The lungs control bicarbonate levels by converting bicarbonate to carbon dioxide and water for excretion. In response to signals from the medulla, the lungs can change the rate and depth of ventilation. Such changes maintain acid-base balance by adjusting the amount of carbon dioxide that's lost. For example, in metabolic alkalosis, which results from excess bicarbonate retention, the rate and depth of ventilation decrease so that carbon dioxide is retained. This increases carbonic acid levels. In metabolic acidosis—a condition resulting from excess acid retention or excess bicarbonate loss—the lungs increase the rate and depth of ventilation to exhale excess carbon dioxide, thereby reducing carbonic acid levels.

A patient with inadequately functioning lungs can experience acid-base imbalances. For example, hypoventilation, which reduces the rate and depth of ventilation of the lungs, results in carbon dioxide retention, causing respiratory acidosis. Conversely, hyperventilation, which increases the rate and depth of ventilation of the lungs, leads to increased exhalation of carbon dioxide and will result in respiratory alkalosis.

Assessment

A complete respiratory assessment will provide you with essential information about the thorax and lungs. The assessment should include obtaining a careful history and performing a complete physical examination. Knowing the basic structures and functions of the respiratory system will help you perform a comprehensive respiratory assessment and recognize abnormalities.

HEALTH HISTORY

Any assessment begins with a health history that includes exploration of the patient's chief complaints. Build the health history by asking open-ended questions. Ask these questions systematically to avoid overlooking important information. If necessary, conduct the interview in several short sessions, depending on the severity of the patient's condition, his expectations, and staffing constraints.

AGE AWARE Most information obtained about a child will come from the family. Sometimes the chief complaint the parent expresses may not be the actual reason she's seeking medical attention.

Always ask the parent if she has other concerns about the child. Asking such questions as "Was there anything else you wanted to ask me today?" or "Do you have any other concerns?" may invite the parent to share her concerns.

The adolescent child usually responds to those who pay attention to him. Showing interest in the adolescent (and not his problem) early in the interview will help build trust and begin a rapport with

13

him. Start the interview by first informally asking about his friends, school, or hobbies. When rapport has been established, you can return to more open-ended questioning.

During the interview, establish a rapport with the patient by explaining who you are and what you'll do. The quantity and quality of the information gathered depends on the relationship you build with the patient. Try to gain his trust by being sensitive to his concerns and feelings. Be alert to nonverbal responses that support or contradict his verbal responses. He may, for example, deny chest pain verbally but reveal it through his facial expressions. If the patient's verbal and nonverbal responses contradict each other, explore this with him to clarify your assessment.

Chief complaint

Ask the patient to tell you about his chief complaint. Use such questions as "When did you first notice you weren't feeling well?" and "What has happened since then that brings you here today?" Because many respiratory disorders are chronic, be sure to ask him how the latest episode compared with the previous episode, and what relief measures were helpful or unhelpful.

Current health history

The current health history includes the patient's biographic data and an analysis of his symptoms. Determine the patient's age, gender, marital status, occupation, education, religion, and ethnic background. These factors provide clues to potential risks and to the patient's interpretation of his respiratory condition. Advanced age, for example, suggests physiologic changes such as decreased vital capacity. Alternatively, the patient's occupation may alert you to problems related to hazardous materials. Ask him for the name, address, and phone number of a relative who can be contacted in an emergency.

After obtaining biographic data, ask the patient to describe his symptoms chronologically. Concentrate on the symptoms':
- onset—the first occurrence of symptoms and if they appeared suddenly or gradually
- incidence—the frequency of his symptoms; for example, if the pain is constant, intermittent, steadily worsening, or crescendo-decrescendo

■ duration—the time period of his symptoms; ask him to use precise terms to describe his answers, such as "30 minutes after meals," "twice per day," or "for 3 hours."

Next, ask the patient to characterize his symptoms. Have him describe:

■ aggravating factors—the cause of increased intensity; for example, if he has dyspnea, ask him how many feet he can walk before he feels short of breath

■ alleviating factors—the relieving measures; determine if he's using any home remedies, such as over-the-counter (OTC) medications, alternative therapies, or a change in sleeping position

■ associated factors—the other symptoms that occur at the same time as the primary symptom

■ location—the area where he experiences the symptom; ask him to pinpoint it and determine if it radiates to other areas

■ quality—the feeling that accompanies the symptom and if he has experienced similar symptoms in the past; ask him to characterize the symptom in his own words and document his description, including the words he chooses to describe pain, for example, sharp, stabbing, or throbbing

■ duration—the length of time symptoms last

■ setting—the place where the patient was when the symptom occurred; ask him what he was doing and who was with him.

Be sure to document your findings.

A patient with a respiratory disorder may complain of dyspnea, fatigue, cough, sputum production, wheezing, and chest pain. Here are some helpful assessment techniques to gain information about each of these signs and symptoms.

DYSPNEA

Dyspnea, or shortness of breath, occurs when breathing is inappropriately difficult for the activity that the patient is performing. When ventilation is disturbed and ventilatory demands exceed the actual or perceived capacity of the lungs to respond, the patient becomes short of breath. In addition, dyspnea is caused by decreased lung compliance, disturbances in the chest bellows system, airway obstruction, or exogenous factors such as obesity.

GRADING DYSPNEA

To assess dyspnea as objectively as possible, ask your patient to briefly describe how various activities affect his breathing. Then document his response using this grading system.

Grade 0—Not troubled by breathlessness except with strenuous exercise

Grade 1—Troubled by shortness of breath when hurrying on a level path or walking up a slight hill

Grade 2—Walks more slowly on a level path because of breathlessness than people of the same age or has to stop to breathe when walking on a level path at his own pace

Grade 3—Stops to breathe after walking about 100 yards (91.4 m) on a level path

Grade 4—Too breathless to leave the house or breathless when dressing or undressing

Obtain the patient's history of dyspnea by using several scales. Ask the patient to rate his usual level of dyspnea on a scale of 0 to 10, in which 0 means no dyspnea and 10 means the worst he has experienced. Then ask him to rate the level that day. Another method to assess dyspnea is to count the number of words the patient speaks between breaths. A normal individual can speak 10 to 12 words. A severely dyspneic patient may speak only 1 to 2 words per breath.

Ask the patient what he does to relieve the dyspnea and how well those measures work. (See *Grading dyspnea*.)

To find out if the dyspnea stems from pulmonary disease, ask the patient about its onset and severity:

- A sudden onset may indicate an acute problem, such as pneumothorax or pulmonary embolus, or may result from anxiety caused by hyperventilation.
- A gradual onset suggests a slow, progressive disorder such as chronic obstructive pulmonary disease (COPD), whereas acute intermittent attacks may indicate asthma.

AGE AWARE Normally, an infant's respirations are abdominal, gradually changing to costal by age 7. Suspect dyspnea in an infant who breathes costally, in an older child who breathes abdominally, or in a child who uses accessory muscles to aid in breathing.

ORTHOPNEA

Orthopnea is increased dyspnea when the patient is in a supine position. It's traditionally measured in "pillows"—as in the number (usually one to three) of pillows needed to prop the patient before dyspnea resolves. A better method is to record the degree of head elevation at which dyspnea is relieved using a goniometer. This device is used by physical therapists to determine range of motion and may be used to measure a patient's orthopnea, for example, "relieved at 35 degrees."

Orthopnea is commonly associated with:

- asthma
- COPD
- diaphragmatic paralysis
- left-sided heart failure
- obesity
- pulmonary hypertension
- fatigue.

Patients with respiratory disorders experience fatigue. Fatigue is subjective and varies with the severity of the disorder and daily activities. Fatigue can be measured by using a scale of 0 to 10, with 0 being no fatigue and 10 being the worst fatigue experienced. Daily activities are prioritized by the daily level of fatigue. Worsening fatigue usually indicates worsening respiratory conditions.

COUGH

If the patient is experiencing a cough, ask him these questions: Is the cough productive? If the cough is a chronic problem, has it changed recently? If so, how? What makes the cough better? What makes it worse?

Also investigate the characteristics of the cough:

- changing sputum, from white to yellow or green—suggesting a bacterial infection
- chronic productive with mucoid sputum—signaling asthma or chronic bronchitis
- congested—suggesting a cold, pneumonia, or bronchitis
- dry—signaling a cardiac condition
- hacking—signaling pneumonia
- increased amounts of mucoid sputum—suggesting acute tracheobronchitis or acute asthma

- occurring in late afternoon—indicating exposure to irritants
- occurring in the early morning—indicating chronic airway inflammation, possibly from cigarette smoke
- occurring in the evening—suggesting chronic postnasal drip or sinusitis
- severe—it disrupts daily activities and causes chest pain or acute respiratory distress.

AGE AWARE In children, evaluate a cough for these characteristics:

- barking, signaling croup
- nonproductive, indicating foreign body obstruction, asthma, pneumonia, acute otitis media, or early cystic fibrosis
- productive, accompanied by thick or excessive secretions, suggesting respiratory distress, asthma, bronchiectasis, bronchitis, cystic fibrosis, or pertussis.

SPUTUM PRODUCTION

When a patient produces sputum, ask him to estimate the amount produced in teaspoons or some other common measurement. Find out what time of day he usually coughs and the color and consistency of his sputum. Ask if his sputum is a chronic problem and if it has recently changed. If it has, ask him how. Also ask if he coughs up blood (hemoptysis); if so, find out how much and how often.

Hemoptysis

Hemoptysis (coughing up blood) may result from violent coughing or from serious disorders, such as pneumonia, lung cancer, lung abscess, tuberculosis (TB), pulmonary embolism, bronchiectasis, and left-sided heart failure. If the hemoptysis is mild (sputum streaked with blood), reassure the patient and be sure to ask when he first noticed it and how often it occurs.

RED FLAG If hemoptysis is severe, causing frank bleeding, place the patient in a semirecumbent position, note pulse rate, blood pressure, and general condition. When the patient's condition stabilizes, ask whether he has ever experienced similar bleeding. (See *Hemoptysis or hematemesis?*)

AGE AWARE If an elderly patient experiences hemoptysis, check his medication history for use of anticoagulants. Changes in diet or medications, including OTC drugs and herbal supplements,

HEMOPTYSIS OR HEMATEMESIS?

If a patient begins bleeding from his mouth, determine if he's experiencing hemoptysis, which is coughing up from the lungs; hematemesis, which is vomiting blood from the stomach; or bleeding from a site in the upper respiratory tract. Compare the conditions based on the signs and symptoms listed here.

Hemoptysis
- Bright red or pink, frothy blood
- Blood mixed with sputum
- Negative litmus paper test of blood (paper remains blue)

Hematemesis
- Dark red blood, possibly with coffee-ground appearance
- Blood mixed with food
- Positive litmus paper test of blood (paper turns pink)

Upper respiratory tract bleeding
Oral sources
- Blood mixed with saliva
- Evidence of mouth or tongue laceration
- Negative litmus paper test of blood

Nasal or sinus source
- Tickling sensation in nasal passages
- Sniffing behavior
- Negative litmus paper test of blood

---

may be necessary because they may alter the anticoagulant effect of Coumadin.

In children, hemoptysis may stem from Goodpasture's syndrome, cystic fibrosis or, rarely, idiopathic primary pulmonary hemosiderosis. In rare cases, pulmonary hemorrhage of unknown cause occurs in the first 2 weeks of life; the prognosis in these patients is poor.

SLEEP DISTURBANCE
Sleep disturbances may be related to obstructive sleep apnea or other sleep disorders requiring additional evaluation.

If the patient complains of being drowsy or irritable in the daytime, ask him how many hours of continuous sleep he gets at night. Ask him if he awakens during the night and if his family complains about his snoring or restlessness.

WHEEZING
If a patient wheezes, initially determine the severity of the condition.

RED FLAG If the patient is in distress, immediately assess his ABCs—airway, breathing, and circulation. Does he have an open airway? Is he breathing? Does he have a pulse? If any of these is absent, call for help and start cardiopulmonary resuscitation.

Next, quickly check for signs of impending crisis:
■ Is the patient having difficulty breathing?
■ Is he using accessory muscles to breathe? If chest excursion is less than the normal 1 ⅛″ to 2″ (3 to 5 cm), he'll use accessory muscles when he breathes. Look for shoulder elevation, intercostal muscle retraction, and use of scalene and sternocleidomastoid muscles.
■ Has his level of consciousness (LOC) diminished?
■ Is he confused, anxious, or agitated?
■ Does he change his body position to ease breathing?
■ Does his skin look pale, diaphoretic, or cyanotic?

If the patient isn't in acute distress, ask him these questions: When does wheezing occur? What makes you wheeze? Do you wheeze loudly enough for others to hear? What helps stop your wheezing?

AGE AWARE Children are especially susceptible to wheezing due to their small airways, which are prone to rapid obstruction.

CHEST PAIN

If the patient has chest pain, ask him where the pain is located. Have the patient rate the pain in a scale from 0 to 10. Ask him what the pain feels like, if it's sharp, stabbing, burning, or aching. Find out if it radiates to another area in his body and, if so, where. Ask the patient how long the pain lasts, what causes it to occur, and what makes it better.

When the patient is describing his chest pain, attempt to determine the type of pain he's experiencing:
■ chest wall pain that's localized and tender (indicates an infection or inflammation of the chest wall, intercostal nerves, or intercostal muscles or, possibly, blunt chest trauma)
■ esophageal pain that's a burning sensation that intensifies with swallowing (indicates local inflammation)
■ pleural pain that's stabbing, knifelike, and increases with deep breathing or coughing (associated with pulmonary infarction, pneumothorax, or pleurisy)

■ substernal pain that's a sharp, stabbing pain in the middle of his chest (indicates pneumonia or spontaneous pneumothorax)

■ tracheal pain that's a burning sensation that intensifies with deep breathing or coughing (suggests oxygen toxicity or aspiration).

Regardless of the type of pain the patient describes, remember to assess associated factors, such as breathing, body position, and ease or difficulty of movement.

Past health history

The information gained from the patient's past health history helps in understanding his current symptoms. It also helps to identify patients at risk for developing respiratory difficulty.

First, focus on identifying previous respiratory problems, such as asthma and COPD. A history of these disorders provides instant clues to the patient's current condition. Then ask about childhood illnesses.

AGE AWARE Infantile eczema, atopic dermatitis, or allergic rhinitis, for example, may precipitate current respiratory problems such as asthma.

Obtain an immunization history, especially of influenza and pneumococcal vaccination, which may provide clues about the potential for respiratory disease. A travel history may be useful and should include dates, destinations, and length of stay.

Next, ask what problems in the past caused the patient to see a health care provider or required hospitalization, paying particular attention to respiratory problems. For example, chronic sinus infection or postnasal discharge may lead to recurrent bronchitis, and repeated episodes of pneumonia involving the same lung lobe may accompany bronchogenic carcinoma.

Ask the patient to describe the prescribed treatment, whether he followed the treatment plan, and whether the treatment helped. Determine whether he has suffered any traumatic injuries. If he has, note when they occurred and how they were treated.

The history should also include brief personal details. Ask the patient if he smokes; if he does, ask when he started and how many packs of cigarettes he smokes per day. By calculating his smoking in pack-years, you can assess his risk of respiratory disease. To estimate pack-years, use this simple formula: number of packs smoked per day multiplied by the number of years the patient has smoked. For example, a patient who has smoked 2 packs of cigarettes per day for 42 years has accumulated 84 pack-years.

Remember to ask about the patient's alcohol use and about his diet because nutritional status commonly influences a patient's risk of respiratory infection.

It's also important to obtain an allergy history. Allergies could include airborne, food, drug, and insect bites. Determine what the allergic reaction is, such as runny nose, sneezing, coughing, or other respiratory complication such as wheezing. Another component of the past health history includes medications the patient is taking. These include prescribed, OTC, herbal, and recreational drugs. All of these have adverse effects, some of them adversely affecting the respiratory system. It's important to note medications that the patient is allergic to. This information needs to be verified and documented properly.

Family history

Obtaining a family history helps determine whether a patient is at risk for hereditary or infectious respiratory diseases. First, ask if any of his immediate blood relatives, such as parents, siblings, and children, have had cancer, sickle cell anemia, heart disease, or a chronic illness, such as asthma and emphysema. Remember that diabetes can lead to cardiac and, possibly, respiratory problems. If an immediate relative has one or more of these disorders, ask for more information about the patient's maternal and paternal grandparents, aunts, and uncles.

Be sure to determine whether the patient lives with anyone who has an infectious disease, such as influenza or TB.

Psychosocial history

Ask the patient about his psychosocial history to assess his lifestyle. Be sure to cover his home, community, and other environmental factors that might influence how he deals with his respiratory problems. For example, people who work in mining, construction, or chemical manufacturing are commonly exposed to environmental irritants. Also ask about interpersonal relationships, mental health status, stress management, and coping style. Keep in mind that a patient's sexual habits or drug use may be connected with pulmonary disorders related to acquired immunodeficiency syndrome.

PHYSICAL ASSESSMENT

Any patient can develop a respiratory disorder. Using a systematic assessment enables the practitioner to detect subtle or obvious respiratory changes. The depth of the assessment will depend on several factors, including the patient's primary health problem and his risk of developing respiratory complications.

A physical examination of the respiratory system follows four steps: inspection, palpation, percussion, and auscultation. Before you begin, make sure the examination room is well lit and warm.

Make a few observations about the patient as soon as you enter the room. Note how he's seated, which will most likely be the position most comfortable for him. Take note of his level of consciousness and general appearance. Does he appear relaxed? Anxious? Uncomfortable? Is he having trouble breathing? Include those observations in your final assessment.

RED FLAG Assess the patient's ability to speak. If he's unable to speak, suspect a complete airway obstruction.

When you're ready to begin the physical assessment, seat the patient in a position that allows access to the anterior and posterior thorax. Provide an examination gown that offers easy access to the chest and back without requiring unnecessary exposure. Make sure the patient isn't cold because shivering can alter breathing patterns.

If the patient can't sit up, place him in the semi-Fowler position to assess the anterior chest wall and the side-lying position to assess the posterior thorax. Keep in mind that these positions may cause some distortion of findings.

AGE AWARE If the patient is an infant or a small child, assess him while he's seated on the parent's lap.

When performing the physical assessment, it may be easier to inspect, palpate, percuss, and auscultate the anterior chest before the posterior. However, this section covers inspection of the entire chest, then palpation, percussion, and auscultation of the entire chest.

Chest inspection

To assess respiratory function, determine the rate, rhythm, and quality of the patient's respirations and inspect his chest configuration, tracheal position, chest symmetry, skin condition, nostrils (for flaring), and accessory muscle use. Accomplish this by observing the patient's breathing and inspecting his anterior and posterior thorax. Note all abnormal findings.

RESPIRATORY PATTERN

To find the patient's respiratory rate, count for 30 seconds and multiply by 2 to give you the rate per minute. If the rhythm is irregular, less than 12 breaths/minute or more than 20 breaths/minute, count for a full minute. Don't tell him what you're doing, or he might alter his natural breathing pattern. Adults normally breathe at a rate of 12 to 20 breaths/minute.

AGE AWARE An infant's respiratory rate may reach about 40 breaths/minute.

The respiratory pattern should be even, coordinated, and regular, with occasional sighs.

AGE AWARE Men, children, and infants usually use abdominal, or diaphragmatic, breathing. Athletes and singers do as well. Most women, however, usually use chest, or intercostal, breathing.

Paradoxical movement of the chest wall may appear as an abnormal collapse of part of the chest wall. The abnormal part of the chest wall contracts (sucks in) during inspiration and expands (pushes out) during exhalation.

Abnormal respiratory patterns

Identifying an abnormal respiratory pattern can help you assess a patient's respiratory status and his overall condition. (See *Recognizing abnormal respiratory patterns*.)

Tachypnea

Tachypnea is a respiratory rate greater than 20 breaths/minute; usually the breaths are shallow. It's commonly seen in patients with restrictive lung disease, pain, sepsis, obesity, anxiety, and respiratory distress. Fever is another possible cause. The respiratory rate my increase by 4 breaths/minute for every 1° F (0.6° C) increase in body temperature.

Recognizing abnormal respiratory patterns

To help you better recognize abnormal respiratory patterns, illustrated below are typical characteristics of the more common ones.

Tachypnea
Shallow breathing with increased respiratory rate

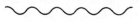

Bradypnea
Decreased rate but regular breathing

Apnea
Absence of breathing; may be periodic

Hyperpnea
Deep breathing at a normal rate

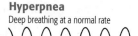

Kussmaul's respirations
Rapid, deep breathing without pauses; in adults, more than 20 breaths/minute; breathing usually sounds labored with deep breaths that resemble sighs

Cheyne-Stokes respirations
Breaths that gradually become faster and deeper than normal, then slower, during a 30- to 170-second period; alternates with 20- to 60-second periods of apnea

Biot's respirations
Rapid, deep breathing with abrupt pauses between each breath; equal depth to each breath

Bradypnea

Bradypnea is a respiratory rate below 12 breaths/minute. It's commonly noted just before a period of apnea or full respiratory arrest.

Patients with bradypnea might have central nervous system (CNS) depression as a result of excessive sedation, tissue damage, diabetic coma, or any situation in which the brain's respiratory center is depressed. Note that the respiratory rate is usually slower during sleep.

Apnea

Apnea is the absence of breathing. Periods of apnea may be short and occur sporadically, such as in Cheyne-Stokes respiration or other abnormal respiratory patterns. This condition may be life threatening if periods of apnea last long enough and should be addressed immediately.

Hyperpnea

Hyperpnea is characterized by deep breathing. It occurs in patients who exercise and those who have metabolic acidosis, are highly anxious, or are experiencing pain.

Kussmaul's respirations

Kussmaul's respirations are rapid and deep, with sighing breaths. This type of breathing occurs in patients with metabolic acidosis, especially when associated with diabetic ketoacidosis, as the respiratory system tries to lower the carbon dioxide level in the blood and restore it to normal pH.

Cheyne-Stokes respirations

Cheyne-Stokes respirations have a regular cycle of change in the rate and depth of breathing. Respirations are initially shallow. They gradually become deeper and then become shallow again before a period of apnea lasting up to 20 seconds. Then the cycle starts again. This respiratory pattern is seen in patients with heart failure, kidney failure, or CNS damage.

 AGE AWARE In children and elderly patients during sleep, Cheyne-Stokes respirations may be normal.

Biot's respirations

Also known as *ataxic respirations,* Biot's respirations involve rapid, deep breaths that alternate with abrupt periods of apnea. It's an ominous sign in the setting of severe CNS damage.

ANTERIOR THORAX

After assessing respiration, inspect the anterior thorax for structural deformities, such as a concave or convex curvature of the anterior chest wall over the sternum. Inspect between and around the ribs for visible sinking of soft tissues (retractions). Assess the patient's respiratory pattern for symmetry. Look for abnormalities in skin color or alterations in muscle tone. For future documentation, note the location of abnormalities according to regions delineated by imaginary lines on the thorax.

Initially inspect the chest wall to identify the shape of the thoracic cage. In an adult, the lateral diameter of the thorax (from side to side) should be twice the anteroposterior diameter (from front to back).

Note the angle between the ribs and the sternum at the point immediately above the xiphoid process. This angle, called the *sternocostal angle,* should be less than 90 degrees in an adult; it widens if the chest wall is chronically expanded, as in cases of increased anteroposterior diameter, or barrel chest.

To inspect the anterior chest for symmetry of movement, have the patient lie in a supine position. Stand at the foot of the bed and carefully observe the patient's quiet and deep breathing for equal expansion of the chest wall.

RED FLAG Watch for abnormal collapse of part of the chest wall during inspiration, along with abnormal expansion of the same area during expiration, which signals paradoxical movement—a loss of normal chest wall function. Also, check whether one portion of the chest wall lags behind the others as the chest moves, which may indicate a progression in the patient's lung disease.

Next, check for the use of accessory muscles for respiration by observing the sternocleidomastoid, scalene, and trapezius muscles in the shoulders and neck. During normal inspiration and expiration, the diaphragm and external intercostal muscles should easily maintain the breathing process.

AGE AWARE In elderly patients, hypertrophy of any of the accessory muscles may indicate frequent abnormal use—although hypertrophy may be normal in a well-conditioned athlete.

Note the position the patient assumes to breathe. A patient who depends on accessory muscles may assume a "tripod position," where he rests his arms on his knees or on the sides of a chair and supports his head.

Observe the patient's skin on the anterior chest for any unusual color, lumps, or lesions, and note the location of any abnormality. Unless the patient has been exposed to significant sun or heat, the skin color of the chest should match the rest of the patient's complexion. A skin abnormality may reflect problems in the underlying structure, so note the location of underlying ribs and other bones, cartilage, and lung lobes. Also, check for any chest wall scars from previous surgeries. If the patient didn't mention past surgery during the health history, ask about it now.

POSTERIOR THORAX

To inspect the posterior thorax, observe the patient's breathing again. If he can't sit in a backless chair or lean forward against a supporting structure, direct him to lie in a lateral position. Be aware that this may distort the findings in some situations. If the patient is obese, findings may be distorted because he may be unable to fully expand the lower lung from the lateral position, leaving breath sounds on that side diminished.

Assess the posterior chest wall for the same characteristics as the anterior: chest structure, respiratory pattern, symmetry of expansion, skin color and muscle tone, and accessory muscle use. During the examination for chest wall abnormalities, keep in mind that the patient might have completely normal lungs and that they might be cramped within the chest. The patient might have a smaller-than-normal lung capacity and limited exercise tolerance, and he may more easily develop respiratory failure from a respiratory tract infection. Other chest wall abnormalities include:

- A barrel chest, which looks like its name implies, is characterized by an abnormally round and bulging chest, with a greater-than-normal front-to-back diameter. It occurs as a result of COPD, indicating that the lungs have lost their elasticity and that the diaphragm is flattened. The patient typically uses accessory muscles when he inhales and easily becomes breathless. You'll also note kyphosis of the thoracic spine, ribs that run horizontally rather than tangentially, and a prominent sternal angle.

  AGE AWARE In infants and elderly patients, barrel chest may be normal.

- Pigeon chest, or pectus carinatum, is characterized by a chest with a sternum that protrudes beyond the front of the abdomen. The displaced sternum increases the front-to-back diameter of the chest.

- Funnel chest, or pectus excavatum, is characterized by a funnel-shaped depression on all or part of the sternum. The shape of the chest may interfere with respiratory and cardiac function. If cardiac compression occurs, you may hear a murmur.

■ Thoracic kyphoscoliosis is characterized by the patient's spine curving to one side with the vertebrae rotated. Because the rotation distorts lung tissues, you may have a more difficult time assessing respiratory status. (See *Identifying chest deformities,* page 30.)

RELATED STRUCTURES

Inspecting the patient's related structures, such as the skin and nails, will provide an overview of the patient's clinical status along with an assessment of his peripheral oxygenation. A dusky or bluish tint (cyanosis) to the patient's skin may indicate a decrease in the oxygen saturation of hemoglobin. Distinguishing central from peripheral cyanosis is important:

■ Central cyanosis results from hypoxemia and may appear in patients with right-to-left cardiac shunting or a pulmonary disease that causes hypoxemia such as chronic bronchitis. It appears on the skin; the mucous membranes of the mouth, lips, and conjunctivae; and in other highly vascular areas, such as the earlobes, tip of the nose, and nail beds.

■ Peripheral cyanosis, typically seen in patients exposed to the cold, results from vasoconstriction, vascular occlusion, or reduced cardiac output. It appears in the nail beds, nose, ears, and fingers. Note that unlike central cyanosis, peripheral cyanosis doesn't affect the mucous membranes. It indicates oxygen depletion in nonperfused areas of the body because deoxygenated hemoglobin hasn't been replaced by fresh oxygenated blood.

A dark-skinned patient may be more difficult to assess for central cyanosis. In this patient, inspect the oral mucous membranes and lips, which will appear ashen gray rather than bluish. Facial skin may appear pale gray or ashen in darker-skinned patients, such as Blacks, and yellowish brown in patients with lighter dark skin such as Hispanics.

Next, assess the patient's finger- and toenail beds for abnormal enlargement. Abnormal enlargement of the patient's nail beds is called *clubbing,* which results from chronic tissue hypoxia. Nail thinning accompanied by an abnormal alteration of the

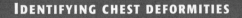

IDENTIFYING CHEST DEFORMITIES

When inspecting the patient's chest, note deviations in size and shape. These illustrations show a normal adult chest, along with four common chest deformities.

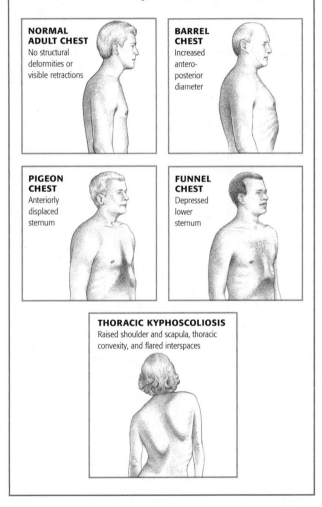

NORMAL ADULT CHEST
No structural deformities or visible retractions

BARREL CHEST
Increased antero-posterior diameter

PIGEON CHEST
Anteriorly displaced sternum

FUNNEL CHEST
Depressed lower sternum

THORACIC KYPHOSCOLIOSIS
Raised shoulder and scapula, thoracic convexity, and flared interspaces

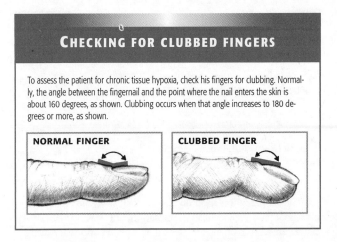

CHECKING FOR CLUBBED FINGERS

To assess the patient for chronic tissue hypoxia, check his fingers for clubbing. Normally, the angle between the fingernail and the point where the nail enters the skin is about 160 degrees, as shown. Clubbing occurs when that angle increases to 180 degrees or more, as shown.

NORMAL FINGER

CLUBBED FINGER

angle of the finger- and toenail bases characterizes clubbing. (See *Checking for clubbed fingers*.)

Chest palpation

Careful palpation of the trachea and the anterior and posterior thorax helps to detect structural and skin abnormalities, areas of pain, and chest asymmetry.

TRACHEA AND ANTERIOR THORAX

First, palpate the trachea for position. (See *Palpating the trachea*, page 32.)

Palpation of the patient's trachea may reveal:
- the trachea isn't midline, possibly resulting from atelectasis (collapsed lung tissue), thyroid enlargement, or pleural effusion (fluid accumulation in the air spaces of the lungs)
- a tumor or pneumothorax (collapsed lung) may have displaced the trachea to one side.

Observe the patient to determine whether he uses accessory neck muscles to breathe. Next, palpate the suprasternal notch. In most patients, the arch of the aorta lies close to the surface just behind the suprasternal notch. Use your fingertips to gently evaluate the strength and regularity of the patient's aortic pulsations in this area. Then palpate the thorax to assess the skin and underlying tissues for density. (See *Palpating the thorax*, page 33.)

PALPATING THE TRACHEA

To palpate the trachea, stand in front of the patient and place one thumb on either side of the trachea above the suprasternal notch. Gently slide both thumbs, at equal speed, along the upper edge of the patient's clavicle until you reach the sternocleidomastoid muscle. Each thumb should cover an equal distance, indicating a midline trachea.

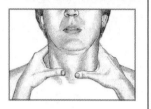

Gentle palpation shouldn't be painful, so assess any complaints of pain for localization, radiation, and severity. Be especially careful to palpate any areas that looked abnormal during inspection. If necessary, support the patient during the procedure with one hand while using the other hand to palpate one side at a time, continuing to compare sides. Note unusual findings, such as masses, crepitus, skin irregularities, and painful areas. The chest wall should feel smooth, warm, and dry.

If the patient has subcutaneous air in the chest, this indicates crepitus, an abnormal condition that feels like puffed-rice cereal crackling under the skin and indicates that air is leaking from the airways or lungs. If a patient has a chest tube, you may find a small amount of subcutaneous air around the insertion site.

RED FLAG If the patient has no chest tube or the area of crepitus is getting larger, immediately alert the health care provider. If the patient complains of chest pain, attempt to determine the cause by palpating the anterior chest.

RED FLAG Increased pain during palpation may be caused by certain conditions—such as musculoskeletal pain, an irritation of the nerves covering the xiphoid process, and an inflammation of the cartilage connecting the bony ribs to the sternum (costochondritis). These conditions may also produce pain during inspiration, causing the patient to breathe shallowly to decrease his discomfort. Keep in mind that palpation doesn't worsen pain caused by cardiac or pulmonary disorders, such as angina and pleurisy.

PALPATING THE THORAX

To palpate the thorax, place the palm of your hand (or hands) lightly over the thorax, as shown. Palpate for tenderness, alignment, bulging, or retractions of the chest and intercostal spaces. Assess the patient for crepitus, especially around drainage sites. Repeat this procedure on the patient's back.

Next, use the pads of your fingers, as shown, to palpate the front and back of the thorax. Pass your fingers over the ribs and any scars, lumps, lesions, or ulcerations. Note the skin temperature, turgor, and moisture. Also note tenderness or bony or subcutaneous crepitus. The muscles should feel firm and smooth.

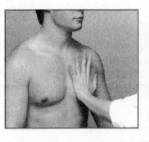
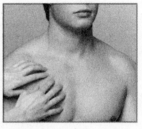

Next, palpate the costal angle. The area around the xiphoid process contains many nerve endings, so be gentle to avoid causing pain.

If a patient frequently uses the internal intercostal muscles to breathe, these muscles will eventually pull the chest cavity upward and outward. If this has occurred, the costal angle will be greater than the normal 90 degrees.

To evaluate how symmetrical the patient's chest wall is and how much it expands, place both hands on the front of the chest wall, with thumbs touching each other at the second intercostal space. As the patient inhales deeply, watch the thumbs. They should separate simultaneously and equally to a distance several centimeters away from the sternum. Repeat the measurement at the fifth intercostal space. The same measurement may be made on the back of the chest near the tenth rib.

During chest palpation, be alert for these findings in the patient's chest:

- asymmetrical expansion possibly due to pleural effusion, atelectasis, pneumonia, or pneumothorax
- decreased expansion at the level of the diaphragm secondary to emphysema, respiratory depression, diaphragm paralysis, atelectasis, obesity, or ascites
- absent or delayed chest movement during respiratory excursion, indicating previous surgical removal of the lung, complete or partial obstruction of the airway or underlying lung, or diaphragmatic dysfunction on the affected side.

POSTERIOR THORAX

Palpate the posterior thorax in a similar manner, using the palmar surface of the fingertips of one or both hands. During the process, identify bony structures, such as the vertebrae and the scapulae.

To determine the location of abnormalities, identify the first thoracic vertebra (with the patient's head tipped forward) and count the number of spinous processes from this landmark to the abnormal finding. Use this reference point for documentation. Also identify the inferior scapular tips and medial borders of both bones to define the margins of the upper and lower lung lobes posteriorly. Locate and describe all abnormalities in relation to these landmarks. Remember to evaluate abnormalities, such as use of accessory muscles and complaints of pain.

Tactile fremitus

Because sound travels more easily through solid structures than through air, checking for tactile fremitus (the palpation of vocalizations) helps you learn about the contents of the patient's lungs. (See *Palpating the thorax for tactile fremitus*.)

The patient's vocalization should produce vibrations of equal intensity on both sides of the chest. Normally, vibrations should occur in the upper chest, close to the bronchi, and then decrease and finally disappear toward the periphery of the lungs.

Conditions that restrict air movement, such as pneumonia, pleural effusion, and COPD with overinflated lungs, cause decreased tactile fremitus. Conditions that consolidate tissue or fluid in a portion of the pleural area, such as a lung tumor, pneumonia, and pulmonary fibrosis, increase tactile fremitus. A

PALPATING THE THORAX FOR TACTILE FREMITUS

When checking the back of the thorax for tactile fremitus, ask the patient to fold his arms across his chest. This movement shifts the scapulae out of the way.

Palpation

Check for tactile fremitus by lightly placing your open palms on both sides of the patient's back, as shown, without touching his back with your fingers. Ask the patient to repeat the phrase "ninety-nine" loud enough to produce palpable vibrations. Then palpate the front of the chest using the same hand positions.

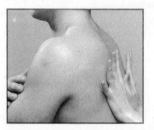

Interpretation

Vibrations that feel more intense on one side than the other indicate tissue consolidation on that side. Less intense vibrations may indicate emphysema, pneumothorax, or pleural effusion. Faint or no vibrations in the upper posterior thorax may indicate bronchial obstruction or a fluid-filled pleural space.

grating feeling when palpating the patient's chest may signify a pleural friction rub.

Chest percussion

Percuss the patient's chest to find the boundaries of the lungs; to determine whether the lungs are filled with air, fluid, or solid material; and to evaluate the distance the diaphragm travels between the patient's inhalation and exhalation. (See *Percussing the chest,* page 36.)

Percussion allows you to assess structures as deep as 3″ (7.6 cm). You'll hear different percussion sounds in different areas of the chest. (See *Percussion sounds,* page 37.)

You may also hear different sounds after certain treatments. For example, if the patient has atelectasis and you percuss his chest before chest physiotherapy, you'll hear a high-pitched, dull, soft sound. After physiotherapy, you should hear a low-pitched, hollow sound. In all cases, make sure you use other assessment techniques to confirm percussion findings.

PERCUSSING THE CHEST

To percuss the chest, hyperextend the middle finger of your left hand if you're right-handed or the middle finger of your right hand if you're left-handed. Place your hand firmly on the patient's chest. Use the tip of the middle finger of your dominant hand—your right hand if you're right-handed, left hand if you're left-handed—to tap on the middle finger of your other hand just below the distal joint (as shown).

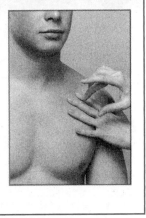

The movement should come from the wrist of your dominant hand, not your elbow or upper arm. Keep the fingernail you use for tapping short so you won't hurt yourself. Follow the standard percussion sequence over the front and back chest walls..

You'll hear resonant sounds over normal lung tissue, which you should find over most of the chest. In the left front chest, from the third or fourth intercostal space at the sternum to the third or fourth intercostal space at the midclavicular line, you should hear a dull sound. Percussion is dull here because that's the space occupied by the heart. Resonance resumes at the sixth intercostal space. The sequence of sounds in the back is slightly different. (See *Percussion sequences,* page 38.)

Hyperresonance during percussion indicates an area of increased air in the lung or pleural space that's associated with pneumothorax, acute asthma, bullous emphysema (large holes in the lungs from alveolar destruction), and gastric distention that pushes up on the diaphragm. Abnormal dullness during percussion indicates areas of decreased air in the lungs that's associated with pleural fluid, consolidation, atelectasis, or a tumor.

Chest percussion also allows assessment of the amount of diaphragmatic movement during inspiration and expiration. The normal diaphragm descends 2″ to 2½″ (5 to 6 cm) when the patient inhales. (See *Measuring diaphragmatic movement,* page 39.) The diaphragm doesn't move as far in a patient with emphyse-

PERCUSSION SOUNDS

This table describes percussion sounds and their clinical significance. To master the different percussion sounds, practice on yourself, your patients, and any other person willing to help.

SOUND	DESCRIPTION	CLINICAL SIGNIFICANCE
Flat	Short, soft, high-pitched, extremely dull, found over the thigh	Consolidation as in atelectasis and extensive pleural effusion
Dull	Medium in intensity and pitch, moderate length, thudlike, found over the liver	Solid area as in pleural effusion, mass, or lobar pneumonia
Resonant	Long, loud, low-pitched, hollow	Normal lung tissue, bronchitis
Hyperresonant	Very loud, lower-pitched, found over the stomach	Hyperinflated lung as in emphysema or pneumothorax
Tympanic	Loud, high-pitched, moderate length, musical, drumlike, found over a puffed-out cheek	Air collection as in a gastric air bubble or air in the intestines or a large pneumothorax

ma, respiratory depression, diaphragm paralysis, atelectasis, obesity, or ascites.

Chest auscultation

As air moves through the bronchial tubes, it creates sound waves that travel to the chest wall. The sounds produced by breathing change as air moves from larger to smaller airways. Sounds also change if they pass through fluid, mucus, or narrowed airways. Chest auscultation helps you to determine the condition of the alveoli and surrounding pleura.

Auscultation sites are the same as percussion sites. Listen to a full inspiration and a full expiration at each site, using the diaphragm of the stethoscope. Ask the patient to breathe through his mouth; nose breathing alters the pitch of breath sounds.

To auscultate for breath sounds, press the stethoscope firmly against the patient's skin. Remember that listening through

PERCUSSION SEQUENCES

When percussing the lungs, follow these percussion sequences to distinguish between normal and abnormal sounds in the patient's lungs. Remember to compare sound variations from one side with the other as you proceed. Carefully document abnormal sounds you hear and include their locations. You'll follow the same sequences for auscultation.

ANTERIOR   **POSTERIOR**

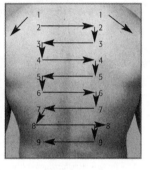

clothing or dry chest hair may result in hearing unusual and deceptive sounds. If the patient has abundant chest hair, mat it down with a damp washcloth so the hair doesn't make sounds like crackles.

NORMAL BREATH SOUNDS

Four types of breath sounds are heard over normal lungs. The type of sound you hear depends on where you listen. (See *Qualities of normal breath sounds*. See also *Locations of normal breath sounds,* page 40.)

- Tracheal breath sounds are harsh, high-pitched, and discontinuous sounds heard over the trachea. They occur when a patient inhales or exhales. Inspiration sounds are equal to expiration sounds.
- Bronchial breath sounds are loud, high-pitched sounds normally heard over the manubrium. They're discontinuous, and they're loudest when the patient exhales. Expiration lasts longer than inspiration.

MEASURING DIAPHRAGMATIC MOVEMENT

You can measure how far the diaphragm moves by first asking the patient to exhale. Percuss the back on one side to locate the upper edge of the diaphragm—the point at which normal lung resonance changes to dullness. Use a pen to mark the spot indicating the position of the diaphragm at full expiration on that side of the back.

Then ask the patient to inhale as deeply as possible. Percuss the back when the patient has breathed in fully until you locate the diaphragm. Use the pen to mark this spot as well. Repeat on the opposite side of the back.

Use a ruler or tape measure to determine the distance between the marks. The distance, normally 1¼" to 2" (3 to 5 cm) long, should be equal on the right and left sides.

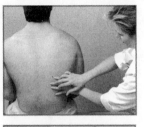
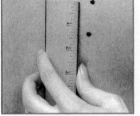

QUALITIES OF NORMAL BREATH SOUNDS

This table outlines the qualities of normal breath sounds, based on sound quality, inspiration-expiration ratio, and location.

BREATH SOUND	QUALITY	INSPIRATION-EXPIRATION RATIO	LOCATION
Tracheal	Harsh, high-pitched	I about = E	Over the trachea
Bronchial	Loud, high-pitched	I < E	Over the manubrium
Broncho-vesicular	Medium in loudness and pitch	I = E	Next to the sternum, between scapulae
Vesicular	Soft, low-pitched	I > E	Over most of both lungs

LOCATIONS OF NORMAL BREATH SOUNDS

These photographs show the normal locations of different types of breath sounds.

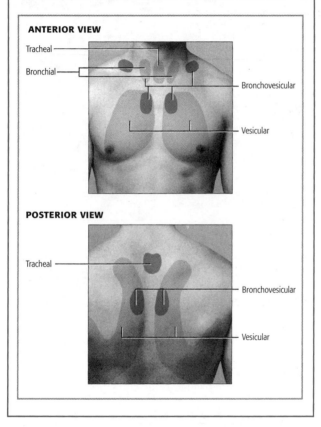

ANTERIOR VIEW

Tracheal

Bronchial

Bronchovesicular

Vesicular

POSTERIOR VIEW

Tracheal

Bronchovesicular

Vesicular

■ Bronchovesicular sounds are medium-pitched, continuous sounds. They're heard when the patient inhales or exhales and are best heard lateral to the upper third of the sternum. Inspiration sounds are equal to expiration sounds.

■ Vesicular sounds are soft, low-pitched sounds heard over the lung fields. They're prolonged when the patient inhales and shortened during exhalation in about a 3:1 ratio.

If you hear diminished but normal breath sounds in both lungs, the patient may have emphysema, atelectasis, severe bronchospasm, or shallow breathing. If breath sounds are heard in one lung only, the patient may have pleural effusion, pneumothorax, a tumor, or mucus plugs in the airways.

Classify each breath sound according to its intensity, location, pitch, duration, and characteristic. Note whether the sound occurs when the patient inhales, exhales, or both. If you hear a sound in an area other than where you would expect to hear it, consider the sound abnormal.

For example, bronchial or bronchovesicular breath sounds found in an area where vesicular breath sounds would normally be heard indicates that the alveoli and small bronchioles in that area might be filled with fluid or exudate, as in pneumonia and atelectasis. You won't hear vesicular sounds in those areas because no air is moving through the small airways.

Examination may reveal abnormal breath sounds, including:
■ louder-than-normal sounds over areas of consolidation because solid tissue transmits sound better than air or fluid
■ quieter-than-normal sounds if pus, fluid, or air fills the pleural space
■ diminished or absent sounds if a foreign body or secretions obstruct a bronchus, over lung tissue located distal to the obstruction
■ adventitious sounds, which include fine and coarse crackles, wheezes, rhonchi, stridor, and pleural friction rub
■ crackles, which are caused by collapsed or fluid-filled alveoli popping open when the patient inhales and are classified as either fine or coarse and usually don't clear with coughing (see *Types of crackles,* page 42)
■ wheezes, which are high-pitched sounds heard on exhalation when airflow is blocked (As severity of the block increases, they may also be heard when the patient inhales. The sound of a wheeze doesn't change with coughing. Patients may wheeze as a result of asthma, infection, heart failure, or airway obstruction from a tumor or foreign body.)

TYPES OF CRACKLES

When assessing the patient's lungs, it's critical to differentiate the characteristics of fine from coarse crackles.

Fine crackles

These characteristics distinguish fine crackles:

- occur when the patient stops inhaling and alveoli "pop" open
- are usually heard in lung bases
- sound like a piece of hair being rubbed between the fingers or like Velcro being pulled apart
- occur in restrictive diseases, such as pulmonary fibrosis, asbestosis, silicosis, atelectasis, congestive heart failure, and pneumonia
- are soft, high-pitched, and very brief sounds unaffected by coughing.

Coarse crackles

These characteristics distinguish coarse crackles:

- are somewhat louder, lower in pitch, and not as brief as fine crackles
- are heard primarily in the trachea and bronchi
- usually clear or diminish after coughing
- occur when the patient starts to inhale; may be present when the patient exhales
- may be heard through the lungs and even at the mouth
- sound more like bubbling or gurgling, as air moves through secretions in larger airways
- occur in chronic obstructive pulmonary disease, bronchiectasis, pulmonary edema, and with severely ill patients who can't cough; also called "death rattle."

RED FLAG If your patient is having an acute asthma attack, the absence of wheezing sounds may not mean that the attack is over. When bronchospasm and mucosal swelling become severe, little air can move through the patient's airways. As a result, you won't hear wheezing. If all other assessment criteria—labored breathing, prolonged expiratory time, accessory muscle use—point to acute bronchial obstruction, maintain the patient's airway and give oxygen, as ordered. The patient may begin wheezing again when the airways open more.

- rhonchi, which are low-pitched, snoring, rattling sounds heard on exhalation, although they may also be heard on in-

halation or may change sound or disappear with coughing
when fluid partially blocks the large airways
■ stridor, which is a loud, high-pitched crowing sound that's
heard during inspiration, usually without a stethoscope
(louder in the neck than over the chest wall), and is caused
by an obstruction in the upper airway; warrants immediate
medical attention
■ pleural friction rub, which is a low-pitched, grating, rubbing
sound heard when the patient inhales and exhales that's
caused by pleural inflammation of the two layers of pleura
rubbing together. (The patient may complain of pain in areas
where the rub is heard.)

VOCAL FREMITUS
Vocal fremitus is the sound that chest vibrations produce as the
patient speaks. Abnormal voice sounds—the most common of
which are bronchophony, egophony, and whispered pectoriloquy—may occur over areas that are consolidated (fluid-filled).
Ask the patient to repeat the words detailed below while you listen. Auscultate over an area where you hear vesicular sounds
and then again over an area where you hear bronchial breath
sounds.

Bronchophony
Ask the patient to say "ninety-nine" or "blue moon." Over normal lung tissue, the words sound muffled. Over consolidated areas, the words sound clear.

Egophony
Ask the patient to say the letter "e." Over normal lung tissue, the
sound is muffled. Over consolidated lung tissue, it will sound
like the letter "a."

Whispered pectoriloquy
Ask the patient to whisper "1, 2, 3." Over normal lung tissue,
the numbers will be almost indistinguishable. Over consolidated
lung tissue, the numbers will be clear.

A patient with abnormal findings during a respiratory assessment may be further evaluated using such diagnostic tests as
arterial blood gas analysis or pulmonary function tests.

ABNORMAL FINDINGS

A patient's chief complaint may stem from any sign or symptom related to the respiratory system. Common findings include coughing, crackles, subcutaneous crepitation, cyanosis, dyspnea, hemoptysis, rhonchi, stridor, and wheezing. The following history, physical assessment, and analysis summaries will help you assess each one quickly and accurately. After obtaining further information, begin to interpret the findings. (See *Respiratory system: Interpreting your findings,* pages 46 to 51.)

Coughing

A cough is a sudden, noisy, forceful expulsion of air from the lungs that may be productive or nonproductive. Coughing is a necessary protective mechanism that clears airway passages. The cough reflex generally occurs when mechanical, chemical, thermal, inflammatory, or psychogenic stimuli activate cough receptors.

HISTORY

Ask the patient when the cough began and whether any body position, time of day, or specific activity affects it. Ask him if there's pain associated with the cough. Ask him to describe the cough, such as harsh, brassy, dry, or hacking.

If the cough is productive, find out how much sputum the patient is coughing up each day. Ask at what time of day he coughs up the most sputum. Find out if sputum production has any relationship to what or when he eats, where he is, or what he's doing. Also ask about the color, odor, and consistency of the sputum.

Ask the patient about cigarette, drug, and alcohol use and whether his weight or appetite has changed. Find out if he has a history of asthma, allergies, or respiratory disorders, and ask about recent illnesses, surgery, or trauma. Find out what medications he's taking and if he works around chemicals or respiratory irritants such as silicone.

AGE AWARE If a child is brought in for medical attention with a barking cough, ask his parents if he has had previous episodes of croup syndrome. Also ask the parents if the coughing improves upon exposure to cold air and what other signs and symptoms the child has.

PHYSICAL ASSESSMENT

Check the depth and rhythm of the patient's respirations, and note if wheezing or "crowing" noises accompany breathing. Feel the patient's skin: is it cold, clammy, or dry?

Check the patient's nose and mouth for congestion, inflammation, drainage, or signs of infection. Note breath odor, as halitosis can be a sign of pulmonary infection. Inspect the neck for vein distention and tracheal deviation, and palpate for masses or enlarged lymph nodes.

Observe the patient's chest for accessory muscle use, retractions, and uneven chest expansion. Percuss for dullness, tympany, or flatness. Finally, auscultate for pleural friction rub and abnormal breath sounds, such as rhonchi, crackles, or wheezes.

ANALYSIS

Coughing usually indicates a respiratory disorder. Evaluating a cough isn't an easy task because the cause can range from trivial (postnasal drip) to life-threatening (severe asthma or lung cancer).

A severe cough can disrupt daily activities and cause chest pain or acute respiratory distress. An early morning cough may indicate chronic airway inflammation, possibly from cigarette smoke. A late afternoon cough may indicate exposure to irritants. An evening cough may suggest chronic postnasal drip or sinusitis. A dry cough may signal a cardiac condition; a hacking cough, pneumonia; and a congested cough, a cold, pneumonia, or bronchitis.

Increasing amounts of mucoid sputum may suggest acute tracheobronchitis or acute asthma. If the patient has a chronic productive cough with mucoid sputum, suspect asthma or chronic bronchitis. If the sputum changes from white to yellow or green, suspect a bacterial infection.

AGE AWARE In children, a barking cough is characteristic of croup. A nonproductive cough may indicate obstruction with a foreign body, asthma, pneumonia, or acute otitis media, or it may be an early indicator of cystic fibrosis. Because a child's airway is narrow,

(Text continues on page 51.)

RESPIRATORY SYSTEM: INTERPRETING YOUR FINDINGS

After you assess the patient, a group of findings may lead you to a particular disorder of the respiratory system. This table shows some common groups of findings for major signs and symptoms related to a respiratory assessment, along with their probable causes.

SIGN/SYMPTOM AND FINDINGS	PROBABLE CAUSE	SIGN/SYMPTOM AND FINDINGS	PROBABLE CAUSE
COUGH		**COUGH** (continued)	
● Nonproductive cough ● Pleuritic chest pain ● Dyspnea ● Tachypnea ● Anxiety ● Decreased vocal fremitus ● Tracheal deviation toward the affected side	Atelectasis	● Decreased chest motion ● Pleural friction rub ● Tachypnea ● Tachycardia ● Flatness on percussion ● Egophony	
		CRACKLES	
● Productive cough with small amounts of purulent (or mucopurulent), blood-streaked sputum or large amounts of frothy sputum ● Dyspnea ● Anorexia ● Fatigue ● Weight loss ● Wheezing ● Clubbing	Lung cancer	● Diffuse, fine to coarse crackles commonly in dependent lung areas ● Cyanosis ● Nasal flaring ● Tachypnea ● Tachycardia ● Grunting respirations ● Rhonchi ● Dyspnea ● Anxiety ● Decreased level of consciousness (LOC)	Acute respiratory distress syndrome (ARDS)
● Nonproductive cough ● Dyspnea ● Pleuritic chest pain	Pleural effusion	● Coarse crackles usually at lung bases ● Prolonged expirations	Chronic bronchitis

RESPIRATORY SYSTEM: INTERPRETING YOUR FINDINGS *(continued)*

SIGN/SYMPTOM AND FINDINGS	PROBABLE CAUSE
CRACKLES *(continued)*	
● Wheezing ● Rhonchi ● Exertional dyspnea ● Tachypnea ● Persistent productive cough ● Clubbing ● Cyanosis	Chronic bronchitis *(continued)*
● Diffuse, fine to coarse, moist crackles ● Productive cough with purulent sputum ● Dyspnea ● Wheezing ● Orthopnea ● Fever ● Malaise ● Mucous membrane irritation	Chemical pneumonitis
● Moist or coarse crackles ● Productive cough ● Chills ● Sore throat ● Slight fever ● Muscle and back pain ● Substernal tightness ● Rhonchi ● Wheezing	Tracheo-bronchitis

SIGN/SYMPTOM AND FINDINGS	PROBABLE CAUSE
CREPITATION	
● Crepitation over eyelid and orbit ● Periorbital ecchymoses ● Swollen eyelid ● Facial edema ● Diplopia ● Hyphema ● Possible dilated or unreactive pupil on affected side	Orbital fracture
● Crepitation in upper chest and neck ● Unilateral chest pain, increasing on inspiration ● Dyspnea ● Anxiety ● Restlessness ● Tachypnea ● Cyanosis ● Tachycardia ● Accessory muscle use ● Asymmetrical chest expansion ● Nonproductive cough	Pneumo-thorax
● Abrupt crepitation of neck and anterior chest wall ● Severe dyspnea with nasal flaring ● Tachycardia ● Accessory muscle use ● Hypotension	Tracheal rupture

(continued)

RESPIRATORY SYSTEM: INTERPRETING YOUR FINDINGS *(continued)*

SIGN/SYMPTOM AND FINDINGS	PROBABLE CAUSE
CREPITATION *(continued)*	
● Cyanosis ● Extreme anxiety ● Hemoptysis ● Mediastinal emphysema	Tracheal rupture *(continued)*
CYANOSIS	
● Central cyanosis, possibly aggravated by exertion ● Exertional dyspnea ● Productive cough with thick sputum ● Anorexia ● Weight loss ● Pursed-lip breathing ● Tachypnea ● Wheezing ● Hyperresonant lung sounds ● Barrel chest ● Clubbing	Chronic obstructive pulmonary disease
● Chronic central cyanosis ● Fever ● Weakness ● Weight loss ● Anorexia ● Dyspnea ● Chest pain ● Hemoptysis ● Possible atelectasis	Lung cancer

SIGN/SYMPTOM AND FINDINGS	PROBABLE CAUSE
CYANOSIS *(continued)*	
● Decreased diaphragmatic excursion ● Asymmetrical chest expansion ● Dullness on percussion ● Diminished breath sounds	
● Acute central cyanosis ● Dyspnea ● Orthopnea ● Frothy blood-tinged sputum ● Tachycardia ● Tachypnea ● Dependent crackles ● Ventricular gallop ● Cold, clammy skin ● Hypotension ● Weak, thready pulse ● Confusion	Pulmonary edema
● Acute peripheral cyanosis in hands and feet ● Cold, clammy pale extremities ● Lethargy ● Confusion ● Increased capillary refill time ● Rapid, weak pulse	Shock

RESPIRATORY SYSTEM: INTERPRETING YOUR FINDINGS *(continued)*

SIGN/SYMPTOM AND FINDINGS	PROBABLE CAUSE	SIGN/SYMPTOM AND FINDINGS	PROBABLE CAUSE
DYSPNEA		**HEMOPTYSIS**	
● Acute dyspnea ● Tachypnea ● Crackles and rhonchi in both lung fields ● Intercostal and suprasternal retractions ● Restlessness ● Anxiety ● Tachycardia	ARDS	● Sputum ranging from pink to dark brown ● Productive cough ● Dyspnea ● Chest pain ● Crackles on auscultation ● Chills ● Fever	Pneumonia
● Progressive exertional dyspnea ● History of smoking ● Barrel chest ● Accessory muscle hypertrophy ● Diminished breath sounds ● Pursed-lip breathing ● Prolonged expiration ● Anorexia ● Weight loss	Emphysema	● Frothy, blood-tinged pink sputum ● Severe dyspnea ● Orthopnea ● Gasping ● Diffuse crackles ● Cold, clammy skin ● Anxiety	Pulmonary edema
● Acute dyspnea ● Pleuritic chest pain ● Tachycardia ● Decreased breath sounds ● Low-grade fever ● Dullness or percussion ● Cool, clammy skin	Pulmonary embolism	● Blood-streaked or blood-tinged sputum ● Chronic productive cough ● Fine crackles after coughing ● Dyspnea ● Dullness to percussion ● Increased tactile fremitus	Pulmonary tuberculosis

(continued)

RESPIRATORY SYSTEM: INTERPRETING YOUR FINDINGS (continued)

SIGN/SYMPTOM AND FINDINGS	PROBABLE CAUSE	SIGN/SYMPTOM AND FINDINGS	PROBABLE CAUSE
RHONCHI		**STRIDOR**	
● Accompanied by crackles ● Rapid, shallow respirations ● Dyspnea ● Hypoxemia ● Retractions ● Diaphoresis ● Restlessness ● Apprehension ● Decreased LOC	ARDS	● Upper airway edema and laryngospasm ● Nasal flaring ● Wheezing ● Accessory muscle use ● Intercostal retractions ● Dyspnea ● Nasal congestion	Anaphylaxis
● Sonorous rhonchi ● Wheezing ● Chills ● Sore throat ● Low-grade fever ● Muscle and back pain ● Substernal tightness	Bronchitis	● Sudden stridor ● Dry paroxysmal coughing ● Gagging or choking ● Hoarseness ● Tachycardia ● Wheezing ● Tachypnea ● Intercostal muscle retractions ● Diminished breath sounds ● Cyanosis ● Shallow respirations	Aspiration of a foreign body
● Sonorous rhonchi with faint, high-pitched wheezing ● Weight loss ● Mild chronic productive cough with scant sputum ● Exertional dyspnea ● Accessory muscle use on inspiration ● Grunting expirations ● Anorexia ● Barrel chest ● Peripheral cyanosis	Emphysema	● Erythematous epiglottiditis ● Fever ● Sore throat ● Crouplike cough	Epiglottiditis

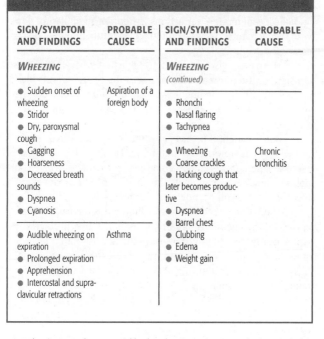

RESPIRATORY SYSTEM: INTERPRETING YOUR FINDINGS (continued)

SIGN/SYMPTOM AND FINDINGS	PROBABLE CAUSE	SIGN/SYMPTOM AND FINDINGS	PROBABLE CAUSE
WHEEZING		**WHEEZING** (continued)	
● Sudden onset of wheezing ● Stridor ● Dry, paroxysmal cough ● Gagging ● Hoarseness ● Decreased breath sounds ● Dyspnea ● Cyanosis	Aspiration of a foreign body	● Rhonchi ● Nasal flaring ● Tachypnea	
● Audible wheezing on expiration ● Prolonged expiration ● Apprehension ● Intercostal and supra-clavicular retractions	Asthma	● Wheezing ● Coarse crackles ● Hacking cough that later becomes productive ● Dyspnea ● Barrel chest ● Clubbing ● Edema ● Weight gain	Chronic bronchitis

a productive cough can quickly develop into airway occlusion and respiratory distress from thick or excessive secretions. Causes include asthma, bronchiectasis, bronchitis, cystic fibrosis, and pertussis.

Crackles

A common finding in patients with certain pulmonary and cardiovascular disorders, crackles are nonmusical clicking or rattling noises heard during auscultation of breath sounds. They usually occur during inspiration and recur constantly from one respiratory cycle to the next. They can be unilateral or bilateral and moist or dry. They're characterized by their pitch, loudness, location, persistence, and occurrence during the respiratory cycle.

HISTORY

Determine if the patient is in acute respiratory distress or is experiencing airway obstruction. Quickly take the patient's vital signs and check the depth and rhythm of respirations. If he's struggling to breathe, check for increased accessory muscle use and chest wall motion, retractions, stridor, or nasal flaring. Provide supplemental oxygen. Endotracheal intubation may be necessary.

If the patient also has a cough, ask when it began and if it's constant or intermittent. Find out what the cough sounds like and whether he's coughing up sputum or blood. If the cough is productive, determine the sputum's consistency, amount, odor, and color.

Ask the patient if he has pain and where it's located. Find out when he first noticed it and if it radiates to other areas. Also ask the patient if movement, coughing, or breathing worsens or helps to relieve his pain. Note the patient's position, for example, if he's lying still or moving about restlessly.

Obtain a brief medical history. Find out if the patient has cancer or any known respiratory or cardiovascular problems. Ask about recent surgery, trauma, or illness. Ask him if he smokes or drinks alcohol. Find out if he's experiencing hoarseness or difficulty swallowing. Ask about the medications he's taking. Also ask about recent weight loss, anorexia, nausea, vomiting, fatigue, weakness, vertigo, and syncope. Find out if the patient has been exposed to irritants, such as vapors, fumes, or smoke.

PHYSICAL ASSESSMENT

Perform a physical examination. Examine the patient's nose and mouth for signs of infection, such as inflammation or increased secretions. Note his breath odor because halitosis could indicate pulmonary infection.

Check his neck for masses, tenderness, swelling, lymphadenopathy, or venous distention. Inspect the patient's chest for abnormal configuration or uneven expansion. Percuss for dullness, tympany, or flatness. Auscultate his lungs for other abnormal, diminished, or absent breath sounds. Listen to his heart for abnormal sounds, and check his hands and feet for edema or clubbing.

ANALYSIS

Crackles indicate abnormal movement of air through fluid-filled airways. They can be irregularly dispersed, as in pneumonia, or localized, as in bronchiectasis. A few basilar crackles can be heard in normal lungs after prolonged shallow breathing. These normal crackles clear with a few deep breaths. Usually, crackles indicate the degree of an underlying illness. When crackles result from a generalized disorder, they usually occur in the less distended and more dependent areas of the lungs, such as the lung bases when the patient is standing. Crackles due to air passing through inflammatory exudate may not be audible if the involved portion of the lung isn't being ventilated because of shallow respirations.

AGE AWARE In infants or children, crackles may indicate a serious respiratory or cardiovascular disorder. Pneumonia produces diffuse, sudden crackles in children. Esophageal atresia and tracheoesophageal fistula can cause bubbling, moist crackles due to the aspiration of food or secretions into the lungs, especially in neonates. Pulmonary edema causes fine crackles at the base of the lungs, and bronchiectasis produces moist crackles. Cystic fibrosis produces widespread, fine to coarse inspiratory crackles and wheezing in infants. Sickle cell anemia may produce crackles when it causes pulmonary infarction or infection.

Crackles that clear after deep breathing may indicate mild basilar atelectasis. In older patients, auscultate lung bases before and after auscultating apices.

Crepitation, subcutaneous

When bubbles of air or other gases, such as carbon dioxide, are trapped in subcutaneous tissue, palpation or stroking of the skin produces a crackling sound called *subcutaneous crepitation* or *subcutaneous emphysema*. The bubbles feel like small, unstable nodules and aren't painful, even though subcutaneous crepitation is commonly associated with painful disorders. Usually, the affected tissue is visibly edematous; this can lead to life-threatening airway occlusion if the edema affects the neck or upper chest.

HISTORY

Because subcutaneous crepitation can indicate a life-threatening disorder, perform a rapid initial evaluation and intervene if necessary. Ask the patient if he's experiencing pain or having difficulty breathing. If he's in pain, find out where the pain is located, how severe it is, and when it began. Ask about recent thoracic surgery, diagnostic tests, respiratory therapy, and a history of trauma or chronic pulmonary disease.

PHYSICAL ASSESSMENT

When the patient's condition permits, palpate the affected skin to evaluate the location and extent of subcutaneous crepitation and to obtain baseline information. Repalpate frequently to determine if the subcutaneous crepitation is increasing.

ANALYSIS

The air or gas bubbles enter the tissues through open wounds from the action of anaerobic microorganisms or from traumatic or spontaneous rupture or perforation of pulmonary or GI organs.

AGE AWARE Children may develop subcutaneous crepitation in the neck from ingestion of corrosive substances that perforate the esophagus.

Cyanosis

Cyanosis—a bluish or bluish-black discoloration of the skin and mucous membranes—results from excessive concentration of unoxygenated hemoglobin in the blood. This common sign may develop abruptly or gradually. It can be classified as central or peripheral, although the two types may coexist.

HISTORY

If cyanosis accompanies less-acute conditions, perform a thorough examination. Begin with a health history, focusing on pulmonary, cardiac, and hematologic disorders. Ask about previous surgeries. Ask the patient if he has a cough and if it's productive. If so, have the patient describe the sputum. Ask about sleep apnea. Find out if the patient sleeps with his head propped up on pillows. Also ask about nausea, anorexia, and weight loss.

RED FLAG If the patient displays sudden, localized cyanosis and other signs of arterial occlusion, protect the affected limb from injury; however, don't massage the limb. If you see central cyanosis stemming from a pulmonary disorder or shock, perform a rapid evaluation. Take immediate steps to maintain ABCs.

PHYSICAL ASSESSMENT

Begin the physical examination by taking the patient's vital signs. Inspect the skin and mucous membranes to determine the extent of cyanosis. Ask the patient when he first noticed the cyanosis and if it subsides and recurs. Find out if it's aggravated by cold, smoking, or stress. Check the skin for coolness, pallor, redness, pain, and ulceration. Also note clubbing.

Next, evaluate the patient's LOC. Ask about headaches, dizziness, or blurred vision, and then test his motor strength. Ask about pain in the arms and legs, especially with walking, and about abnormal sensations, such as numbness, tingling, and coldness.

Ask the patient about chest pain and its severity. Ask him to identify any aggravating and alleviating factors. Palpate peripheral pulses, and test capillary refill time. Also, note edema. Auscultate heart rate and rhythm, especially noting gallops and murmurs, and auscultate the abdominal aorta and femoral arteries to detect any bruits.

Evaluate respiratory rate and rhythm. Check for nasal flaring and use of accessory muscles. Inspect the patient for asymmetrical chest expansion or barrel chest. Percuss the lungs for dullness or hyperresonance, and auscultate for decreased or adventitious breath sounds.

Inspect the abdomen for ascites, and test for shifting dullness or fluid wave. Percuss and palpate for liver enlargement and tenderness.

ANALYSIS

Central cyanosis reflects inadequate oxygenation of systemic arterial blood caused by right-to-left cardiac shunting, pulmonary disease, or hematologic disorders. It may occur anywhere on the skin especially on the mucous membranes of the mouth.

Peripheral cyanosis reflects sluggish peripheral circulation caused by vasoconstriction, reduced cardiac output, or vascular occlusion. It may be widespread or may occur locally in one extremity; however, it doesn't affect mucous membranes. Typically, peripheral cyanosis appears on exposed areas, such as the fingers, nail beds, feet, nose, and ears.

Although cyanosis is an important sign of pulmonary and cardiovascular disorders, it isn't always an accurate gauge of oxygenation. Several factors contribute to its development: hemoglobin concentration and oxygen saturation, cardiac output, and partial pressure of arterial oxygen (PaO_2). Cyanosis is usually undetectable until the oxygen saturation of hemoglobin falls below 80%. Severe cyanosis is obvious, whereas mild cyanosis is more difficult to detect, even in natural, bright light.

In dark-skinned patients, cyanosis is most apparent in the mucous membranes and nail beds.

Transient, nonpathologic cyanosis may result from environmental factors. For example, peripheral cyanosis may result from cutaneous vasoconstriction following a brief exposure to cold air or water. Central cyanosis may result from reduced PaO_2 at high altitudes.

AGE AWARE Children are afflicted with many of the same pulmonary disorders responsible for cyanosis in adults. In addition, central cyanosis may result from cystic fibrosis, asthma, airway obstruction by a foreign body, acute laryngotracheobronchitis, or epiglottiditis. It may also result from a congenital heart defect such as transposition of the great vessels, which causes right-to-left intracardiac shunting. In children, circumoral cyanosis may precede generalized cyanosis. In infants, acrocyanosis (also called *glove and bootie cyanosis*) may occur due to excessive crying or exposure to cold.

Elderly patients commonly have reduced tissue perfusion; therefore, peripheral cyanosis can develop with just a slight decrease in cardiac output or systemic blood pressure.

Dyspnea

Commonly a symptom of cardiopulmonary dysfunction, dyspnea is the sensation of difficult or uncomfortable breathing. It's usually reported as shortness of breath. The severity varies greatly and is typically unrelated to the severity of the underlying cause.

Dyspnea may arise suddenly or slowly and may subside rapidly or persist for years.

HISTORY

If the patient complains of dyspnea, ask if it began suddenly or gradually. Find out if it's constant or intermittent and when the attack began. Ask if it occurs during activity or while at rest. If the patient has had dyspneic attacks before, ask if they're increasing in severity. Ask him to identify what aggravates or alleviates these attacks. Find out if he has a productive or nonproductive cough or chest pain.

Ask about recent trauma, and note a history of upper respiratory tract infections, deep vein phlebitis, or other disorders. Ask the patient if he smokes or is exposed to toxic fumes or irritants in his occupation.

Find out if he has orthopnea (dyspnea when in a supine position), paroxysmal nocturnal dyspnea (dyspnea during sleep), or progressive fatigue.

PHYSICAL ASSESSMENT

During the physical examination, look for signs of chronic dyspnea, such as accessory muscle hypertrophy, especially in the shoulders and neck. Also look for pursed-lip exhalation, clubbing, peripheral edema, barrel chest, diaphoresis, and jugular vein distention. Auscultate for adventitious breath sounds, abnormal heart sounds or rhythms, egophony, bronchophony, and whispered pectoriloquy. Then palpate the abdomen for hepatomegaly.

ANALYSIS

Most people normally experience dyspnea when they overexert themselves, and its severity depends on their physical condition. In a healthy person, dyspnea is quickly relieved by rest. Pathologic causes of dyspnea include pulmonary, cardiac, neuromuscular, and allergic disorders. In addition, anxiety may cause dyspnea.

Dyspnea occurs when ventilation is disturbed. When ventilatory demands exceed the actual or perceived capacity of the lungs to respond, the patient becomes short of breath. Decreased lung compliance, a disturbance in the chest bellows system, an airway obstruction, or obesity can increase the work of breathing.

When evaluating dyspnea, determine whether it stems from pulmonary or cardiac disease; then evaluate the degree of impairment the dyspnea has caused.

Your questions about the onset and severity of your patient's dyspnea should prove helpful. A sudden onset may indicate an acute problem, such as pneumothorax or pulmonary embolus. Sudden dyspnea may also result from anxiety caused by hyperventilation. A gradual onset suggests a slow, progressive disorder, such as COPD, whereas acute intermittent attacks may indicate asthma.

Precipitating factors also help pinpoint the cause. For example, paroxysmal nocturnal dyspnea or orthopnea may stem from a chronic lung disorder or a cardiac disorder such as left-sided heart failure. Dyspnea aggravated by activity suggests poor ventilation and perfusion or inefficient breathing mechanisms.

AGE AWARE Elderly patients with dyspnea related to chronic illness may not initially be aware of a significant change in their breathing pattern.

Hemoptysis

Hemoptysis is the expectoration of blood or bloody sputum from the lungs or tracheobronchial tree. It's sometimes confused with bleeding from the mouth, throat, nasopharynx, or GI tract.

HISTORY

If your patient complains of hemoptysis, ask if it's mild and when it began. Find out if the patient has ever coughed up blood before. Ask him about how much blood he's coughing up now and how often.

Ask about a history of pulmonary, cardiac, or bleeding disorders. If he's receiving anticoagulant therapy, find out the drug, its dosage and schedule, and the duration of therapy. Find out if he's taking other prescription or nonprescription drugs, if he smokes, or if he has a history of TB.

PHYSICAL ASSESSMENT

Examine the patient's nose, mouth, and pharynx to determine the source of the bleeding. Inspect the configuration of his chest, and look for abnormal movement during breathing, use of accessory muscles, and retractions. Observe respiratory rate, depth, and rhythm. Examine the skin for lesions.

Next, palpate the patient's chest for diaphragm level and for tenderness, respiratory excursion, fremitus, and abnormal pulsations; then percuss for flatness, dullness, resonance, hyperresonance, and tympany. Finally, auscultate the lungs, noting especially the quality and intensity of breath sounds. Assess for the presence of a pleural friction rub. Also auscultate for heart murmurs and bruits.

Obtain a sputum sample and examine it for overall quantity, for the amount of blood it contains, and for its color, odor, and consistency.

ANALYSIS

Commonly frothy because it's mixed with air, hemoptysis is typically bright red with an alkaline pH. Expectoration of 200 ml of blood in a single episode suggests severe bleeding, whereas expectoration of 400 ml in 3 hours or more than 600 ml in 16 hours signals a life-threatening crisis.

Hemoptysis usually results from TB, chronic bronchitis, lung cancer, or bronchiectasis. However, it may also result from inflammatory, infectious, cardiovascular, and coagulation disorders or, in rare cases, from a ruptured aortic aneurysm. In up to 15% of patients, the cause is unknown. The most common causes of massive hemoptysis are lung cancer, bronchiectasis, active TB, and cavitary pulmonary disease from necrotic infections or TB.

Rhonchi

Rhonchi are continuous adventitious breath sounds detected by auscultation. They're usually louder and lower pitched than crackles—more like a hoarse moan or a deep snore—though they may be described as rattling, sonorous, bubbling, rumbling, or musical. However, sibilant rhonchi, or wheezes, are high pitched.

HISTORY

When obtaining the health history, ask these related questions: Does the patient smoke? If so, obtain a history in pack-years.

Has he recently lost weight or felt tired or weak? Does he have asthma or other pulmonary disorder? Is he taking any prescription or OTC drugs?

PHYSICAL ASSESSMENT

If you auscultate rhonchi, take the patient's vital signs, including oxygen saturation, and be alert for signs of respiratory distress. Characterize the patient's respirations as rapid or slow, shallow or deep, and regular or irregular. Inspect the chest, noting the use of accessory muscles. Observe if the patient is audibly wheezing or gurgling. Auscultate for other abnormal breath sounds, such as crackles and a pleural friction rub. If you detect these sounds, note their location. Note if breath sounds are diminished or absent.

Next, percuss the chest. If the patient has a cough, note its frequency and characterize its sound. If it's productive, examine the sputum for color, odor, amount, consistency, and blood.

RED FLAG During the examination, keep in mind that thick or excessive secretions, bronchospasm, or inflammation of mucous membranes may lead to airway obstruction. If necessary, suction the patient and keep equipment available for inserting an artificial airway. Keep a bronchodilator available to treat bronchospasm.

ANALYSIS

Rhonchi are heard over large airways, such as the trachea. They can occur in a patient with a pulmonary disorder when air flows through passages that have been narrowed by secretions, a tumor or foreign body, bronchospasm, or mucosal thickening. The resulting vibration of airway walls produces the rhonchi.

AGE AWARE In children, rhonchi can result from bacterial pneumonia, cystic fibrosis, and croup. Because a respiratory tract disorder may begin abruptly and progress rapidly in an infant or a child, observe closely for signs of airway obstruction.

Stridor

A loud, harsh, musical respiratory sound, stridor results from an obstruction in the trachea or larynx. Usually heard during inspiration, this sign may also occur during expiration in severe upper airway obstruction.

HISTORY

When the patient's condition permits, obtain a health history from him or a family member. First, find out when the stridor began and if he has had it before. Ask if he has had an upper respiratory tract infection and, if so, how long he has had it.

Ask about a history of allergies, tumors, and respiratory and vascular disorders. Note recent exposure to smoke or noxious fumes or gases. Next, explore associated signs and symptoms. Find out if the stridor occurs with pain or a cough.

RED FLAG If you hear stridor, quickly check the patient's vital signs, including oxygen saturation, and examine him for other signs of partial airway obstruction—choking or gagging, tachypnea, dyspnea, shallow respirations, intercostal retractions, nasal flaring, tachycardia, cyanosis, and diaphoresis. Be aware that abrupt cessation of stridor signals complete obstruction in which the patient has inspiratory chest movement but absent breath sounds. He may be unable to talk and can quickly become lethargic and lose conscious-ness. In this case, begin measures to clear the obstruction. Initiate cardiopulmonary resuscitation.

PHYSICAL ASSESSMENT

Examine the patient's mouth for excessive secretions, foreign matter, inflammation, and swelling. Assess his neck for swelling, masses, subcutaneous crepitation, and scars. Observe the pa-tient's chest for delayed, decreased, or asymmetrical chest ex-pansion. Auscultate for adventitious breath sounds. Percuss for dullness, tympany, or flatness. Finally, note any burns or signs of trauma, such as ecchymoses and lacerations.

ANALYSIS

Stridor may begin as low-pitched "croaking" and progress to high-pitched "crowing" as respirations become more vigorous. Life-threatening upper airway obstruction can stem from foreign-body aspiration, increased secretions, intraluminal tu-mor, localized edema or muscle spasms, and external compres-sion by a tumor or aneurysm.

AGE AWARE In children, stridor is a major sign of airway ob-struction. Quick intervention is needed to prevent total airway obstruction. This emergency can happen more rapidly in a child be-cause his airway is narrower than an adult's. Causes of stridor include foreign-body aspiration, croup syndrome, laryngeal diphtheria, pertussis, retropharyngeal abscess, and congenital abnormalities of the larynx.

Wheezing

Wheezes are adventitious breath sounds with a high-pitched, musical, squealing, creaking, or groaning quality. When they originate in the large airways, they can be heard by placing an unaided ear over the chest wall or at the mouth. When they originate in the smaller airways, they can be heard by placing a stethoscope over the anterior or posterior chest. Unlike rhonchi, wheezes can't be cleared by coughing.

HISTORY

Ask the patient what triggers his wheezing. Find out if he has asthma or allergies, if he smokes or has a history of pulmonary, cardiac, or circulatory disorders, or if he has cancer.

Ask the patient if he has recently had surgery, illness, or trauma, or changes in appetite, weight, exercise tolerance, or sleep patterns. Find out which drugs he's currently taking and which he has taken in the past. Also find out if he has been exposed to toxic fumes or respiratory irritants.

If he has a cough, ask how it sounds, when it occurs, and how often it occurs. Find out if he has paroxysms of coughing and if the cough is dry, sputum producing, or bloody.

Ask the patient if he's experiencing chest pain. If so, determine its quality, onset, duration, intensity, and radiation. Find out if it increases with breathing, coughing, or certain positions.

PHYSICAL ASSESSMENT

Examine the patient's nose and mouth for congestion, drainage, or signs of infection such as halitosis. If he produces sputum, obtain a sample for examination. Check for cyanosis, pallor, clamminess, masses, tenderness, swelling, jugular vein distention, and enlarged lymph nodes. Inspect his chest for abnormal configuration and asymmetrical motion, and determine if the trachea is midline. Percuss for dullness or hyperresonance, and auscultate for adventitious breath sounds. Note absent or hypoactive breath sounds, abnormal heart sounds, gallops, or murmurs. Also note arrhythmias, bradycardia, or tachycardia.

ANALYSIS

Usually, prolonged wheezing occurs during expiration when bronchi are shortened and narrowed. Causes of airway narrowing include bronchospasm; mucosal thickening or edema; partial obstruction from a tumor, foreign body, or secretions; and extrinsic pressure, as in tension pneumothorax or goiter. With airway obstruction, wheezing occurs during inspiration.

AGE AWARE Children are especially susceptible to wheezing because their small airways allow rapid obstruction. Primary causes of wheezing include bronchospasm, mucosal edema, and accumulation of secretions. These may occur with such disorders as cystic fibrosis, acute bronchiolitis, and pulmonary hemosiderosis, or foreign-body aspiration.

3

Diagnostic tests and procedures

If the patient's history and physical examination reveal evidence of pulmonary dysfunction, diagnostic tests will help identify and evaluate the dysfunction. These tests include blood, sputum, and pleural studies; endoscopic and imaging tests; biopsies; and various other tests, including pulmonary function tests, pulse oximetry, and thoracentesis.

BLOOD STUDIES

Blood studies used to diagnose respiratory disorders include arterial blood gas (ABG) analysis, arterial-to-alveolar oxygen ratio, white blood cell (WBC) count, and WBC differential.

Arterial blood gas analysis

ABG analysis is one of the first tests ordered to assess respiratory status because it helps evaluate gas exchange in the lungs by measuring:

- pH—an indication of hydrogen ion concentration in the blood, which shows the blood's acidity or alkalinity (see *Balancing pH*)
- partial pressure of arterial carbon dioxide ($PaCO_2$)—known as the *respiratory parameter,* reflects the adequacy of the lungs' ventilation and carbon dioxide (CO_2) elimination
- partial pressure of arterial oxygen (PaO_2)—reflects the body's ability to pick up oxygen from the lungs
- bicarbonate level (HCO_3^-)—known as the *metabolic parameter,* reflects the kidneys' ability to retain and excrete bicarbonate. (See *Understanding acid-base disorders,* pages 66 and 67.)

BALANCING pH

To measure the acidity or alkalinity of a solution, chemists use a pH scale of 1 to 15 that measures hydrogen ion concentrations. As hydrogen ions and acidity increase, pH falls below 7.0, which is neutral. Conversely, when hydrogen ions decrease, pH and alkalinity increase. Acid-base balance, or homeostasis of hydrogen ions, is necessary if the body's enzyme systems are to work properly.

The slightest change in ionic hydrogen concentration alters the rate of cellular chemical reactions; a sufficiently severe change can be fatal. To maintain a normal blood pH—generally between 7.35 and 7.45—the body relies on three mechanisms.

Buffers

Chemically composed of two substances, buffers prevent radical pH changes by replacing strong acids added to a solution (such as blood) with weaker ones. For example, strong acids capable of yielding many hydrogen ions are replaced by weaker ones that yield fewer hydrogen ions. Because of the principal buffer coupling of bicarbonate and carbonic acid—normally in a ratio of 20:1—the plasma acid-base level rarely fluctuates. Increased bicarbonate, however, indicates alkalosis, whereas decreased bicarbonate points to acidosis. Increased carbonic acid indicates acidosis, and decreased carbonic acid indicates alkalosis.

Respiration

Respiration is important in maintaining blood pH. The lungs convert carbonic acid to carbon dioxide and water. With every expiration, carbon dioxide and water leave the body, decreasing the carbonic acid content of the blood. Consequently, fewer hydrogen ions are formed, and blood pH increases. When the blood's hydrogen ion or carbonic acid content increases, neurons in the respiratory center stimulate respiration.

Hyperventilation eliminates carbon dioxide and hence carbonic acid from the body, reduces hydrogen ion formation, and increases pH. Conversely, increased blood pH from alkalosis—decreased hydrogen ion concentration—causes hypoventilation, which restores blood pH to its normal level by retaining carbon dioxide and thus increasing hydrogen ion formation.

Urinary excretion

The third factor in acid-base balance is urine excretion. Because the kidneys excrete varying amounts of acids and bases, they control urine pH, which in turn affects blood pH. For example, when blood pH is decreased, the distal and collecting tubules remove excessive hydrogen ions (carbonic acid forms in the tubular cells and dissociates into hydrogen and bicarbonate) and displaces them in urine, thereby eliminating hydrogen from the body. In exchange, basic ions in the urine—usually sodium—diffuse into the tubular cells, where they combine with bicarbonate. This sodium bicarbonate is then reabsorbed in the blood, resulting in decreased urine pH and, more important, increased blood pH.

UNDERSTANDING ACID-BASE DISORDERS

This table outlines acid-base disorders, along with laboratory values associated with the disorder.

DISORDERS AND ABG FINDINGS	POSSIBLE CAUSES	SIGNS AND SYMPTOMS
RESPIRATORY ACIDOSIS (EXCESS CO_2 RETENTION)		
pH < 7.35 (SI, < 7.35) HCO_3^- > 26 mEq/L (SI, > 26 mmol/L) (if compensating) $Paco_2$ > 45 mm Hg (SI, > 5.3 kPa)	● Central nervous system depression from drugs, injury, or disease ● Asphyxia ● Hypoventilation due to pulmonary, cardiac, musculoskeletal, or neuromuscular disease ● Obesity ● Postoperative pain ● Abdominal distention	Diaphoresis, headache, tachycardia, confusion, restlessness, apprehension
RESPIRATORY ALKALOSIS (EXCESS CO_2 EXCRETION)		
pH > 7.45 (SI, > 7.45) HCO_3^- < 22 mEq/L (SI, < 22 mmol/L) (if compensating) $Paco_2$ < 35 mm Hg (SI, < 4.7 kPa)	● Hyperventilation due to anxiety, pain, or improper ventilator settings ● Respiratory stimulation caused by drugs, disease, hypoxia, fever, or high room temperature ● Gram-negative bacteremia ● Compensation for metabolic acidosis (chronic renal failure)	Rapid, deep breathing; paresthesia; lightheadedness; twitching; anxiety; fear
METABOLIC ACIDOSIS (HCO_3^- LOSS, ACID RETENTION)		
pH < 7.35 (SI, < 7.35) HCO_3^- < 22 mEq/L (SI, < 22 mmol/L) $Paco_2$ < 35 mm Hg (SI, < 4.7 kPa) (if compensating)	● HCO_3^- depletion due to renal disease, diarrhea, or small-bowel fistulas ● Excessive production of organic acids due to hepatic disease and endocrine disorders, including diabetes mellitus, hypoxia, shock, and drug intoxication ● Inadequate excretion of acids due to renal disease	Rapid, deep breathing; fruity breath; fatigue; headache; lethargy; drowsiness; nausea; vomiting; coma (if severe)

UNDERSTANDING ACID-BASE DISORDERS *(continued)*

DISORDERS AND ABG FINDINGS	POSSIBLE CAUSES	SIGNS AND SYMPTOMS
METABOLIC ALKALOSIS (HCO_3^- RETENTION, ACID LOSS)		
pH > 7.45 (SI, > 7.45) HCO_3^- > 26 mEq/L (SI, > 26 mmol/L) $PaCO_2$ > 45 mm Hg (SI, > 5.3 kPa)	● Loss of hydrochloric acid from prolonged vomiting or gastric suctioning ● Loss of potassium due to increased renal excretion (as in diuretic therapy) or steroid overdose ● Excessive alkali ingestion ● Compensation for chronic respiratory acidosis	Slow, shallow breathing; hypertonic muscles; restlessness; twitching; confusion; irritability; apathy; tetany; seizures; coma (if severe)

The respiratory and metabolic systems work together to keep the body's acid-base balance within normal limits. For example, if respiratory acidosis develops, the kidneys try to compensate by conserving HCO_3^-. Therefore, if respiratory acidosis is present, expect to see the HCO_3^- value rise above normal. Similarly, if metabolic acidosis develops, the lungs try to compensate by increasing the respiratory rate and depth to eliminate CO_2. Therefore, if metabolic acidosis is present, expect to see the $PaCO_2$ level fall below normal.

NURSING CONSIDERATIONS

■ Blood for an ABG analysis should be drawn from an arterial line if the patient has one. If a percutaneous puncture must be done, the site must be chosen carefully. The brachial, radial, and femoral arteries can be used.

■ After the sample is obtained, apply pressure to the puncture site for 5 minutes and tape a gauze pad firmly in place. (Don't apply tape around the arm; it could restrict circulation.) Regularly monitor the site for bleeding and check the arm for signs of complications (such as swelling, discoloration, pain, numbness, and tingling).

■ Make sure it's noted if the patient is breathing room air or oxygen. If oxygen, document the number of liters and delivery device. If the patient is receiving mechanical ventilation, the fraction of inspired oxygen should be documented.

■ Keep in mind that certain actions may interfere with test results—for example, exposing the sample to air or failing to properly heparinize the syringe before drawing a blood sample. Venous blood in the sample may lower PaO_2 levels and elevate $PaCO_2$ levels.

■ Wait at least 20 minutes before drawing blood for ABGs in the following situations:
  – after starting, changing, or stopping oxygen therapy
  – after starting or changing settings of mechanical ventilation
  – after extubation.

■ Tell the patient which site—radial, brachial, or femoral artery—has been selected for the puncture.

■ Instruct the patient to breathe normally during the test, and warn him that he may feel brief cramping or throbbing pain at the puncture site.

■ Monitor vital signs and observe for signs of circulatory impairment, such as swelling, discoloration, pain, numbness, or tingling in the bandaged arm or leg.

Arterial-to-alveolar oxygen ratio

By using calculations based on the patient's laboratory values, the arterial-to-alveolar (a/A) oxygen ratio test can help identify the cause of hypoxemia and intrapulmonary shunting by providing an approximation of the partial pressure of oxygenation of the alveoli and arteries. It may help differentiate the cause as ventilated alveoli but no perfusion, unventilated alveoli with perfusion, or collapse of the alveoli and capillaries.

NURSING CONSIDERATIONS

■ Explain to the patient that the a/A ratio test is used to evaluate how well the lungs are delivering oxygen to the blood and eliminating carbon dioxide.

■ Tell the patient that the test requires a blood sample. Explain who will perform the arterial puncture and when.

■ Inform the patient that he need not restrict food and fluids.

- Instruct the patient to breathe normally during the test, and warn him that he may experience cramping or throbbing pain at the puncture site.
- Perform an arterial puncture or draw blood from an arterial line using a heparinized blood gas syringe.
- Eliminate all air from the sample and place it on ice immediately.
- Apply pressure to the puncture for 5 minutes or until bleeding stops.
- Place a gauze pad over the site and tape it in place, but don't tape the entire circumference.
- Monitor vital signs and observe for signs of circulatory impairment, such as swelling, discoloration, pain, numbness, and tingling distal to the puncture site.
- Watch for bleeding from the puncture site.
- The arterial sample is analyzed for partial pressure of arterial oxygen (PaO_2) and partial pressure of arterial carbon dioxide ($PaCO_2$). Also examined are barometric pressure (Pb), water vapor pressure (PH_2O), and fractional concentration of inspired oxygen (FIO_2) (21% for room air). From these values, the alveolar oxygen tension (PAO_2), the a/A ratio, and the alveolar-to-arterial oxygen gradient ($A\text{-}aDO_2$) are derived by solving these mathematical formulas:

$$PaO_2 = FIO_2 (Pb - PH_2O) - 1.25 (PaCO_2)$$
$$\text{a/A ratio} = PaO_2 \div PAO_2$$
$$A\text{-}aDO_2 = PAO_2 - PaO_2$$

- Based on the results of the formulas, appropriate interventions to correct patient problems are initiated.

White blood cell count

The white blood cell (WBC), or leukocyte, count measures the number of WBCs in a microliter of whole blood. This is done through the use of electronic devices. A WBC count can be useful in diagnosing infection and inflammation as well as in monitoring a patient's response to chemotherapy or radiation therapy. WBC counts can also help determine whether further tests are needed.

An elevated WBC count (leukocytosis) commonly signals infection, such as an abscess, meningitis, appendicitis, or tonsillitis. A high count may indicate leukemia or tissue necrosis caused by burns, myocardial infarction, or gangrene.

NURSING CONSIDERATIONS
- Tell the patient that he should avoid strenuous exercise for 24 hours before the test to avoid altered readings and that he also should avoid ingesting a large meal before the test.
- Perform a venipuncture and collect the sample in a 7-ml tube containing EDTA.
- Completely fill the sample collection tube, and invert it gently several times to mix the sample and anticoagulant adequately.

White blood cell differential

A white blood cell (WBC) differential can provide specific information about a patient's immune system. In a WBC differential, the laboratory classifies 100 or more WBCs in a stained film of blood according to five major types of leukocytes: neutrophils, eosinophils, basophils, lymphocytes, and monocytes, and determines the percentage of each type.

Abnormally high levels of WBCs are associated with such things as infections, allergic reactions and parasitic infections. After the normal values for the patient have been determined, an assessment can be made.

NURSING CONSIDERATIONS
- Tell the patient to avoid strenuous exercise before a WBC count to ensure accurate results.
- Perform a venipuncture, and collect the sample in a 7-ml tube containing EDTA.
- Completely fill the collection tube and invert it gently several times to mix the sample and anticoagulant adequately.

SPUTUM AND PLEURAL FLUID STUDIES

Sputum studies include sputum analysis, nasopharyngeal culture, and throat culture. Pleural fluid studies include thoracentesis.

Sputum analysis

Analysis of a sputum specimen (the material expectorated from a patient's lungs and bronchi during deep coughing) helps diagnose respiratory disease, determine the cause of respiratory infection (including viral and bacterial causes), identify abnormal lung cells, and manage lung disease.

A sputum specimen is stained and examined under a microscope and, depending on the patient's condition, sometimes cultured. Culture and sensitivity testing identifies a specific microorganism and its antibiotic sensitivities. A negative culture may suggest a viral infection.

Flora commonly found in the respiratory tract include alpha-hemolytic streptococci, *Neisseria* species, diphtheroids, some *Haemophilus* species, pneumococci, staphylococci, and yeasts such as *Candida*. However, the presence of normal flora doesn't rule out infection. A culture isolate must be interpreted in light of the patient's overall clinical condition.

Pathogenic organisms most often found in sputum include *Streptococcus pneumoniae, Mycobacterium tuberculosis, Klebsiella pneumoniae* (and other Enterobacteriaceae), *H. influenzae, Staphylococcus aureus,* and *Pseudomonas aeruginosa.* Other pathogens, such as *Pneumocystis carinii, Legionella* species, *Mycoplasma pneumoniae,* and respiratory viruses, may exist in the sputum and can cause lung disease, but they usually require serologic or histologic diagnosis rather than diagnosis by sputum culture.

NURSING CONSIDERATIONS

- Encourage the patient to increase his fluid intake the night before sputum collection to aid expectoration.
- When the patient is ready to expectorate, instruct him to take three deep breaths and force a deep cough.
- Before sending the specimen to the laboratory, make sure the specimen is sputum, not saliva. Saliva has a thinner consistency and more bubbles (froth) than sputum.
- Explain to the patient that this test requires sputum, not saliva. Teach him how to expectorate.

Expectoration

- Put on gloves and a mask.

- Instruct the patient to cough deeply and expectorate into the container.
- If the cough is nonproductive, use chest physiotherapy or nebulization to induce sputum, as ordered.
- Using aseptic technique, close the container securely and place it in a leakproof bag before sending it to the laboratory.

Tracheal suctioning

- Give the patient oxygen, as needed.
- Using sterile gloves, lubricate the catheter with normal saline solution and pass the catheter through the nostril, without suction. (The patient will cough when the catheter passes through the larynx.)
- Advance the catheter into the trachea.
- Apply suction for no longer than 15 seconds to obtain the specimen.
- Stop suction and gently remove the catheter.
- Discard the catheter and gloves.
- Detach the in-line sputum trap from the suction apparatus and cap the opening.
- If the patient becomes hypoxic or cyanotic, remove the catheter immediately and give oxygen. (See *Using an in-line trap*.)

Bronchoscopy

- Secretions are collected with a bronchial brush or aspirated through the inner channel of the scope, using an irrigating solution, such as normal saline solution, if necessary.
- After the specimen is obtained, the bronchoscope is removed.
- After bronchoscopy, observe the patient carefully for signs of hypoxemia, laryngospasm, bronchospasm, pneumothorax, perforation of the trachea or bronchus (subcutaneous crepitus), or trauma to respiratory structures.
- Check for difficulty breathing or swallowing.
- *Don't* give liquids until the gag reflex returns.
- In a patient with asthma or chronic bronchitis, watch for aggravated bronchospasms.
- Include on the laboratory slip the nature and origin of the specimen, the date and time of collection, the initial diagnosis, and any antibiotics the patient is currently taking.

USING AN IN-LINE TRAP

When using an in-line trap, put on sterile gloves, push the suction tubing onto the male adapter of the trap, and follow these three steps:

1. Insert the suction catheter into the rubber tubing of the trap. Then suction the patient.

2. After suctioning, disconnect the in-line trap from the suction tubing and catheter.

3. To seal the container, connect the rubber tubing to the female adapter of the trap.

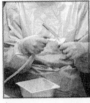

■ Send the specimen to the laboratory immediately.

Nasopharyngeal culture

Direct microscopic inspection of a Gram-stained smear of the nasopharyngeal specimen provides preliminary identification of organisms, which may guide clinical management and determine the need for additional testing. Streaking a culture plate with the swab to allow any organisms present to grow permits isolation and identification of pathogens. Cultured pathogens may require susceptibility testing to determine the appropriate antimicrobial agent.

Flora commonly found in the nasopharynx include non-hemolytic streptococci, alpha-hemolytic streptococci, *Neisseria* species (except *N. meningitidis* and *N. gonorrhoeae*), *Staphylococcus epidermidis* and, occasionally, *S. aureus*.

NURSING CONSIDERATIONS

■ Inform the patient how and where the specimen will be obtained and that he may experience slight discomfort and may gag.

OBTAINING A NASOPHARYNGEAL SPECIMEN

Gather the sterile swab and specimen container. Explain the procedure to the patient. Gently but quickly rotate the sterile swab in the nasopharynx to collect the specimen. Remove the swab, being careful not to injure the nasal mucous membrane.

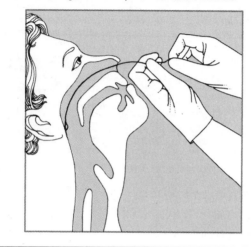

- Put on gloves. Moisten the swab with sterile water or normal saline solution. Ask the patient to cough before you begin collecting the specimen, and then position the patient with his head tilted back.
- Using a penlight and a tongue blade, inspect the nasopharyngeal area. Next, without touching the sides of the patient's nostril, gently pass the swab through the nostril and into the nasopharynx, keeping the swab near the septum and floor of the nose. (See *Obtaining a nasopharyngeal specimen*.)
- If *Bordetella pertussis* is suspected, Dacron or calcium alginate minitipped swabs should be used for collection.
- If the specimen is for isolation of a virus, verify the laboratory's recommended collection and refrigeration techniques.
- Note recent antimicrobial therapy or chemotherapy on the laboratory request.

CHARACTERISTICS OF PULMONARY TRANSUDATE AND EXUDATE

These characteristics help classify pleural fluid as either a transudate or an exudate.

CHARACTERISTIC	TRANSUDATE	EXUDATE
Appearance	Clear	Cloudy, turbid
Specific gravity	< 1.016	> 1.016
Clot (fibrinogen)	Absent	Present
Protein	< 3 g/dl (SI, < 30 g/L)	> 3 g/dl (SI, > 30 g/L)
White blood cells	Few lymphocytes	Many lymphocytes; may be purulent
Red blood cells	Few	Variable
Glucose level	Equal to serum level	May be less than serum level
Lactate dehydrogenase	Low	High

- Tell the laboratory if *Corynebacterium diphtheriae* or *B. pertussis* is suspected; these organisms need special growth media.
- Keep the container upright.

Thoracentesis

Thoracentesis, also known as pleural fluid aspiration, is used to obtain a sample of pleural fluid for analysis, relieve lung compression and, occasionally, obtain a lung tissue biopsy specimen.

The pleural cavity should contain less than 20 ml of serous fluid. Pleural effusion results from the abnormal formation or reabsorption of pleural fluid. Certain characteristics classify pleural fluid as either a transudate or an exudate. (See *Characteristics of pulmonary transudate and exudate.*)

Pleural fluid may contain blood, chyle, or pus and necrotic tissue. A high percentage of neutrophils suggest septic inflammation. Pleural fluid glucose levels that are 30 to 40 mg/dl (SI,

1.5 to 2 mmol/L) lower than blood glucose levels may indicate cancer, bacterial infection, nonseptic inflammation, or metastasis. Increased amylase levels occur with pleural effusions associated with pancreatitis.

NURSING CONSIDERATIONS
- Check the patient's history for bleeding disorders or anticoagulant therapy.
- Explain that a chest X-ray or ultrasound study may precede the test.
- Tell the patient that his vital signs will be taken and then the area around the needle insertion site will be shaved.
- The physician will clean the needle insertion site with a cold antiseptic solution, and then inject a local anesthetic. He may feel a burning sensation as the physician injects the anesthetic.
- Explain to him that after his skin is numb, the physician will insert the needle. He'll feel pressure during needle insertion and withdrawal. He'll need to remain still during the test to avoid the risk of lung injury. He should try to relax and breathe normally during the test and shouldn't cough, breathe deeply, or move. (See *Positioning the patient for thoracentesis.*)
- Monitor the patient's vital signs every 30 minutes for 2 hours, and then every 4 hours until they're stable.
- Watch for signs and symptoms of complications. (See *Recognizing complications of thoracentesis,* page 78.)
- Emphasize that he should tell the physician if he experiences dyspnea, palpitations, wheezing, dizziness, weakness, or diaphoresis, as these symptoms may indicate respiratory distress. After withdrawing the needle, the physician will apply slight pressure to the site and then an adhesive bandage.
- Tell the patient to report fluid or blood leakage from the needle insertion site as well as signs and symptoms of respiratory distress.

Throat culture
A throat culture requires swabbing the throat, streaking a culture plate, and allowing the organisms to grow for isolation and identification of pathogens. A Gram-stained smear may provide

POSITIONING THE PATIENT FOR THORACENTESIS

To prepare a patient for thoracentesis, place him in one of these positions shown below. These positions serve to widen the intercostal spaces and permit easy access to the pleural cavity. Using pillows (as shown) will make the patient more comfortable.

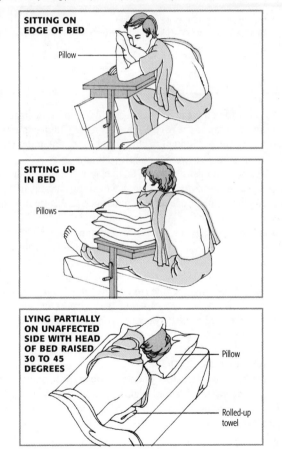

SITTING ON EDGE OF BED

Pillow

SITTING UP IN BED

Pillows

LYING PARTIALLY ON UNAFFECTED SIDE WITH HEAD OF BED RAISED 30 TO 45 DEGREES

Pillow

Rolled-up towel

RECOGNIZING COMPLICATIONS OF THORACENTESIS

You can identify complications of thoracentesis by watching for characteristic signs and symptoms:

- *pneumothorax*–apprehension, increased restlessness, cyanosis, sudden breathlessness, tachycardia, chest pain
- *tension pneumothorax*–dyspnea, chest pain, tachycardia, hypotension, absent or diminished breath sounds on the affected side
- *subcutaneous emphysema*–local tissue swelling, crackling on palpation of site
- *infection*–fever, rapid pulse rate, pain
- *mediastinal shift*–labored breathing, cardiac arrhythmias, pulmonary edema.

preliminary identification, which may guide clinical management and determine the need for further tests. Culture results must be interpreted in light of clinical status, recent antimicrobial therapy, and the amount of normal flora.

Possible pathogens cultured include group A beta-hemolytic streptococci (*Streptococcus pyogenes*), which can cause scarlet fever or pharyngitis; *Candida albicans*, which can cause thrush; *Corynebacterium diphtheriae*, which can cause diphtheria; and *Bordetella pertussis*, which can cause whooping cough. Other cultured bacteria include *Legionella* species, *Mycobacterium pneumoniae*, *Staphylococcus aureus*, *Streptococcus pneumoniae*, and *Hemophilus influenzae*. It's also used to screen for carriers of *Neisseria meningitidis*. Fungi include *Histoplasma capsulatum*, *Coccidioides immitis*, and *Blastomyces dermatitidis*. Viruses include adenovirus, enterovirus, herpesvirus, rhinovirus, influenza virus, and parainfluenza virus.

NURSING CONSIDERATIONS

- Check for a recent history of antimicrobial therapy and obtain the throat specimen before beginning antimicrobial therapy.
- Explain to the patient that this test helps identify the microorganisms and takes about 30 seconds. Tell him he may gag during swabbing.

- Use gloves when performing the procedure and while handling specimens.
- Have the patient tilt his head back and close his eyes. With the throat well illuminated, check for inflamed areas using a tongue blade.
- Swab the tonsillar areas from side to side; include inflamed or purulent sites. Don't touch the tongue, cheeks, or teeth with the swab.
- Immediately place the swab in the culture tube. If a commercial sterile collection and transport system is used, crush the ampule and force the swab into the medium to keep it moist.
- Note recent antimicrobial therapy on the laboratory request. Also, indicate the suspected organism.
- Send the specimen to the laboratory immediately; keep the container upright during transport. Don't refrigerate specimens.

ENDOSCOPIC AND IMAGING TESTS

Endoscopic and imaging tests include bronchoscopy, chest X-ray, direct laryngoscopy, fluoroscopy, mediastinoscopy, magnetic resonance imaging, pulmonary angiography, paranasal sinus radiography, thoracic computed tomography scan, thoracoscopy, and ventilation-perfusion scan.

Bronchoscopy

Bronchoscopy is direct inspection of the larynx, trachea, and bronchi through a flexible fiber-optic or rigid metal bronchoscope. A more recent approach is the use of virtual bronchoscopy. (See *Virtual bronchoscopy,* page 80.) Although a flexible fiber-optic bronchoscope allows a wider view and is used more commonly, the rigid metal bronchoscope is required to remove foreign objects, excise endobronchial lesions, and control massive hemoptysis. A brush biopsy forceps or catheter may be passed through the bronchoscope to obtain specimens for cytologic examination.

VIRTUAL BRONCHOSCOPY

Using a computer and data from a spiral computed tomography (CT) scan, physicians can now examine the respiratory tract noninvasively with virtual bronchoscopy. Although still in its early stages, researchers believe that this test can enhance screening, diagnosis, preoperative planning, surgical technique, and postoperative follow-up.

Unlike its counterpart–conventional bronchoscopy–virtual bronchoscopy is noninvasive, doesn't require sedation, and provides images for examination beyond the segmental bronchi, thus allowing for possible diagnosis of areas that may be stenosed, obstructed, or compressed from an external source. The images obtained from the CT scan include views of the airways and lung parenchyma. Anatomic structures and abnormalities can be precisely identified and,

therefore, can be helpful in locating potential biopsy sites to be obtained with conventional bronchoscopy and provide simulation for planning the optimal surgical approach.

Virtual bronchoscopy does have disadvantages. This technique doesn't allow for actual biopsies to be obtained from tissue sources. It also can't demonstrate details of the mucosal surface, such as color or texture. Also, if an area contains viscous secretions, such as mucus or blood, visualization becomes difficult.

More research on this technique is needed. However, researchers believe that virtual bronchoscopy may play a major role in the screening and early detection of certain cancers, thus allowing for treatment at an earlier, possibly curable stage.

NURSING CONSIDERATIONS

- Tell the patient that he'll receive a sedative, such as diazepam (Valium) or midazolam (Versed).
- Explain that the physician will introduce the bronchoscope tube through the patient's nose or mouth into the airway. Then he'll flush small amounts of anesthetic through the tube to suppress coughing and gagging.
- Explain to the patient that he'll be asked to lie on his side or sit with his head elevated at least 30 degrees until his gag reflex returns. Food, fluid, and oral drugs will be withheld during this time. Hoarseness or a sore throat is temporary, and when his gag reflex returns, he can have throat lozenges or a gargle.
- Report bloody mucus, dyspnea, wheezing, or chest pain to the physician immediately. A chest X-ray will be taken after the procedure and the patient may receive an aerosolized bronchodilator treatment.

- Watch for subcutaneous crepitus around the patient's face and neck, which may indicate tracheal or bronchial perforation.
- Monitor the patient for breathing problems from laryngeal edema or laryngospasm; call the physician immediately if you note labored breathing.
- Observe the patient for signs of hypoxia, pneumothorax, bronchospasm, or bleeding.
- Keep resuscitative equipment and a tracheostomy tray available during the procedure and for 24 hours afterward.

Chest X-ray

Because normal pulmonary tissue is radiolucent, foreign bodies, infiltrates, fluids, tumors, and other abnormalities appear as densities (white areas) on a chest X-ray. Films are most useful when compared with the patient's previous studies, which allows the radiologist to detect changes.

By itself, a chest X-ray film may not provide information for a definitive diagnosis. For example, it may not reveal mild to moderate obstructive pulmonary disease. Even so, it can show the location and size of lesions and identify structural abnormalities that influence ventilation and diffusion. Examples of abnormalities visible on X-ray include pneumothorax, fibrosis, atelectasis, and infiltrates. (See *Selected clinical implications of chest X-ray films,* pages 82 to 84.)

NURSING CONSIDERATIONS

- Tell the patient that he must wear a gown without snaps and must remove all jewelry from his neck and chest; however, he doesn't need to remove his pants, socks, and shoes.
- If the test is performed in the radiology department, tell the patient that he'll stand or sit in front of a machine. If it's performed at the bedside, someone will help him to a sitting position, and a cold, hard film plate will be placed behind his back. He'll be asked to take a deep breath and to hold it for a few seconds while the X-ray is taken. He should remain still for those few seconds.
- Reassure the patient that the amount of radiation exposure is minimal. Facility personnel will leave the area when the tech-
(Text continues on page 84.)

SELECTED CLINICAL IMPLICATIONS OF CHEST X-RAY FILMS

This table shows the normal anatomic location and appearance of chest X-ray film, along with possible abnormalities and implications.

NORMAL LOCATION AND APPEARANCE	POSSIBLE ABNORMALITY	IMPLICATIONS
TRACHEA Visible midline in the anterior mediastinal cavity; translucent tubelike appearance	● Deviation from midline	● Tension pneumothorax, atelectasis, pleural effusion, consolidation, mediastinal nodes or, in children, enlarged thymus
	● Narrowing with hourglass appearance and deviation to one side	● Substernal thyroid or stenosis secondary to trauma
HEART Visible in the anterior left mediastinal cavity; solid appearance due to blood contents; edges may be clear in contrast with surrounding air density of the lung	● Shift ● Hypertrophy of right heart ● Cardiac borders obscured by stringy densities ("shaggy heart")	● Atelectasis, pneumothorax ● Cor pulmonale, heart failure ● Cystic fibrosis
AORTIC KNOB Visible as water density; formed by the arch of the aorta	● Solid densities, possibly indicating calcifications ● Tortuous shape	● Atherosclerosis ● Atherosclerosis
MEDIASTINUM Visible as the space between the lungs; shadowy appearance that widens at the hilum of the lungs	● Deviation to nondiseased side; deviation to diseased side by traction ● Gross widening	● Pleural effusion or tumor, fibrosis or collapsed lung ● Neoplasms of esophagus, bronchi, lungs, thyroid, thymus, peripheral nerves, lymphoid tissue; aortic aneurysm; mediastinitis; cor pulmonale

SELECTED CLINICAL IMPLICATIONS OF CHEST X-RAY FILMS *(continued)*

NORMAL LOCATION AND APPEARANCE	POSSIBLE ABNORMALITY	IMPLICATIONS
RIBS Visible as thoracic cavity encasement	• Break or misalignment • Widening of intercostal spaces	• Fractured sternum or ribs • Emphysema
SPINE Visible midline in the posterior chest; straight bony structure	• Spinal curvature • Break or misalignment	• Scoliosis, kyphosis • Fractures
CLAVICLES Visible in upper thorax; intact and equidistant in properly centered X-ray films	• Break or misalignment	• Fractures
HILA (LUNG ROOTS) Visible above the heart, where pulmonary vessels, bronchi, and lymph nodes join the lungs; appear as small, white, bilateral densities	• Shift to one side • Accentuated shadows	• Atelectasis • Pneumothorax, emphysema, pulmonary abscess, tumor, enlarged lymph nodes
MAINSTEM BRONCHUS Visible; part of the hila with translucent tubelike appearance	• Spherical or oval density	• Bronchogenic cyst
BRONCHI Usually not visible	• Visible	• Bronchial pneumonia

(continued)

SELECTED CLINICAL IMPLICATIONS OF CHEST X-RAY FILMS *(continued)*

NORMAL LOCATION AND APPEARANCE	POSSIBLE ABNORMALITY	IMPLICATIONS
LUNG FIELDS Usually not visible throughout, except for the blood vessels	● Visible ● Irregular	● Atelectasis ● Resolving pneumonia, infiltrates, silicosis, fibrosis, metastatic neoplasm
HEMIDIAPHRAGM Rounded, visible; right side ⅜″ to ¾″ (1 to 2 cm)	● Elevation of diaphragm (difference in elevation can be measured on inspiration and expiration to detect movement) ● Flattening of diaphragm ● Unilateral elevation of either side ● Unilateral elevation of left side only	● Active tuberculosis, pneumonia, pleurisy, acute bronchitis, active disease of the abdominal viscera, bilateral phrenic nerve involvement, atelectasis ● Asthma, emphysema ● Possible unilateral phrenic nerve paresis ● Perforated ulcer (rare), gas distention of stomach or splenic flexure of colon, free air in abdomen

nician takes the X-ray because they're potentially exposed to radiation many times each day.

■ Explain that female patients of childbearing age will wear a lead apron. Males will be given a protective shield for the testes.

Direct laryngoscopy

Direct laryngoscopy allows visualization of the larynx by the use of a fiber-optic endoscope or laryngoscope passed through the mouth or nose and pharynx to the larynx. It's indicated for patients requiring direct visualization or specimen samples for diagnosis, such as those with strong gag reflexes due to anatomical abnormalities, and for patients who have had no response to short-term therapy for symptoms of pharyngeal or laryngeal disease, such as stridor and hemoptysis. Secretions or tissue may be removed during this procedure for further study. The test is usually contraindicated in patients with epiglottiditis but may be performed on them in an operating room with resuscitative equipment available.

NURSING CONSIDERATIONS

- Explain to the patient that direct laryngoscopy is used to detect laryngeal abnormalities.
- Instruct the patient to fast for 6 hours before the test.
- Tell the patient who will perform the procedure and where it will be done.
- Inform the patient that he'll receive a sedative to help him relax, medication to reduce secretions and, during the procedure, a general or local anesthetic. Reassure him that this procedure won't obstruct his airway.
- Make sure that the patient or a responsible family member has signed an informed consent form.
- Check the patient's history for hypersensitivity to the anesthetic.
- Obtain the patient's baseline vital signs.
- Give the sedative and other medication (usually 30 minutes to 1 hour before the test), as ordered.
- Instruct the patient to remove dentures, contact lenses, and jewelry and to void before giving him a sedative.
- Place the conscious patient in semi-Fowler's position; place the unconscious patient on his side with his head slightly elevated to prevent aspiration.
- Check the patient's vital signs according to your facility's protocol, or every 15 minutes until the patient is stable and then every 30 minutes for 2 hours, every hour for the next 4 hours, and then every 4 hours for 24 hours. Immediately report to the physician any adverse reaction to the anesthetic or sedative (tachycardia, palpitations, hypertension, euphoria, excitation, and rapid, deep respirations).

 RED FLAG Sedation given to patients with respiratory insufficiency may precipitate respiratory arrest.

- Apply an ice collar to minimize laryngeal edema.

- Provide an emesis basin, and instruct the patient to spit out saliva rather than swallow it. Observe sputum for blood and report excessive bleeding immediately.
- Instruct the patient to refrain from clearing his throat and coughing to prevent hemorrhaging at the biopsy site.
- Advise the patient to avoid smoking until his vital signs are stable and there's no evidence of complications.
- Immediately report subcutaneous crepitus around the patient's face and neck, which may indicate tracheal perforation.
- Listen to the patient's neck with a stethoscope for signs of stridor and airway obstruction.

RED FLAG Observe the patient with epiglottiditis for signs of airway obstruction and immediately report signs of respiratory difficulty. Keep emergency resuscitation equipment available; keep a tracheotomy tray nearby for 24 hours.

- Restrict food and fluids to avoid aspiration until the gag reflex returns (usually within 2 hours). Then the patient may resume his usual diet, beginning with sips of water.
- Reassure the patient that voice loss, hoarseness, and sore throat are temporary. Provide throat lozenges or a soothing liquid gargle when his gag reflex returns.

Fluoroscopy

In fluoroscopy, a continuous stream of X-rays passes through the patient, casting shadows of the heart, lungs, and diaphragm on a fluorescent screen. Because fluoroscopy exposes the patient to high levels of radiation and reveals less detail than does standard chest radiography, it's indicated only when diagnosis requires visualization of physiologic or pathologic motion of thoracic contents—for example, to rule out paralysis in patients with diaphragmatic elevation. Normal diaphragmatic movement is synchronous and symmetrical. Normal diaphragmatic excursion ranges from $3/4''$ to $1 5/8''$ (2 to 4 cm).

Diminished diaphragmatic movement may indicate pulmonary disease. Increased lung translucency (not transparent but permitting light passage) may indicate elasticity loss or bronchiolar obstruction. In elderly people, the lowest part of the trachea may be displaced to the right by an elongated aorta. Diminished or paradoxical diaphragmatic movement may indicate diaphragmatic paralysis, which sometimes occurs after open-heart surgery. However, fluoroscopy may not detect such paralysis if the patient compensates for diminished diaphragm function by forcefully contracting abdominal muscles to aid expiration.

Fluoroscopy may also be used to assist with invasive procedures, such as chest needle biopsy or transbronchial biopsy.

NURSING CONSIDERATIONS

- Describe the procedure to the patient and explain that this test assesses respiratory structures and their motions.
- Instruct the patient to remove all metallic objects, including jewelry, in the X-ray field.
- If necessary, assist with patient positioning. Move cardiac monitoring cables, I.V. tubing from subclavian lines, pulmonary artery catheter lines, and safety pins as far as possible from the X-ray field. During the test, cardiopulmonary motion is observed on a screen.
- If the patient is intubated, check that no tubes have been dislodged during positioning.
- To avoid exposure to radiation, leave the room or the immediate area during the test; if you must stay, wear a lead-lined apron.

Mediastinoscopy

Mediastinoscopy is performed under general anesthesia and involves insertion of a mirrored-lens instrument that's similar to a bronchoscope but is inserted through an incision at the base of the anterior neck. A biopsy of mediastinal lymph nodes is obtained. Because mediastinal lymph nodes drain lymphatic fluid from the lungs, specimens can identify carcinoma, granulomatous infection, sarcoidosis, coccidioidomycosis, or histoplasmosis. It can also be used to stage lung cancer or determine the extent of lung tumor metastasis.

NURSING CONSIDERATIONS

- Explain to the patient that this is a surgical procedure that requires general anesthesia.
- Tell the patient that he can't eat or drink anything for 8 or more hours before the test.
- Make certain that the patient has signed a consent form.

- Inform the patient that a lighted instrument will be introduced through the anterior portion of his neck to obtain a biopsy of lymph nodes.
- Explain to the patient that this test will help identify disease, stage his lung cancer, or determine the extent of lung tumor metastasis.
- After the procedure, evaluate the patient's breathing and lung sounds and check the wound site for bleeding and hematoma.

Magnetic resonance imaging

Magnetic resonance imaging (MRI) is a noninvasive test that uses a powerful magnet, radio waves, and a computer to help diagnose respiratory disorders. It provides high-resolution, cross-sectional images of lung structures and traces blood flow. The greatest advantage of an MRI is its ability to "see through" bone and to delineate fluid-filled soft tissue in great detail, without using ionizing radiation or contrast media.

NURSING CONSIDERATIONS

- Tell the patient that he must remove all jewelry and take everything out of his pockets. No metal can be in the test room. The powerful magnet may demagnetize the magnetic strip on a credit card or stop a watch from ticking. If the patient has any metal inside his body, such as a pacemaker, orthopedic pins or disks, and bullets or shrapnel fragments, he must notify his physician.
- Explain to the patient that he'll be asked to lie on a table that slides into an 8′ (2.4-m) tunnel inside the magnet.
- Tell him to breathe normally but not talk or move during the test to avoid distorting the results; the test usually takes 15 to 30 minutes but may take up to 45 minutes.
- Warn the patient that the machinery will be noisy with sounds ranging from a constant ping to a loud bang. He may feel claustrophobic or bored. Suggest that he try to relax and concentrate on breathing or a favorite subject or image.
- Medication may be given to the patient who's claustrophobic if open MRI isn't available.

Paranasal sinus radiography

The paranasal sinuses—air-filled cavities lined with mucous membranes—lie within the maxillary, ethmoid, sphenoid, and frontal bones. Sinus abnormalities resulting from inflammation, trauma, cysts, mucoceles, granulomatosis, and other conditions may include distorted bony sinus walls, altered mucous membranes, and fluid or masses within the cavities. In paranasal sinus radiography, X-rays or electromagnetic waves penetrate the paranasal sinuses and react on specially sensitized film, forming a film image that differentiates sinus structures.

When surrounding facial structures that are superimposed on the paranasal sinuses interfere with visualization of relevant areas, computed tomography scanning may be performed to provide further information. (See *Abnormal findings in paranasal sinus radiography,* page 90.)

NURSING CONSIDERATIONS

- Explain to the patient that paranasal sinus radiography helps evaluate abnormalities of the paranasal sinuses.
- Describe the test, including who will perform it and when and where it will take place.
- Tell the patient that his head may be immobilized in a foam vise during the test to help him maintain the correct position, but that the vise doesn't hurt.
- Explain to the patient that he'll be asked to sit upright and avoid moving while the X-rays are being taken to prevent blurring of the image and to allow visualization of air-fluid levels, if present. Emphasize the importance of his cooperation.
- Instruct the patient to remove dentures, all jewelry, and metallic objects in the X-ray field.

Pulmonary angiography

Pulmonary angiography, also called pulmonary arteriography, allows radiographic examination of the pulmonary circulation. After injecting a radioactive contrast dye through a catheter inserted into the pulmonary artery or one of its branches, a series of X-rays is taken to detect blood flow abnormalities, possibly caused by emboli or pulmonary infarction. This test provides

ABNORMAL FINDINGS IN PARANASAL SINUS RADIOGRAPHY

This table outlines disorders and abnormalities found in paranasal sinus radiography.

DISORDER	ABNORMAL FINDINGS
Paranasal sinus trauma or fracture	● Edema or hemorrhage in mucous membrane lining or sinus cavity ● Clouded sinus air cells ● Air-fluid level ● Radiolucent, linear bone defects ● Irregular, overriding bone edges ● Depression or displacement of bone fragments ● Foreign bodies
Acute sinusitis	● Swollen, inflamed mucous membrane ● Inflammatory exudate ● Hazy to opaque sinus air cells ● Air-fluid level
Chronic sinusitis	● Thickening or sclerosis of bony wall of affected sinus
Wegener's granulomatosis	● Clouded to opaque sinus air cells ● Destruction of bony sinus wall
Malignant neoplasm	● Rounded or lobulated soft-tissue mass, projecting into sinus ● Destruction of bony sinus wall
Benign bone tumor	● Distortion of bony sinus wall in specific patterns
Cyst, polyp, or benign tumor	● Rounded or lobulated soft-tissue mass, projecting into sinus
Mucocele	● Clouded sinus air cells ● Destruction of bony sinus wall resulting in various degrees of radiolucency

more reliable results than a ventilation-perfusion scan but carries higher risks, including cardiac arrhythmias.

NURSING CONSIDERATIONS

- Tell the patient who will perform the test and where and when it will be done. Explain that the test takes about 1 hour and allows confirmation of pulmonary emboli.
- Tell the patient he must fast for 6 hours before the test, or as ordered. He may continue his prescribed drug regimen unless the physician orders otherwise.
- Explain that he'll be given a sedative, such as diazepam (Valium), as ordered. Diphenhydramine (Benadryl) may also be given to reduce the risk of a reaction to the dye.
- Explain the procedure to the patient. The physician will make a percutaneous needle puncture in an antecubital, femoral, jugular, or subclavian vein. The patient may feel pressure at the site. The physician will then insert and advance a catheter.
- After catheter insertion, check the pressure dressing for bleeding and assess for arterial occlusion by checking the patient's temperature, sensation, color, and peripheral pulse distal to the insertion site.
- After the test, monitor the patient for hypersensitivity to the contrast medium or the local anesthetic. Keep emergency equipment nearby and watch for dyspnea.

Thoracic CT scan

A thoracic computed tomography (CT) scan provides cross-sectional views of the chest by passing an X-ray beam from a computerized scanner through the body at different angles and depths. The CT scan provides a three-dimensional image of the lung, allowing the physician to assess abnormalities in the configuration of the trachea or major bronchi and evaluate masses or lesions, such as tumors and abscesses, and abnormal lung shadows. A contrast agent is sometimes used to highlight blood vessels and to allow greater visual discrimination.

NURSING CONSIDERATIONS

- Tell the patient that, if a contrast dye will be used, he should fast for 4 hours before the test.

- Explain that he'll lie on a large, noisy, tunnel-shaped machine. When the dye is injected into his arm vein, he may experience transient nausea, flushing, warmth, and a salty taste.
- Tell him that the equipment may make him feel claustrophobic. He shouldn't move during the test but try to relax and breathe normally. Movement may invalidate the results and require repeat testing.
- Reassure the patient that radiation exposure during the test is minimal.
- Encourage fluid intake if a contrast agent was used.

Thoracoscopy

A thoracoscopy is an invasive diagnostic procedure that uses a fiber-optic endoscope to examine the thoracic cavity. Video assist may also be a part of the test. Thoracoscopy allows visualization of the visceral and parietal pleura, pleural spaces, mediastinum, thoracic walls, and pericardium. It can also be used to perform laser procedures, to assess pleural effusion, tumor growth, emphysema, inflammatory disease, and conditions that would predispose the patient to pneumothorax. Biopsies of the pleura, mediastinal lymph nodes, and lungs can also be obtained through thoracoscopy.

NURSING CONSIDERATIONS

- Obtain ordered laboratory tests as well as urinalysis and chest X-ray.
- Make sure that the patient has signed a consent form.
- Explain to the patient that he must fast from food or drink for at least 6 hours before the test.
- Explain to the patient that this is a surgical procedure and that he'll receive general anesthesia.
- Obtain a postoperative chest X-ray as ordered to check for abnormal air or fluid in the chest cavity.
- Monitor the patient's vital signs and amount and color of chest tube drainage.
- Encourage the patient to frequently cough and deep breathe.
- Assist the patient in splinting his incision during coughing and deep breathing to reduce discomfort.

V̇/Q̇ scan

Although less reliable than pulmonary angiography, a ventilation-perfusion (V̇/Q̇) scan carries fewer risks. This test indicates lung perfusion and ventilation. It's used to evaluate V̇/Q̇ mismatch, to detect pulmonary emboli, atelectasis, obstructing tumors, and chronic obstructive pulmonary disease and to evaluate pulmonary function, particularly in preoperative patients with marginal lung reserves.

Usually in a V̇/Q̇ scan, two radionuclides are administered. One is technetium 99m, which is used for the perfusion part of the study and is injected intravenously. If there's decreased uptake of radioactivity in an area of the lung, it corresponds to a decreased blood flow to an area where embolization has occurred.

For the ventilation portion of the test, the other radionuclide commonly used is xenon 133 gas. This test, as the name implies, requires the patient to "ventilate" or breathe the radioactive particles into his lungs. Decreased areas of radioactivity correspond to irregular lung function.

NURSING CONSIDERATIONS

- Tell the patient that, like pulmonary angiography, a V̇/Q̇ scan requires injection of a radioactive contrast dye. Explain that he'll lie in a supine position on a table as a radioactive protein substance is injected into an arm vein.
- While he remains in the supine position, a large camera will take pictures, continuing as he lies on his side, lies prone, and sits up. When he's prone, more dye will be injected.
- Also, inform the patient that during the ventilation part of the test, he will be asked to inhale a radioactive gas. He will be again asked to remain still as a machine scans his chest after he inhales the gas and again as he exhales it. (See *Comparing normal and abnormal ventilation scans,* page 94.)
- Reassure the patient that the amount of radioactivity in the dye is minimal. However, he may experience some discomfort from the venipuncture and from lying on a cold, hard table. He may also feel claustrophobic when surrounded by the camera equipment.

COMPARING NORMAL AND ABNORMAL VENTILATION SCANS

The normal ventilation scan, taken 30 minutes to 1 hour after the washout phase, shows equal gas distribution. The abnormal scan, taken 1½ to 2 hours after the start of the washout phase, shows unequal gas distribution, represented by the area of poor washout on both the left and right sides.

NORMAL SCAN

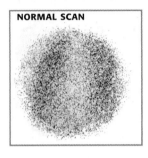

ABNORMAL SCAN

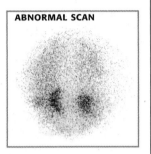

BIOPSIES

Biopsies include lung and pleural biopsies.

Lung biopsy

In a lung biopsy, a specimen of pulmonary tissue is excised for examination, using either the closed or open technique. The closed technique, performed under local anesthesia, includes both needle and transbronchial biopsies. The open technique, performed under general anesthesia in the operating room, includes both limited and standard thoracotomies.

Needle biopsy is appropriate when the lesion is readily accessible. This procedure provides a much smaller specimen than the open technique. Transbronchial biopsy, the removal of multiple tissue specimens through a fiber-optic bronchoscope, is appropriate for some lung abnormalities or when the patient's condition won't tolerate an open biopsy.

Examination of lung tissue specimens can reveal squamous cell or oat cell carcinoma and adenocarcinoma.

NURSING CONSIDERATIONS

- Describe the test to the patient and tell him that the test takes 30 to 60 minutes. Instruct him to fast after midnight or 6 hours before the procedure.
- Make sure the patient has signed a consent form. Check his history for hypersensitivity to the local anesthetic.
- Explain to the patient that a mild sedative will be administered 30 minutes before the biopsy to help him relax.
- Explain to the patient that after the biopsy site is selected, lead markers are placed on the patient's skin, and X-rays are ordered to verify the markers' correct placement.
- During biopsy, observe for signs of respiratory distress—shortness of breath, elevated pulse rate, and cyanosis (late sign); if such signs develop, report them immediately.
- Check vital signs every 15 minutes for 1 hour, every 30 minutes for 2 hours, every hour for 4 hours, and then every 4 hours for 24 hours.
- Assess for bleeding, shortness of breath, increased pulse, diminished breath sounds on the biopsy side and, eventually, cyanosis.
- Make sure the chest X-ray is repeated immediately after the biopsy.

Pleural biopsy

Pleural biopsy is the removal of pleural tissue, by needle biopsy or open biopsy, for examination. Performed under local anesthesia, pleural biopsy usually follows thoracentesis—aspiration of pleural fluid—that's performed when the cause of the effusion is unknown. However, it can be performed separately.

Open pleural biopsy, performed in the absence of pleural effusion, permits direct visualization of the pleura and the underlying lung. It's performed in the operating room.

Microscopic examination of the tissue specimen can reveal malignant disease, tuberculosis, or viral, fungal, parasitic, or collagen vascular disease. Primary tumors of the pleura are commonly fibrous and epithelial.

NURSING CONSIDERATIONS

▪ Explain the procedure to the patient and tell him that it typically takes 30 to 45 minutes.

▪ Advise the patient that blood studies will be necessary before the biopsy and that chest X-rays will be taken before and after the biopsy.

▪ Make sure the patient has signed a consent form. Check the patient history for hypersensitivity to the local anesthetic. Just before the procedure, record his vital signs.

▪ Explain to the patient that he'll be sitting on the side of the bed, with his feet resting on a stool and his arms supported by the overbed table or his upper body. If he can't sit up, place him in a side-lying position with the side to be biopsied facing up.

▪ The specimen is immediately put in a special solution in a labeled specimen bottle. Then the skin around the biopsy site is cleaned, and an adhesive bandage is applied.

▪ After the biopsy, check the patient's vital signs every 15 minutes for 1 hour, every 30 minutes for 2 hours, and then every hour for 4 hours or until his condition is stable.

▪ Make sure the chest X-ray is repeated immediately after the biopsy. Instruct the patient to lie on his unaffected side to promote healing of the biopsy site.

▪ Watch for signs of respiratory distress (shortness of breath), shoulder pain, and such other complications as pneumothorax (immediate) and pneumonia (delayed).

▪ Send the specimen to the laboratory immediately.

▪ Pleural biopsy is contraindicated in patients with severe bleeding disorders.

OTHER DIAGNOSTIC TESTS

Other diagnostic tests include end-tidal carbon dioxide and mixed venous oxygen saturation monitoring, pulmonary function tests, pulse oximetry, and sweat testing.

End-tidal carbon dioxide monitoring

End-tidal carbon dioxide monitoring ($ETCO_2$) is used to measure the carbon dioxide concentration at end expiration. An

$ETCO_2$ monitor may be a separate monitor or part of the patient's bedside hemodynamic monitoring system.

Indications for $ETCO_2$ monitoring include:

- monitoring patency of the airway in acute airway obstruction
- monitoring for apnea and respiratory function
- early detection of changes in carbon dioxide production and elimination with hyperventilation therapy, or hypercapnia or hyperthermia states
- assessing effectiveness of interventions, such as mechanical ventilation or neuromuscular blockade used with mechanical ventilation and prone positioning.

In $ETCO_2$ monitoring, a photodetector measures the amount of infrared light absorbed by the airway during inspiration and expiration. (Light absorption increases along with the carbon dioxide concentration.) The monitor converts these data to a carbon dioxide value and a corresponding waveform, or capnogram if capnography is used. (See *Understanding $ETCO_2$ monitoring,* page 98.)

Values are obtained by monitoring samples of expired gas from an endotracheal (ET) tube or an oral or nasopharyngeal airway. Although the values are similar, the $ETCO_2$ values are usually 2 to 5 mm Hg lower than the partial pressure of arterial carbon dioxide value.

Capnograms and $ETCO_2$ monitoring reduce the need for frequent arterial blood gas sampling.

NURSING CONSIDERATIONS

- Explain the procedure to the patient and his family.
- Assess the patient's respiratory status, vital signs, oxygen saturation, and $ETCO_2$ readings. Observe waveform quality and trends of $ETCO_2$ readings for suddenly increased readings (which may indicate hypoventilation, partial airway obstruction, or respiratory depressant effects from drugs), or decreased readings (due to complete airway obstruction, dislodged ET tube, or ventilator malfunction). Notify the physician of a 10% increase or decrease in readings.

Mixed venous oxygen saturation monitoring

Mixed venous oxygen saturation ($S\overline{v}O_2$) reflects the oxygen saturation level of venous blood. It's determined by measuring the

UNDERSTANDING ETCO₂ MONITORING

The optical portion of an end-tidal carbon dioxide (ETCO₂) monitor contains an infrared light source, a sample chamber, a special carbon dioxide (CO_2) filter, and a photodetector.

In ETCO₂ monitoring, the infrared light passes through the sample chamber and is absorbed in varying amounts, depending on the amount of CO_2 the patient just exhaled. The photodetector measures CO_2 content and relays this information to the microprocessor in the monitor, which displays the CO_2 value and waveform.

Capnogram reading

The CO_2 waveform, or *capnogram*, produced in ETCO₂ monitoring reflects the course of CO_2 elimination during exhalation. A normal capnogram (shown below) consists of several segments, which reflect the various stages of exhalation and inhalation.

Normally, any gas eliminated from the airway during early exhalation is dead-space gas that hasn't undergone exchange at the alveolocapillary membrane. Measurements taken during this period contain no CO_2. As exhalation continues, CO_2 concentration increases sharply and rapidly. The sensor now detects gas that

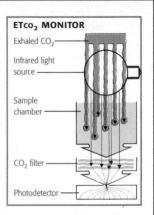

ETCO₂ MONITOR

Exhaled CO_2

Infrared light source

Sample chamber

CO_2 filter

Photodetector

has undergone exchange, producing measurable quantities of CO_2.

The final stages of alveolar emptying occur during late exhalation. During the alveolar plateau phase, CO_2 concentration increases gradually because alveolar emptying is relatively constant.

The point at which the ETCO₂ value is derived is the end of exhalation, when CO_2 concentration peaks. However, this value doesn't accurately reflect alveolar CO_2 if no alveolar plateau is present. During inhalation, the CO_2 concentration declines sharply to zero.

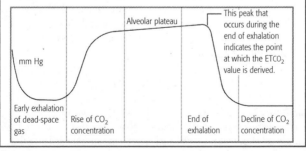

Alveolar plateau

This peak that occurs during the end of exhalation indicates the point at which the ETCO₂ value is derived.

mm Hg

| Early exhalation of dead-space gas | Rise of CO_2 concentration | End of exhalation | Decline of CO_2 concentration |

amount of oxygen extracted and used or consumed by the body's tissues.

In a healthy adult, an $S\bar{v}O_2$ level between 60% and 80% indicates adequate tissue perfusion. Values less than 60% indicate increased oxygen extraction by the tissues. A decrease in oxygen delivery or an increase in tissue demands can cause this. Values greater than 80% may occur in states of increased oxygen delivery or may indicate decreased oxygen extraction by the tissues (when tissue hypoxia exists despite the availability of oxygen).

Ideally, the $S\bar{v}O_2$ sample is obtained from the most distal port of the pulmonary artery (PA) catheter, which contains the ideal mix of all venous blood in the heart. Samples may be drawn from a central catheter if a PA catheter isn't available.

Continuous $S\bar{v}O_2$ monitoring is done using the $S\bar{v}O_2$ or oximetric PA catheter. This specialized PA catheter calculates oxygen saturation of hemoglobin by measuring the wavelengths of reflected light through fiberoptic bundles.

The information is exhibited on a bedside computer and may be displayed numerically and graphically. The manufacturer's instructions for catheter calibration must be followed to ensure accurate readings.

NURSING CONSIDERATIONS

- Explain the procedure to the patient and his family. Make sure they understand the expected outcomes and risks of the procedure related to catheter placement, pneumothorax, cardiac arrhythmias, and infection.
- If you assist with catheter insertion, monitor the patient's vital signs and heart rhythm as you assess for changes in ventilatory function.
- Apply a sterile dressing or sterile transparent dressing over the catheter insertion site. Follow your facility's policy for changing the dressing and pulmonary artery monitoring system (tubing and solution).
- Document the date and time of catheter insertion, initial $S\bar{v}O_2$ readings, and changes in the patient's condition. Monitor the pulmonary artery pressure and $S\bar{v}O_2$ readings, and document hourly or according to your facility's policy.
- Closely monitor the patient's hemodynamic status. Troubleshoot the catheter for problems that can interfere with ac-

curate testing, such as loose connections, balloon rupture, or clot formation on the tip of the catheter.

Pulmonary function tests

There are two types of pulmonary function tests (PFTs): volume and capacity. These tests aid diagnosis in patients with suspected respiratory dysfunction. The physician orders these tests to:
- evaluate ventilatory function through spirometric measurements
- determine the cause of dyspnea
- assess the effectiveness of medications, such as bronchodilators and steroids
- determine whether a respiratory abnormality stems from an obstructive or restrictive disease process
- evaluate the extent of dysfunction.

Of the five pulmonary volume tests, tidal volume and expiratory reserve volume are measurements obtained through direct spirography. Minute volume, inspiratory reserve volume, and residual volume are calculated from the results of other PFTs.

Of the pulmonary capacity tests, functional residual capacity, total lung capacity, and maximal midexpiratory flow must be calculated. Vital capacity and inspiratory capacity may be measured directly or calculated indirectly. Direct spirographic measurements include forced vital capacity, forced expiratory volume, and maximal voluntary ventilation. The amount of carbon monoxide exhaled permits calculation of the diffusing capacity for carbon monoxide. (See *Interpreting pulmonary function tests,* pages 102 to 107.)

Nursing considerations
- For some tests, the patient will sit upright and wear a noseclip. For others, he may sit in a small airtight box called a body plethysmograph and not need a noseclip. In this case, warn him that he may experience claustrophobia. Reassure him that he won't suffocate and that he'll be able to communicate with the technician through the window in the box.
- Explain that he may receive an aerosolized bronchodilator. Administration of the bronchodilator may be repeated to evaluate the drug's effectiveness.

PULSE OXIMETRY LEVELS

Pulse oximetry may be intermittent or continuous, and is used to monitor arterial oxygen saturation. Normal oxygen saturation levels are 95% to 100% for adults and 94% to 100% for full-term neonates. Lower levels may indicate hypoxemia and warrant intervention.

Interfering factors

Certain factors can interfere with accuracy. For example, an elevated bilirubin level may falsely lower oxygen saturation readings, whereas elevated carboxyhemoglobin or methemoglobin levels can falsely elevate oxygen saturation readings.

Certain intravascular substances, such as lipid emulsions and dyes, may also affect readings. Other interfering factors include excessive light (such as from phototherapy or direct sunlight), excessive patient movement, excessive ear pigment, severe peripheral vascular disease, hypothermia, hypotension, and vasoconstriction.

In addition, anemic conditions, vasoconstriction, certain drugs (such as vasopressors), hypotension, vessel obstruction, nail polish or false nails, and lipid emulsions may interfere with test results.

■ Emphasize that the test will proceed quickly if the patient follows directions, tries hard, and keeps a tight seal around the mouthpiece or tube to ensure accurate results.

■ Instruct the patient to loosen tight clothing so he can breathe freely. Tell him he must not smoke or eat a large meal for 4 hours before the test.

■ Keep in mind that anxiety can affect test accuracy. Also, remember that medications, such as analgesics and bronchodilators, may produce misleading results. You may be asked to withhold bronchodilators and other respiratory treatments before the test. If the patient receives a bronchodilator during the test, don't give another dose for 4 hours.

Pulse oximetry

Pulse oximetry is a noninvasive study of arterial blood oxygen saturation using a clip or probe attached to a sensor site (usually an earlobe or a fingertip). The percentage expressed is the ratio of oxygen to hemoglobin. Pulse oximetry can be measured intermittently or continuously. (See *Pulse oximetry levels*.)

(Text continues on page 106.)

INTERPRETING PULMONARY FUNCTION TESTS

Pulmonary function tests are interpreted after data are collected and calculated. The implications are reviewed in this table.

PULMONARY FUNCTION TEST	METHOD OF CALCULATION
TIDAL VOLUME (V_T) Amount of air inhaled or exhaled during normal breathing	Determining the spirographic measurement for 10 breaths and then dividing by 10
MINUTE VOLUME (MV) Total amount of air expired per minute	Multiplying V_T by the respiratory rate
CARBON DIOXIDE (CO_2) RESPONSE Increase or decrease in MV after breathing various CO_2 concentrations	Plotting changes in MV against increasing inspired CO_2 concentrations
INSPIRATORY RESERVE VOLUME (IRV) Amount of air inspired over above-normal inspiration	Subtracting V_T from IC
EXPIRATORY RESERVE VOLUME (ERV) Amount of air exhaled after normal expiration	Direct spirographic measurement
RESIDUAL VOLUME (RV) Amount of air remaining in the lungs after forced expiration	Subtracting ERV from FRC
VITAL CAPACITY (VC) Total volume of air that can be exhaled after maximum inspiration	Direct spirographic measurement or adding V_T, IRV, and ERV
INSPIRATORY CAPACITY (IC) Amount of air that can be inhaled after normal expiration	Direct spirographic measurement or adding IRV and V_T

IMPLICATIONS

Decreased V_T may indicate restrictive disease and requires further testing, such as full pulmonary function studies or chest X-rays.

Normal MV can occur in emphysema; decreased MV may indicate other diseases such as pulmonary edema. Increased MV can occur with acidosis, increased CO_2, decreased partial pressure of arterial oxygen, exercise, and low compliance states.

Reduced CO_2 response may occur in emphysema, myxedema, obesity, hypoventilation syndrome, and sleep apnea.

Abnormal IRV alone doesn't indicate respiratory dysfunction; IRV decreases during normal exercise.

ERV varies, even in healthy people, but usually decreases in obese people.

RV >35% of TLC after maximal expiratory effort may indicate obstructive disease.

Normal or increased VC with decreased flow rates may indicate any condition that causes a reduction in functional pulmonary tissue such as pulmonary edema. Decreased VC with normal or increased flow rates may indicate decreased respiratory effort resulting from neuromuscular disease, drug overdose, or head injury; decreased thoracic expansion; or limited diaphragm movement.

Decreased IC indicates restrictive disease.

(continued)

INTERPRETING PULMONARY FUNCTION TESTS *(continued)*

PULMONARY FUNCTION TEST	METHOD OF CALCULATION
THORACIC GAS VOLUME (TGV) Total volume of gas in the lungs from ventilated and nonventilated airways	Body plethysmography
FUNCTIONAL RESIDUAL CAPACITY (FRC) Amount of air remaining in the lungs after normal expiration	Nitrogen washout, helium dilution technique, or adding ERV and RV
TOTAL LUNG CAPACITY (TLC) Total volume of the lungs when maximally inflated	Adding V_T, IRV, ERV, and RV; FRC and IC; or VC and RV
FORCED VITAL CAPACITY (FVC) Amount of air exhaled forcefully and quickly after maximum inspiration	Direct spirographic measurement; expressed as a percentage of the total volume of gas exhaled
FLOW-VOLUME CURVE (ALSO CALLED FLOW-VOLUME LOOP) Greatest rate of flow (V_{max}) during FVC maneuvers versus lung volume change	Direct spirographic measurement at 1-second intervals; calculated from flow rates (expressed in L/second) and lung volume changes (expressed in liters) during maximal inspiratory and expiratory maneuvers
FORCED EXPIRATORY VOLUME (FEV) Volume of air expired in the 1st, 2nd, or 3rd second of an FVC maneuver	Direct spirographic measurement; expressed as a percentage of FVC
FORCED EXPIRATORY FLOW (FEF) Average rate of flow during the middle half of FVC	Calculated from the flow rate and the time needed for expiration of the middle 50% of FVC

IMPLICATIONS

Increased TGV indicates air trapping, which may result from obstructive disease.

Increased FRC indicates overdistention of the lungs, which may result from obstructive pulmonary disease.

Low TLC indicates restrictive disease; high TLC indicates overdistended lungs caused by obstructive disease.

Decreased FVC indicates flow resistance in the respiratory system from obstructive disease such as chronic bronchitis, or from restrictive disease such as pulmonary fibrosis.

Decreased flow rates at all volumes during expiration indicate obstructive disease of the small airways such as emphysema. A plateau of expiratory flow near TLC, a plateau of inspiratory flow at mid-VC, and a square wave pattern through most of VC indicate obstructive disease of large airways. Normal or increased PEFR, decreased flow with decreasing lung volumes, and markedly decreased VC indicate restrictive disease.

Decreased FEV_1 and increased FEV_2 and FEV_3 may indicate obstructive disease; decreased or normal FEV_1 may indicate restrictive disease.

Low FEF (25% to 75%) indicates obstructive disease of the small and medium-sized airways.

(continued)

INTERPRETING PULMONARY FUNCTION TESTS *(continued)*

PULMONARY FUNCTION TEST	METHOD OF CALCULATION
PEAK EXPIRATORY FLOW RATE (PEFR) V_{max} during forced expiration	Calculated from the flow-volume curve or by direct spirographic measurement using a pneumotachometer or electronic tachometer with a transducer to convert flow to electrical output display
MAXIMAL VOLUNTARY VENTILATION (MVV) (ALSO CALLED MAXIMUM BREATHING CAPACITY) Greatest volume of air breathed per unit of time	Direct spirographic measurement
DIFFUSING CAPACITY FOR CARBON MONOXIDE (DLCO) Milliliters of carbon monoxide diffused per minute across the alveolocapillary membrane	Calculated from analysis of the amount of carbon monoxide exhaled compared with the amount inhaled

NURSING CONSIDERATIONS

- Explain to the patient that this test assesses oxygen content in the hemoglobin.
- Make sure the patient has no false fingernails or nail polish.
- Place the probe or clip over the finger or other intended sensor site so that the light beams and sensors are opposite each other.
- Intermittent pulse oximetry is measured with a probe that looks similar to a clothes pin.
- Protect the transducer from exposure to strong light. Check the transducer site frequently to make sure the device is in place and examine the skin for abrasion and circulatory impairment.
- Rotate the transducer at least every 4 hours to avoid skin irritation.
- If oximetry has been performed properly, the oxygen saturation readings are usually within 2% of arterial blood gas values when saturations range between 84% and 98%.

IMPLICATIONS

Decreased PEFR may indicate a mechanical problem, such as upper airway obstruction, or obstructive disease. PEFR is usually normal in restrictive disease but decreases in severe cases. Because PEFR is effort dependent, it's also low in a person who has poor expiratory effort or doesn't understand the procedure.

Decreased MVV may indicate obstructive disease; normal or decreased MVV may indicate restrictive disease such as myasthenia gravis.

Decreased DLco due to a thickened alveolocapillary membrane occurs in interstitial pulmonary diseases, such as pulmonary fibrosis, asbestosis, and sarcoidosis; DLco is reduced in emphysema because of alveolocapillary membrane loss.

Sweat test

The sweat test is a quantitative measurement of electrolyte concentrations (primarily sodium and chloride) in sweat, usually performed using pilocarpine iontophoresis (pilocarpine is a sweat inducer). Although this test is primarily used to confirm cystic fibrosis (CF) in children, it's also performed in adults to determine if they're homozygous or heterozygous for CF. Genetic testing for CF also has become available. (See *Tag-It Cystic Fibrosis Kit,* page 108.)

NURSING CONSIDERATIONS
- Explain the sweat test to the child, if he's old enough to understand, using clear, simple terms.
- Inform the child and his parents that there are no restrictions on diet, medication, or activity before the test.
- Tell the child who will perform the test and where it will be done.

TAG-IT CYSTIC FIBROSIS KIT

The U.S. Food and Drug Administration approved the use of a deoxyribonucleic acid (DNA) test for diagnosing cystic fibrosis (CF). The test, called the *Tag-It Cystic Fibrosis Kit*, is a blood test that screens for genetic mutations and variations in the cystic fibrosis transmembrane conductance regulator (CFTR) gene. This test identifies 23 genetic mutations and 4 variations in the CFTR gene. It also screens for 16 additional mutations in the gene that are involved in many cases of CF.

The test is recommended for use in detecting and identifying these mutations and variations in the gene as a means for determining carrier status in adults, screening neonates, and for confirming diagnostic testing in neonates and children. More than 1,300 genetic variations in the CFTR gene are responsible for causing CF. Therefore, the test isn't recommended as the only means for diagnosing CF. Test results need to be viewed along with the patient's condition, ethnic background, and family history. Additionally, genetic counseling is suggested to help patients understand the results and their implications.

- Tell the child that he may feel a slight tickling sensation during the procedure but won't feel any pain.
- Encourage the parents to assist with preparations and to stay with their child during the test. Their presence will minimize the child's anxiety.
- Try to distract the child with a book, television, toy, or another diversion if he becomes nervous or frightened during the test.
- Wash the area that underwent iontophoresis with soap and water and dry it thoroughly. If the area looks red, reassure the patient that this is normal and will disappear within a few hours.
- Tell the patient or his parents that he may resume his usual activities.

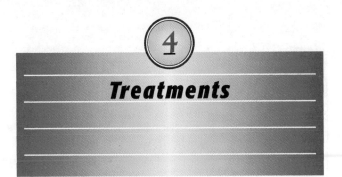

Treatments

Respiratory disorders interfere with airway clearance, breathing patterns, and gas exchange. If not corrected, these disorders can adversely affect many other body systems and can be life-threatening. Treatments for respiratory disorders include drug therapy, inhalation therapy, surgery, and other types of therapies.

DRUG THERAPY

Drugs are used for airway management in patients with such disorders as acute respiratory failure, acute respiratory distress syndrome, asthma, emphysema, chronic bronchitis, and chronic obstructive pulmonary disease (COPD).

Drug categories
Types of drugs used to improve respiratory function include:
- aerosol anti-infectives
- antitussives
- beta$_2$-adrenergic agonists
- corticosteroids
- decongestants
- expectorants
- leukotriene modifiers
- mast cell stabilizers
- mucus inhibitors
- xanthines.

AEROSOL ANTI-INFECTIVES

Aerosol inhalation provides direct, targeted local airway delivery of anti-infectives with minimal systemic blood levels. Aerosol anti-infectives, especially antibiotics, should be given with high flow rate nebulizers that deliver flow rates of 10 to 12 L/minute. Four inhaled anti-infectives are available: pentamidine (Nebupent), ribavirin (Virazole), tobramycin (TOBI), and zanamivir (Relenza).

Pentamidine is an antiprotozoal recommended as a second-line drug for the prevention of *Pneumocystis carinii* pneumonia (PCP) in high-risk human immunodeficiency virus-infected patients who have a history of one or more episodes of PCP or a CD4+ lymphocyte count of less than or equal to 200/μl. This drug should be given in isolation and through an environmental containment system such as a negative-pressure room. The nebulizer system should have one-way valves and scavenging filters that prevent or reduce environmental contamination.

Ribavirin is an antiviral recommended for the treatment of respiratory syncytial virus (RSV) or in patients who are at risk for severe infection. RSV is a common seasonal respiratory infection that occurs in young infants and children. Adverse reactions include bronchospasm, skin rash, eyelid erythema, and conjunctivitis.

Tobramycin is used to treat *Pseudomonas aeruginosa* in patients with cystic fibrosis. This drug should be given after other cystic fibrosis therapies such as other inhaled drugs. It should be given under containment to prevent environmental saturation of the antibiotic into other hospital areas, which in turn helps prevent the development of resistant organisms. Possible adverse reactions include auditory and vestibular damage with the potential for deafness and nephrotoxicity. Women who are pregnant should avoid inhalant exposure because of fetal harm resulting from aminoglycosides.

Zanamivir is used to treat uncomplicated cases of influenza in adults and adolescents ages 12 and older who have had symptoms lasting no longer than 2 years. Adverse reactions include diarrhea, vomiting, bronchitis, cough, sinusitis, dizziness, and headaches.

Nursing considerations
- Monitor the patient for bronchospasm and reduction of lung function, especially if the patient has asthma or COPD.
- Make sure that the patient understands how to use the aerosol correctly.
- Caution the patient to report adverse effects immediately.
- Advise the patient taking inhaled tobramycin to report episodes of tinnitus, changes in hearing, or voice alteration.

ANTITUSSIVES
Antitussive drugs suppress or inhibit coughing. They are given orally as a liquid and are typically used to treat dry, nonproductive coughs. The major antitussives include:
- benzonatate (Tessalon)
- codeine
- dextromethorphan hydrobromide (Robitussin)
- hydrocodone (Vicodin).

The uses and actions of these drugs differ, but each is used to treat a nonproductive cough that interferes with a patient's ability to rest or carry out activities of daily living.

Benzonatate acts by anesthetizing stretch receptors throughout the bronchi, alveoli, and pleura. Benzonatate relieves coughs caused by pneumonia, bronchitis, the common cold, and chronic pulmonary diseases such as emphysema. It can also be used during bronchial diagnostic tests, such as bronchoscopy, when the patient must avoid coughing.

Codeine, dextromethorphan, and hydrocodone suppress the cough reflex by direct action on the cough center in the medulla of the brain, thus lowering the cough threshold.

Nursing considerations
- Obtain a history of the patient's cough before giving the drug, and reassess the patient after giving the drug.
- Look for adverse reactions and drug reactions.
- Assess the patient's and his family's knowledge of drug therapy.

BETA₂-ADRENERGIC AGONISTS
Beta₂-adrenergic agonists are used to treat symptoms associated with asthma and COPD. These drugs increase levels of cyclic

adenosine monophosphate through the stimulation of the $beta_2$-adrenergic receptors in the smooth muscle, resulting in bronchodilation. Inhaled $beta_2$-adrenergic agonists are preferred because they act locally in the lung, resulting in fewer adverse reactions than systemic drugs.

Drugs in this class may be short or long acting. A short-acting inhaled $beta_2$-adrenergic agonist, such as albuterol (Proventil) or pirbuterol (Maxair), is used to quickly relieve symptoms in patients with asthma or COPD. Some COPD patients may use these drugs around-the-clock on a specified schedule.

A long-acting $beta_2$-adrenergic agonist is best used in combination with anti-inflammatories—namely, the inhaled corticosteroids—to provide maintenance therapy to control asthma. Salmeterol (Serevent) is the only long-acting $beta_2$-adrenergic agonist currently approved in the United States. Because of its prolonged onset, it must be given on a scheduled basis.

Nursing considerations
- Caution the patient about possible adverse reactions, which may include tremors, nervousness, dizziness, headache, nausea, tachycardia, palpitations, electrocardiogram (ECG) changes, bronchospasm, and cough.
- Make sure that the patient taking a long-acting $beta_2$-adrenergic agonist knows that he can't use this drug to treat acute symptoms because the onset isn't quick enough.
- Excessive use of a short-acting $beta_2$-adrenergic agonist may indicate poor asthma control, requiring reassessment of the patient's therapeutic regimen.

CORTICOSTEROIDS
Corticosteroids are anti-inflammatory drugs that are available in inhaled and systemic forms for the short- and long-term control of asthma symptoms. Many different products are available and have various potencies. (See *Understanding corticosteroids*.)

Corticosteroids are the most effective drugs available for the long-term treatment of patients with reversible airflow obstruction. They work to prevent asthma exacerbations by suppressing immune responses and reducing inflammation.

Systemic corticosteroids are commonly reserved for moderate to severe acute exacerbations but are also used for severe

UNDERSTANDING CORTICOSTEROIDS

Use this table to learn about the indications, adverse reactions, and practice pointers associated with corticosteroids.

DRUG	INDICATIONS	ADVERSE REACTIONS	PRACTICE POINTERS
SYSTEMIC CORTICOSTEROIDS ● Dexamethasone (Decadron) ● Methylprednisolone (Medrol) ● Prednisone (Prednisone)	● Anti-inflammatory in acute respiratory failure, acute respiratory distress syndrome, and chronic obstructive pulmonary disease ● Anti-inflammatory and immunosuppressor in asthma	● Heart failure, cardiac arrhythmias, edema, circulatory collapse, thromboembolism, pancreatitis, peptic ulcer	● Use cautiously in patients with recent myocardial infarction, hypertension, renal disease, and GI ulcer. ● Monitor blood pressure and blood glucose levels.
INHALED CORTICOSTEROIDS ● Beclomethasone (Qvar) ● Budesonide (Pulmicort) ● Flunisolide (Aerobid) ● Fluticasone (Flonase) ● Triamcinolone (Azmacort)	● Long-term asthma control	● Hoarseness, dry mouth, wheezing, bronchospasm, oral candidiasis	● *Don't* use to treat an acute asthma attack. ● Use a spacer to reduce adverse effects. ● Rinse mouth after use to prevent oral fungal infection.

asthma that's refractory to other measures. Systemic corticosteroids, such as dexamethasone (Decadron), methylprednisolone (Medrol), and prednisone, are given to manage an acute respiratory event, such as acute respiratory failure or exacerbations of COPD. These drugs should be used at the lowest effective dose and for the shortest period possible to avoid adverse reactions. These drugs are initially given I.V. and, when the patient stabilizes, the dosage is tapered and an oral form may be substituted.

Inhaled corticosteroids remain the mainstay of therapy to prevent flare-ups in those with mild to severe asthma. Patients commonly use beclomethasone (Qvar), budesonide (Pulmicort Turbuhaler), flunisolide (AeroBid), fluticasone (Flovent), and triamcinolone (Azmacort). Use of these drugs reduces the need for systemic steroids in many patients, thus reducing the risk of serious long-term adverse effects.

Nursing considerations
- To reduce the risk of adverse effects occurring with inhaled drugs, use the lowest possible doses to maintain control.
- Advise the patient to rinse his mouth with water after each dose to prevent oropharyngeal fungal infections.
- Caution the patient that inhaled corticosteroids may cause hoarseness, throat and nose irritation, dry mouth, and headache or dizziness.
- Monitor the patient for serious adverse effects, which may include dyspnea, wheezing, or bronchospasm.

DECONGESTANTS
Decongestants may be classified as systemic or topical. Both types of decongestants are used to relieve the symptoms of swollen nasal membranes resulting from hay fever, allergic rhinitis, vasomotor rhinitis, acute coryza, sinusitis, and the common cold.

Systemic decongestants activate the sympathetic division of the autonomic nervous system to reduce swelling of the respiratory tract's vascular network. Topical decongestants are powerful vasoconstrictors that provide immediate relief from nasal congestion and swollen mucous membranes when applied directly to the nasal mucosa. Absorption of the topical form of the drug is negligible.

Nursing considerations
- Discourage the use of over-the-counter decongestants in a patient who's hypersensitive to other sympathomimetic amines. Such a patient may also be hypersensitive to decongestants.
- Monitor the patient's blood pressure, pulse, and ECG, as instructed, particularly noting hypertension and an irregular heartbeat or tachycardia.

■ Maintain seizure precautions during decongestant therapy.
■ Note if the patient uses drugs that alter urine pH because alkaline urine increases renal tubular reabsorption of sympathomimetic amines.
■ Don't give a monoamine oxidase inhibitor, a beta-adrenergic blocker, methyldopa (Aldomet), reserpine (Hiserpia), or guanethidine (Ismelin) at the same time as a topical decongestant.
■ Warn the patient that transient burning and stinging of the nasal mucosa may occur during administration of the topical decongestant.
■ Monitor the patient receiving a topical decongestant for signs of rebound nasal congestion such as red, swollen, boggy nasal mucosa. If rebound nasal congestion occurs, withhold the drug and notify the prescriber.
■ Encourage the patient taking a decongestant to report difficulty urinating, which is especially common in the patient with prostatic hypertrophy.

EXPECTORANTS

By increasing production of respiratory tract fluids, expectorants reduce the viscosity, thickness, adhesiveness, and surface tension of mucus, making it easier to clear from the airways. Expectorants also soothe mucous membranes of the respiratory tract and result in a more productive cough. The most commonly used oral expectorant is guaifenesin (Robitussin).

Nursing considerations

■ Caution the patient that the drug may produce vomiting if taken in doses larger than necessary for the expectorant action. Administer with a full glass of water.
■ Monitor the patient for dyspnea or ineffective cough. Instruct him to cough effectively.
■ Teach the patient about the prescribed drug.
■ Monitor the patient for adverse effects, such as diarrhea, drowsiness, nausea, vomiting, and abdominal pain.

LEUKOTRIENE MODIFIERS

The leukotriene modifiers (zafirlukast [Accolate] and montelukast [Singulair]) are primarily used for the prevention and long-term control of mild asthma. They may also be used as steroid-sparing drugs in some patients.

Leukotrienes are substances released from mast cells, eosinophils, and basophils. They can result in smooth muscle contraction of the airways, increased permeability of the vasculature, increased secretions, and activation of other inflammatory mediators.

The leukotriene receptor antagonists (zafirlukast, montelukast) are competitive inhibitors of the leukotriene receptors, inhibiting leukotriene from interacting with its receptor, thereby blocking its action.

Nursing considerations

- Zafirlukast's absorption is decreased by food (especially high-fat or high-protein meals); therefore, give the dose 1 hour before or 2 hours after meals.
- Headache is the most common adverse reaction experienced with these drugs. Asthenia, dizziness, dyspepsia, gastroenteritis, and fever may also occur.
- The drug isn't used to treat acute bronchospasm.
- The drug is used in conjunction with corticosteroids and other antiasthmatics.
- Patients with liver impairment may require a dosage adjustment if taking zafirlukast. Monitor the patient closely for adverse reactions. Monitor liver enzyme levels in the patient taking zafirlukast because the drug may cause an increase in these levels.

MAST CELL STABILIZERS

Mast cell stabilizers are used to prevent asthma attacks, especially in pediatric patients and those with mild disease. They're given in inhalation or intranasal form. Some examples are nedocromil (Alocril) and cromolyn (Intal).

The mechanism of these drugs is poorly understood, but they inhibit the release of inflammatory mediators by stabilizing the mast cell membrane, possibly through the inhibition of chloride channels.

These drugs are used for the prevention and long-term control of asthma symptoms by controlling the inflammatory process. They're also useful for the prevention of exercise-induced asthma.

Adverse reactions may include throat irritation, bad taste in the mouth, cough, and nausea. Severe reactions, such as wheezing or bronchospasm after inhalation of powder, may also occur.

Nursing considerations

- Mast cell stabilizers shouldn't be used for an acute asthmatic attack.
- These drugs are used in combination with an inhaled beta$_2$-adrenergic agonist or inhaled corticosteroid.
- Reduce dosage gradually to the lowest effective dosage.
- Discontinue the drug if eosinophilic pneumonia or pulmonary infiltrates with eosinophilia occur.
- Instruct the patient to follow his practitioner's and the manufacturer's directions closely.

MUCUS INHIBITORS

Mucus inhibitors, or mucolytics, act directly on mucus, breaking down thick, tenacious secretions so they're more easily eliminated. The most commonly used mucolytic is acetylcysteine (Mucomyst). Mucus-controlling drugs are given by inhalation.

Another type of mucolytic, called *dornase alpha* (Pulmozyme), is a genetically engineered clone of natural human pancreatic DNase enzyme. It's a proteolytic enzyme that can break down the deoxyribonucleic acid material found in purulent secretions. For that reason, it's more effective than acetylcysteine in reducing the viscosity of infected mucus in cystic fibrosis.

Acetylcysteine decreases the thickness of respiratory tract secretions by altering the molecular composition of mucus and irritates the mucosa to stimulate clearance.

Mucolytics are used with other therapies to treat patients with abnormal or thick mucus secretions and may benefit patients with bronchitis, pulmonary complications related to cystic fibrosis, and atelectasis caused by mucus obstruction, as may occur in pneumonia, bronchiectasis, or chronic bronchitis.

Mucolytics may also be used to prepare patients for bronchial studies.

Nursing considerations

■ Warn the patient about the drug's "rotten egg" smell, which may cause nausea.

■ Give acetylcysteine via nebulizer. Because acetylcysteine reacts with iron, copper, and rubber, frequently monitor the patient's nebulizer equipment for reactive effects. The drug doesn't react with glass, plastic, aluminum, or stainless steel.

■ Be ready to give a beta$_2$-adrenergic agonist by aerosol, as prescribed, if the patient experiences bronchospasm.

■ Use 10% and 20% acetylcysteine solutions undiluted, as prescribed. If further dilution is needed, use normal saline solution or sterile water for injection.

■ Avoid contamination of the solution, and refrigerate an opened vial. Discard opened vials after 96 hours.

■ Assess the patient's respiratory status before and after each dose, particularly noting any breathing difficulty, unproductive cough, wheezing, or dyspnea. Follow acetylcysteine administration with chest physiotherapy and postural drainage, as prescribed, and encourage coughing and deep breathing to facilitate removal of respiratory secretions. Suction the patient as needed.

■ Have the patient gargle after administration to relieve the unpleasant odor and dryness; wash the patient's face to eliminate stickiness caused by the drug.

■ Monitor the patient closely for signs of stomatitis, such as swollen, tender gums that bleed easily, papulovesicular ulcers in the mouth and throat, malaise, irritability, and fever.

XANTHINES

Xanthines, also called *methylxanthines* (theophylline [Theo-Dur] and derivatives), are adrenergics that dilate bronchial passages and reduce airway resistance, making it easier for the patient to breathe. They can be given orally or inhaled.

Xanthines decrease airway reactivity and relieve bronchospasm by relaxing bronchial smooth muscle. Theophylline relaxes smooth muscle in addition to decreasing inflammatory mediators (such as mast cells, T cells, and eosinophils), possibly through the inhibition of phosphodiesterase.

In nonreversible obstructive airway disease (chronic bronchitis, emphysema, and apnea), xanthines appear to increase the sensitivity of the brain's respiratory center to carbon dioxide and to stimulate the respiratory drive.

In chronic bronchitis and emphysema, these drugs decrease fatigue of the diaphragm, the respiratory muscle that separates the abdomen from the thoracic cavity. They also improve ventricular function and, therefore, the heart's pumping action.

Theophylline is used as a second- or third-line drug for the long-term control and prevention of symptoms related to:

■ asthma

■ chronic bronchitis

■ emphysema.

Theophylline levels need to be monitored to evaluate efficacy and avoid toxicity. Levels need to be assessed when a dose is started or changed and when drugs are added or removed from the patient's regimen.

Especially high serum levels of theophylline may cause nausea, vomiting, diarrhea, and central nervous system effects, such as irritability, insomnia, anxiety, headache and, with very high levels, seizures. Adverse effects may also include abdominal cramping, epigastric pain, anorexia, and diarrhea.

Nursing considerations

■ Instruct the patient that smoking cigarettes or marijuana increases theophylline elimination, decreasing its serum level and effectiveness.

■ Advise the patient that taking adrenergic stimulants or drinking caffeinated beverages may result in additive adverse effects to theophylline or signs and symptoms of xanthine toxicity.

■ Instruct the patient about possible adverse effects, including cardiovascular effects, such as tachycardia and palpitations, and to notify the physician if they occur.

■ Monitor the patient's theophylline level during treatment.

AGE AWARE When theophylline is given to a neonate, monitor serum theophylline and caffeine levels because theophylline metabolizes to caffeine in the neonate.

DELIVERY METHODS

Some inhalant drugs may be dispensed into the respiratory tract through aerosol treatments (using metered-dose inhalers [MDIs] and turbo-inhalers) and nebulizer therapy (using large- or small-volume, ultrasonic, or in-line devices).

AEROSOL TREATMENTS

Aerosol treatment can be delivered through handheld nebulizers or MDIs. These devices deliver topical medications to the respiratory tract, producing local and systemic effects. The mucosal lining of the respiratory tract absorbs the inhalant almost immediately.

Common inhalants are bronchodilators, used to improve airway patency and facilitate mucus drainage; mucolytics, to achieve a high local concentration to liquefy tenacious bronchial secretions; and corticosteroids, to decrease inflammation.

MDIs are handheld inhalers that use air under pressure to produce a mist containing medication. Drugs delivered in this form, such as bronchodilators and mucolytics, can travel deep into the lungs. MDIs are portable, compact, and relatively easy to use. (See *Types of handheld inhalers.*)

The pressurized MDI canisters contain a micronized powder form of medication. The drug is dissolved or suspended in one or more liquid propellants along with oily, viscous substances called *surfactants,* which are used to keep the drug suspended in the propellants. The surfactant also lubricates the valve mechanism of the MDI. Hand-breath coordination is needed to successfully deliver the aerosol during the patient's inhalation.

Newer devices called *flow-triggered MDIs* eliminate the need for hand-breath coordination. They automatically trigger the medication in response to the patient's inspiratory effort.

Inhalers with a special attachment called a *spacer* provide greater therapeutic benefits for children and patients with poor coordination. The spacer attachment, an extension to the inhaler's mouthpiece, provides more dead-air space for mixing medication.

Turbo-inhalers deliver dry powder medication without the use of propellants and don't require hand-breath coordination. Used to dispense terbutaline (Brethine) or budesonide (Pulmicort), the inhaler contains 200 doses of medication.

The patient holds the turbo-inhaler in the upright position and twists the lower ring to load the medication. He then ex-

TYPES OF HANDHELD INHALERS

Handheld inhalers use air under pressure to produce a mist containing tiny droplets of medication. Drugs delivered in this form (such as mucolytics and bronchodilators) can travel deep into the lungs.

Metered-dose inhaler

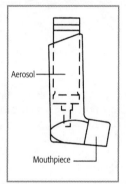

- Aerosol
- Mouthpiece

Inhaler with built-in spacer

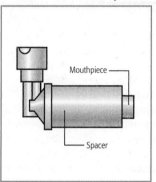

- Mouthpiece
- Spacer

Turbo-inhaler

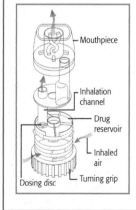

- Mouthpiece
- Inhalation channel
- Drug reservoir
- Inhaled air
- Dosing disc
- Turning grip

Diskus dry powder inhaler

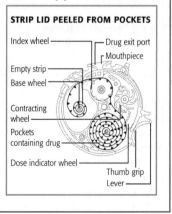

STRIP LID PEELED FROM POCKETS

- Index wheel
- Drug exit port
- Mouthpiece
- Empty strip
- Base wheel
- Contracting wheel
- Pockets containing drug
- Dose indicator wheel
- Thumb grip
- Lever

hales and places his mouth over the dispenser and inhales the medication. The dispenser has a dose counter so that the patient knows when he has 20 doses remaining.

Another device, such as the Advair or Serevent metered inhaler incorporates a disk that contains 60 sealed pockets on an aluminum foil strip within the disk. A lever that the patient activates advances the strip. As the drug pocket reaches the mouthpiece, the cover is peeled away and the medication is dispensed and ready for inhalation.

Patient preparation

- Instruct the patient how to use the device, and encourage him to practice before actually using it to develop hand-breath coordination.
- Inform the patient of possible adverse reactions to each drug.
- Instruct the patient to rinse his mouth after drug administration to prevent stomatitis.
- If the patient is using a steroid inhaler along with a bronchodilator, instruct him to use the bronchodilator first, wait 5 minutes, and then use the steroid inhaler.
- Instruct the patient to exhale completely before using the inhaler. This increases his inspiratory effort, giving him better drug administration and distribution.

Monitoring and aftercare

- Monitor the effectiveness of the medication.
- Because proper drug dosage depends on the correct use of the equipment, assess the patient's ability to perform the medication administration.
- Assess the patient's breath sounds before and after inhaler use.

NEBULIZER THERAPY

An established component of respiratory care, nebulizer therapy helps bronchial hygiene by restoring and maintaining the continuity of the mucosal lining; hydrating dried, retained secretions; promoting expectoration of secretions; humidifying inspired oxygen; and delivering medications. Treatment may be given through nebulizers that have a large or small volume, are ultrasonic, or are placed inside ventilator tubing.

Large-volume nebulizers are used to provide humidity for an artificial airway, such as a tracheostomy, and small-volume nebulizers are used to deliver medications such as bronchodilators. Ultrasonic nebulizers are electrically driven and use high-frequency vibrations to break up surface water into particles. The resultant dense mist can penetrate smaller airways and is useful for hydrating secretions and inducing a cough. In-line nebulizers are used to deliver medications to patients who are being mechanically ventilated. In this case, the nebulizer is placed in the inspiratory side of the ventilatory circuit as close to the endotracheal tube as possible. (See *Comparing nebulizers,* page 124.)

Patient preparation
- Explain the procedure to the patient.
- Take the patient's vital signs and auscultate his lung fields to establish a baseline. If possible, place the patient in a sitting or high Fowler's position to encourage full lung expansion and promote aerosol dispersion. Encourage the patient to take slow, even breaths during the treatment.
- Before using an ultrasonic nebulizer, give an inhaled bronchodilator (MDI or small-volume nebulizer) to prevent bronchospasm.

Monitoring and aftercare
- Check the patient frequently during the procedure to observe for adverse reactions. Watch for labored respirations because ultrasonic nebulizer therapy may hydrate retained secretions and obstruct airways. Monitor the patient's vital signs and auscultate his lung fields for adventitious breath sounds and effectiveness of therapy.
- Encourage the patient to cough and expectorate, or suction as needed.
- Check the water level in a large-volume nebulizer at frequent intervals and refill or replace as indicated. When refilling a reusable container, discard the old water to prevent infection from bacterial or fungal growth, and refill the container to the indicator line with sterile distilled water.
- Change the nebulizer unit and tubing according to your facility's policy to prevent bacterial contamination.

COMPARING NEBULIZERS

NEBULIZER	CHARACTERISTICS
ULTRASONIC	Uses high-frequency sound waves to create an aerosol mist *Advantages* ● Provides 100% humidity ● About 20% of its particles reach the lower airways ● Loosens secretions *Disadvantages* ● May cause bronchospasm in patients with asthma ● Increases risk of overhydration (in infants)
LARGE VOLUME (VENTURI JET)	Works by passing air through a Venturi opening, drawing liquid up through feeding tubes, and nebulizing the solution *Advantages* ● Provides 100% humidity with cool or heated devices ● Provides oxygen and aerosol therapy ● Can be used for long-term therapy *Disadvantages* ● Increases the risk of bacterial growth (in reusable units) ● Causes a collection of condensate in large-bore tubing ● May cause mucosal irritation from breathing hot, dry air (if water level isn't maintained correctly in reservoir) ● Increases the risk of overhydration from mist (in infants) ● Uses a handheld device to deliver aerosolized medication
SMALL VOLUME (MINI-NEBULIZER, MAXI-MIST)	Handheld device that disperses a moisturizing agent into microscopic droplets and delivers it to the lungs with inhalation *Advantages* ● Allows the patient to inhale and exhale on his own ● Can cause less air trapping than drug given by intermittent positive-pressure breathing ● May be used with compressed air, oxygen, or compressor pump ● Allows for portability and disposability *Disadvantages* ● Increases the time of the procedure if the patient needs your assistance ● Distributes medication unevenly if the patient doesn't breathe properly

NEBULIZER THERAPY IN CHILDREN

When using high-output nebulizers, such as an ultrasonic nebulizer, on pediatric patients or patients with a delicate fluid balance, be alert for signs of overhydration (exhibited by unexplained weight gain occurring over several days after the beginning of therapy), pulmonary edema, crackles, and electrolyte imbalance.

Young children may be frightened by the mask used to deliver the medication and may become fatigued from fighting. Because of this, they may appear worse after the medication has been dispensed. Allow the child to calm down before assessing his breath sounds after the treatment.

- If the nebulizer is heated, tell the patient to report warmth, discomfort, or hot tubing because these may indicate a heater malfunction.
- Be especially careful when using ultrasonic nebulization in children. Monitor the child's weight and note any changes. (See *Nebulizer therapy in children*.)
- Nebulized particles can irritate the mucosa in some patients and result in bronchospasm and dyspnea. Other complications include airway burns (when heating elements are used), infection from contaminated equipment (although rare), and adverse reactions from medications.

INHALATION THERAPY

Inhalation therapy uses carefully controlled ventilation techniques to help the patient maintain optimal oxygenation in the event of respiratory failure. Techniques include continuous positive airway pressure (CPAP), endotracheal (ET) intubation, mechanical ventilation, and oxygen therapy.

Continuous positive airway pressure

As its name suggests, CPAP ventilation maintains positive pressure in the airways throughout the patient's respiratory cycle. Originally delivered only with a ventilator, CPAP may now be delivered to intubated or nonintubated patients through an arti-

Using nasal CPAP

This illustration shows the continuous positive-airway pressure (CPAP) apparatus used to apply positive pressure to the airway to prevent obstruction during inspiration in the patient with sleep apnea.

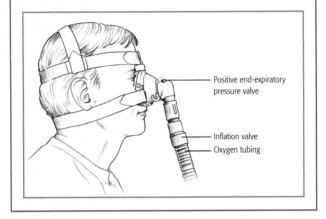

Positive end-expiratory pressure valve

Inflation valve
Oxygen tubing

ficial airway, a mask, or nasal prongs by means of a ventilator or a separate high-flow generating system. (See *Using nasal CPAP.*)

CPAP is available as a continuous-flow and as a demand system. In the continuous-flow system, an air-oxygen blend flows through a humidifier and a reservoir bag into a T-piece. In the demand system, a valve opens in response to the patient's inspiratory flow.

In addition to treating acute respiratory distress syndrome (ARDS), CPAP has been used successfully in pulmonary edema, pulmonary embolism, bronchiolitis, fat embolism, pneumonitis, viral pneumonia, and postoperative atelectasis. In mild to moderate cases of these disorders, CPAP provides an alternative to intubation and mechanical ventilation. It increases the functional residual capacity by distending collapsed alveoli, which improves partial pressure of arterial oxygen and decreases intrapulmonary shunting and oxygen consumption. It reduces the work of breathing. CPAP can also be used to help wean a patient from mechanical ventilation.

Nasal CPAP has proved successful for the long-term treatment of obstructive sleep apnea. In this type of CPAP, high-flow compressed air is directed into a mask that covers only the patient's nose. The pressure supplied through the mask serves as a back-pressure splint, preventing the unstable upper airway from collapsing during inspiration.

CPAP may cause gastric distress if the patient swallows air during the treatment (most common when CPAP is delivered without intubation). He may also feel claustrophobic because of the mask. Because mask CPAP can cause nausea and vomiting, it shouldn't be used in an unresponsive patient or in a patient at risk for vomiting and aspiration. Rarely does CPAP cause barotrauma or lower cardiac output.

PATIENT PREPARATION

- If the patient is intubated or has a tracheostomy, you can accomplish CPAP with a mechanical ventilator by adjusting the settings. Assess his vital signs, oxygen saturation, and breath sounds during CPAP.
- If CPAP is delivered through a mask, a respiratory therapist usually sets up the system and fits the mask. The mask should be transparent and lightweight, with a soft, pliable seal. A tight seal isn't required as long as pressure can be maintained. Measure arterial blood gas (ABG) analysis and bedside pulmonary function studies to establish a baseline.

MONITORING AND AFTERCARE

- Check for decreased cardiac output, which may result from increased intrathoracic pressure associated with CPAP.
- Watch closely for changes in respiratory rate, rhythm, and effort. Uncoordinated breathing patterns may indicate severe respiratory muscle fatigue that can't be helped by CPAP. Report this to the physician; the patient may need mechanical ventilation.
- Check the CPAP system for pressure fluctuations, which may affect oxygenation.
- Keep in mind that high airway pressures increase the risk of pneumothorax; monitor the patient for chest pain and decreased breath sounds.

- Use oximetry, if possible, to monitor oxygen saturation, especially when the CPAP mask is removed to provide routine care.
- If the patient is stable, remove his mask briefly every 2 to 4 hours to provide mouth and skin care along with fluids. Don't apply oils or lotions under the mask—they may react with the mask seal material. Increase the length of time the mask is off as the patient's ability to maintain oxygenation without CPAP improves.
- Check closely for air leaks around the mask near the eyes (an area difficult to seal); escaping air can dry the eyes, causing conjunctivitis or other problems.
- If the patient is using a nasal CPAP device for sleep apnea, watch for decreased snoring and mouth breathing while he sleeps. If these symptoms don't subside, notify the physician; either the system is leaking or the pressure is inadequate to provide relief.

Endotracheal intubation

ET intubation involves insertion of a tube into the lungs through the mouth or nose to establish a patent airway. It protects patients from aspiration by sealing off the trachea from the digestive tract and permits removal of tracheobronchial secretions in patients who can't cough effectively. ET intubation also provides a route for mechanical ventilation.

Drawbacks of ET intubation are that it bypasses normal respiratory defenses against infection, reduces cough effectiveness, may be uncomfortable, and prevents verbal communication.

Potential complications of ET intubation include:
- bronchospasm or laryngospasm
- cardiac arrhythmias
- hypoxemia (if attempts at intubation are prolonged or oxygen delivery is interrupted)
- injury to the lips, mouth, pharynx, or vocal cords
- tooth damage or loss
- tracheal stenosis, erosion, and necrosis.

In orotracheal intubation, the tube is inserted through the mouth. This type of intubation is preferred in emergencies because it's easier and faster. However, maintaining exact tube placement is more difficult because the tube must be well secured to avoid kinking and prevent bronchial obstruction or accidental extubation. It's also uncomfortable for conscious patients because it stimulates salivation, coughing, and retching. Orotracheal intubation is contraindicated in patients with orofacial injuries, acute cervical spinal injury, and degenerative spinal disorders.

In nasal intubation, the tube is inserted through a nasal passage. Nasal intubation is preferred for elective insertion when the patient can breathe on his own for a short period. Nasal intubation is more comfortable than oral intubation and is typically used in a conscious patient who's at risk for respiratory arrest or who has a cervical spinal injury. It's contraindicated in a patient with a facial or basilar skull fracture.

Nasal intubation is more difficult to perform than oral intubation. Because the tube passes blindly through the nasal cavity, it causes more tissue damage, increases the risk of infection by nasal bacteria introduced into the trachea, and increases the risk of pressure necrosis of the nasal mucosa.

PATIENT PREPARATION

- If possible, explain the procedure to the patient and his family.
- Obtain the correct size ET tube. The typical size for an oral ET tube for women is 7.5 mm (indicates the size of the lumen) and 8 mm for men.
- Give medication as ordered to decrease respiratory secretions, induce amnesia or analgesia, and help calm and relax the conscious patient. Remove dentures and bridgework, if present, to prevent aspiration.

MONITORING AND AFTERCARE

- After securing the ET tube, reconfirm tube placement by noting bilateral breath sounds and end-tidal carbon dioxide ($ETCO_2$) readings. (See *Securing an ET tube,* page 130.)
- Auscultate breath sounds and watch for chest movement to ensure correct tube placement and full lung ventilation.
- A chest X-ray may be ordered to confirm tube placement.
- Disposable $ETCO_2$ detectors are commonly used to confirm tube placement in emergency departments, postanesthesia care units, and critical care units that don't use continuous $ETCO_2$ monitoring. Follow the manufacturer's instructions for proper use of the device. Don't use the detector with a heated

SECURING AN ET TUBE

Before securing an endotracheal (ET) tube, make sure that the patient's face is clean, dry, and free from beard stubble. If possible, suction his mouth and dry the ET tube just before taping. Check the reference mark on the tube to ensure correct placement. After securing, always check for bilateral breath sounds to ensure that the ET tube hasn't been displaced by manipulation. To secure the tube, use one of the methods described here.

Method 1

● Cut one piece of 1″ cloth adhesive tape long enough to wrap around the patient's head and overlap in front, and then cut an 8″ (20.3-cm) piece of tape and center it on the longer piece, sticky sides together.

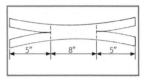

● Cut a 5″ (12.7-cm) slit in each end of the longer tape (as shown).

● Apply benzoin tincture to the patient's cheeks, under his nose, and under the lower lip. (Don't spray benzoin directly on the patient's face; the vapors can be irritating if inhaled and can harm the eyes.)

● Place the top half of one end of the tape under the patient's nose and wrap the lower half around the ET tube. Place the lower half of the other end of the tape along his lower lip and wrap the top half around the tube.

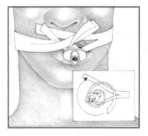

Method 2

● ET tube holders are available that can help secure an ET tube.

● Made of hard plastic or of softer material, the tube holder secures the ET tube in place. The tube holder is available in adult and pediatric sizes. Some models come with bite blocks attached.

● Place the strap around the patient's neck and secure it around the tube with Velcro fasteners (as shown).

● Because each model is different, check the manufacturer's guidelines for correct placement and care.

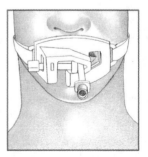

ANALYZING CO₂ LEVELS

Depending on the end-tidal carbon dioxide (ETco₂) detector you use, the meaning of color changes within the detector dome may differ from the analysis for the Easy Cap detector described here.

● The rim of the Easy Cap is divided into sections A, B, and C. Their control colors range from purple (in section A), signifying the absence of carbon dioxide (CO_2), to beige, tan and, finally, yellow (in section C). The numbers in the sections range from 0.03 to 5 and indicate the percentage of exhaled CO_2.

● The color in the center rectangle reflects the patient's CO_2 level. It should fluctuate during ventilation from purple (matching section A) during inspiration to yellow (matching section C) at the end of expiration. This indicates that the ETco₂ levels are adequate—above 2%.

● An end-expiratory color change from the C range to the B range may be the first sign of hemodynamic instability.

● During cardiopulmonary resuscitation (CPR), an end-expiratory color change from the A or B range to the C range may mean the return of spontaneous ventilation.

● During prolonged cardiac arrest, inadequate pulmonary perfusion leads to inadequate gas exchange. The patient exhales little or no CO_2, so the color stays in the purple range even with proper intubation. Ineffective CPR also leads to inadequate pulmonary perfusion.

COLOR INDICATORS ON ETco₂ DETECTOR

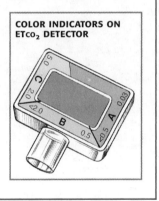

humidifier or nebulizer because humidity, heat, and moisture can interfere with device function. (See *Analyzing CO₂ levels*.)

■ Follow standard precautions, and suction through the ET tube as the patient's condition indicates, to clear secretions and prevent mucus plugs from obstructing the tube.

■ After suctioning, hyperoxygenate the patient being maintained on a ventilator with the handheld resuscitation bag.

■ If available, use a closed tracheal suctioning system, which permits the ventilated patient to remain on the ventilator during suctioning. (See *Closed tracheal suctioning*, pages 132 and 133.)

CLOSED TRACHEAL SUCTIONING

The closed tracheal suction system can ease removal of secretions and reduce patient complications. Consisting of a sterile suction catheter in a clear plastic sleeve, the system permits the patient to remain connected to the ventilator during suctioning. With this system, the patient can maintain the tidal volume, oxygen concentration, and positive end-expiratory pressure delivered by the ventilator while being suctioned. In turn, this reduces the occurrence of suction-induced hypoxemia.

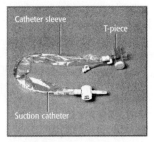

Catheter sleeve
T-piece
Suction catheter

Because the catheter remains in a protective sleeve, another advantage of this system is a reduced risk of infection, even when the same catheter is used many times. The caregiver doesn't need to touch the catheter and the ventilator circuit remains closed.

In patients receiving intermittent mandatory mechanical ventilation, closed tracheal suctioning may reduce arterial desaturation and eliminate the need for preoxygenation.

Because suction catheters are considered contaminated after a single use, researchers studied whether closed tracheal suctioning increased the rate of health care-associated pneumonia in mechanically ventilated patients. They found that patients receiving closed tracheal suctioning had lower rates of health care-associated pneumonia than those receiving open suctioning. Moreover, researchers found that changing closed tracheal suction catheters as needed was just as effective in preventing ventilator-associated pneumonia as daily catheter changes.

On the negative side, closed tracheal suctioning has been found to produce increased negative airway pressure when certain ventilatory modes are used, increasing the risk of atelectasis and hypoxemia.

Implementation

To perform the procedure, gather the closed suction system that consists of a control valve, a T-piece to connect the artificial airway to the ventilator breathing circuit, and a catheter sleeve that encloses the catheter and has connections at each end for the control valve and the T-piece. Then follow these steps:
● Wash your hands.

Mechanical ventilation

Mechanical ventilation involves the use of a machine to move air into a patient's lungs. Mechanical ventilators use either positive or negative pressure to ventilate the patient. Reasons for use of mechanical ventilation include:

● Remove the closed suction system from its wrapping. Attach the control valve to the connecting tubing.

● Depress the thumb suction control valve and keep it depressed while setting the suction pressure to the desired level.

● Connect the T-piece to the ventilator breathing circuit; make sure that the irrigation port is closed. Then connect the T-piece to the patient's endotracheal or tracheostomy tube (as shown below).

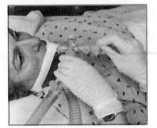

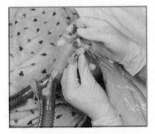

● Hyperoxygenate and hyperinflate the patient using the ventilator.

● Put on clean gloves. Steadying the T-piece, use the thumb and index finger of the other hand to advance the catheter through the tube and into the patient's tracheobronchial tree (as shown at top of next column). It may be necessary to gently retract the catheter sleeve as you advance the catheter.

● While continuing to hold the T-piece and control valve, apply continuous suction and withdraw the catheter until it reaches its fully extended length in the sleeve. Repeat the procedure only if necessary.

● After you've finished suctioning, flush the catheter by maintaining suction while slowly introducing normal saline solution or sterile water into the irrigation port.

● Place the thumb control valve in the off position.

● Dispose of and replace the suction equipment and supplies according to your facility's policy.

● Remove your gloves and wash your hands.

● Change the closed suction system every 24 hours to minimize the risk of infection.

▪ acute respiratory failure caused by ARDS, pneumonia, acute exacerbations of chronic obstructive pulmonary disease, pulmonary embolism, heart failure, trauma, tumors, or drug overdose

VENTILATOR MODES

Positive-pressure ventilators are categorized as volume or pressure ventilators and have various modes and options.

Volume modes

Volume modes include controlled ventilation (CV) or controlled mandatory ventilation (CMV), assist-control (A/C) or assisted mandatory ventilation (AMV), and intermittent mandatory ventilation (IMV) and synchronized intermittent mandatory ventilation (SIMV).

CV or CMV

In the CV or CMV mode, the ventilator supplies all ventilation for the patient. The respiratory rate, tidal volume (V_T), inspiratory time, and positive end-expiratory pressure (PEEP) are preset. This mode is usually used when a patient can't initiate spontaneous breaths, such as when he's paralyzed from a spinal cord injury or neuromuscular disease or chemically paralyzed with neuromuscular blocking agents.

A/C or AMV

In the A/C or AMV mode, the basic respiratory rate is set along with the V_T, inspiratory time, and PEEP, but the patient is allowed to breathe faster than the preset rate. The sensitivity is set so that when the patient initiates a spontaneous breath, a full V_T is delivered so that all breaths are the same V_T, whether triggered by the patient or delivered at the set rate. If the patient tires and his drive to breathe is negated, the ventilator continues to deliver breaths at the preset rate.

IMV or SIMV

IMV and SIMV modes require preset respiratory rate, V_T, inspiratory time, sensitivity, and PEEP. Mandatory breaths are delivered at a set rate and V_T. In between the mandatory breaths, the patient can breathe

■ respiratory center depression caused by stroke, brain injury, or trauma

■ neuromuscular diseases, such as Guillain-Barré syndrome, multiple sclerosis, and myasthenia gravis; trauma, including spinal cord injury; or central nervous system depression.

Positive-pressure ventilators exert a positive pressure on the airway, which causes inspiration while increasing tidal volume. A high-frequency ventilator uses high respiratory rates and low tidal volume to maintain alveolar ventilation. The inspiratory cycles of these ventilators may be adjusted for volume, pressure, or time:

■ A volume-cycled ventilator, the type used most commonly, delivers a preset volume of air each time, regardless of the amount of lung resistance.

spontaneously at his own rate and V_T. The V_T of these spontaneous breaths can vary because the breaths are determined by the patient's ability to generate negative pressure in his chest. With SIMV, the ventilator synchronizes the mandatory breaths with the patient's inspirations.

Pressure modes

Pressure modes include pressure-support ventilation (PSV), pressure-controlled ventilation (PCV), and pressure-controlled/inverse ratio ventilation (PC/IRV).

PSV

The PSV mode augments inspiration for a spontaneously breathing patient. The inspiratory pressure level, PEEP, and sensitivity are preset. When the patient initiates a breath, the breath is delivered at the preset pressure level and is maintained throughout inspiration. The patient determines the V_T, respiratory rate, and inspiratory time.

PCV

In the PCV mode, inspiratory pressure, inspiratory time, respiratory rate, and PEEP are preset. V_T varies with the patient's airway pressure and compliance.

PC/IRV

PC/IRV combines pressure-limited ventilation with an inverse ratio of inspiration to expiration. In this mode, the inspiratory pressure, respiratory rate, inspiratory time (1:1, 2:1, 3:1, or 4:1), and PEEP are preset. PCV and PC/IRV modes may be used in patients with acute respiratory distress syndrome.

- A pressure-cycled ventilator generates flow until the machine reaches a preset pressure, regardless of the volume delivered or the time required to achieve the pressure.
- A time-cycled ventilator generates flow for a preset amount of time.

Several different modes of ventilatory control are found on the ventilator. The choice of mode depends on the patient's respiratory condition. (See *Ventilator modes.*)

Negative-pressure ventilators work by creating negative pressure, which pulls the thorax outward and allows air to flow into the lungs. They're used primarily to treat patients with neuromuscular disorders. Examples of such ventilators include the iron lung, the cuirass (chest shell), and the body wrap.

RESPONDING TO VENTILATOR ALARMS

SIGNAL	POSSIBLE CAUSE
LOW-PRESSURE ALARM	● Tube disconnected from ventilator
	● Endotracheal (ET) tube displaced above vocal cords or tracheostomy tube extubated
	● Leaking tidal volume from low cuff pressure (from an underinflated or ruptured cuff or a leak in the cuff or one-way valve)
	● Ventilator malfunction
	● Leak in ventilator circuitry (from loose connection or hole in tubing, loss of temperature-sensitive device, or cracked humidification jar)
HIGH-PRESSURE ALARM	● Increased airway pressure or decreased lung compliance caused by worsening disease
	● Patient biting on oral ET tube
	● Secretions in airway
	● Condensate in large-bore tubing
	● Intubation of right mainstem bronchus
	● Patient coughing, gagging, or attempting to talk
	● Chest wall resistance
	● Failure of high-pressure relief valve
	● Bronchospasm

NURSING CONSIDERATIONS

■ Provide emotional support to the patient during all phases of mechanical ventilation to reduce anxiety and promote successful treatment. Even if the patient is unresponsive, continue to explain all procedures and treatments.

■ Make sure the ventilator alarms are on at all times to alert you to potentially hazardous conditions and changes in the patient's status. If an alarm sounds and the problem can't be easily identified, disconnect the patient from the ventilator and use a handheld resuscitation bag to ventilate him. (See *Responding to ventilator alarms.*)

INTERVENTIONS

- Reconnect the tube to the ventilator.
- Check tube placement and reposition, if needed. If extubation or displacement has occurred, ventilate the patient manually and call the physician immediately.
- Listen for a whooshing sound around the tube, indicating an air leak. If you hear one, check the cuff pressure. If you can't maintain pressure, call the physician; he may need to insert a new tube.
- Disconnect the patient from the ventilator and ventilate him manually, if necessary. Obtain another ventilator.
- Make sure all connections are intact. Check for holes or leaks in the tubing and replace, if necessary. Check the humidification jar and replace, if cracked.

- Auscultate the lungs for evidence of increasing lung consolidation, barotrauma, or wheezing. Call the physician if indicated.
- Insert a bite block if needed.
- Look for secretions in the airway. To remove them, suction the patient or have him cough.
- Check tubing for condensate and remove any fluid.
- Check tube position. If it has slipped, call the physician, who may need to reposition it.
- If the patient fights the ventilator, the physician may order a sedative or neuromuscular blocking agent.
- Reposition the patient to see if doing so improves chest expansion. If repositioning doesn't help, administer the prescribed analgesic.
- Have the faulty equipment replaced.
- Assess the patient for the cause. Report to the physician and treat the patient, as ordered.

- Assess cardiopulmonary status frequently, at least every 2 to 4 hours, or more often, if indicated. Also assess vital signs and auscultate breath sounds. Monitor pulse oximetry or $ETCO_2$ levels and hemodynamic parameters, as ordered. Monitor intake and output and assess for fluid volume imbalances.
- Unless contraindicated, turn the patient from side to side every 1 to 2 hours to aid lung expansion and removal of secretions. Perform active or passive range-of-motion exercises for all extremities to reduce the hazards of immobility.
- Because intubation and mechanical ventilation impair the patient's ability to speak, place the call bell within the patient's

UNDERSTANDING MANUAL VENTILATION

A handheld resuscitation bag is an inflatable device that can be attached to a face mask or directly to a tracheostomy or an endotracheal (ET) tube to allow manual delivery of oxygen or room air to the lungs of a patient who can't breathe by himself.

Although usually used in an emergency, manual ventilation can also be performed while the patient is disconnected temporarily from a mechanical ventilator, such as during a tubing change, during transport, or before suctioning. In such instances, the use of the handheld resuscitation bag maintains ventilation. Oxygen administration with a resuscitation bag can help improve a compromised cardiorespiratory system.

Ventilation guidelines

To manually ventilate a patient with an ET or a tracheostomy tube, follow these guidelines:

● If oxygen is readily available, connect the handheld resuscitation bag to the oxygen. Attach one end of the tubing to the bottom of the bag and the other end to the nipple adapter on the flowmeter of the oxygen source.
● Turn on the oxygen and adjust the flow rate according to the patient's condition.
● Before attaching the handheld resuscitation bag, suction the ET or tracheostomy tube to remove any secretions that may obstruct the airway.
● Remove the mask from the ventilation bag and attach the handheld resuscitation bag directly to the tube.
● Keeping your nondominant hand on the connection of the bag to the tube, exert downward pressure to seal the mask against his face. For an adult patient, use your dominant hand to compress the bag every 5 seconds to deliver approximately 1 L of air.

reach and establish a method of communication such as a communication board.

■ Give a sedative or neuromuscular blocker, as ordered, to relax the patient or eliminate spontaneous breathing efforts that can interfere with the ventilator's action.

■ Remember that the patient receiving a neuromuscular blocker requires close observation because he can't breathe or communicate. In addition, if the patient is receiving a neuromuscular blocker, make sure he also receives a sedative. Neuromuscular blockers cause paralysis without altering the patient's level of consciousness (LOC). Reassure the patient and his family that the paralysis is temporary. Provide routine eye care and instill artificial tears because the patient can't blink.

■ Make sure emergency equipment is available in case the ventilator malfunctions or the patient is extubated accidentally. If

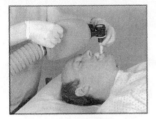

● Deliver breaths with the patient's inspiratory effort if any is present. Don't attempt to deliver a breath as the patient exhales.
● Observe the patient's chest to ensure that it rises and falls with each compression. If ventilation fails to occur, check the connection and the patency of the patient's airway; if necessary, reposition his head and suction.
● Be alert for possible underventilation, which commonly occurs because the handheld resuscitation bag is difficult to keep positioned while ensuring an open airway. In addition, the volume of air delivered to the patient varies with the type of bag used and the hand size of the person compressing the bag. An adult with a small- or medium-sized hand may not consistently deliver 1 L of air. For these reasons, have someone assist with the procedure if possible.
● Keep in mind that air is forced into the patient's stomach with manual ventilation, placing the patient at risk for aspiration of vomitus (possibly resulting in pneumonia) and gastric distention.
● Record the date and time of the procedure, reason and length of time the patient was disconnected from mechanical ventilation and received manual ventilation, any complications and the nursing action taken, and the patient's tolerance of the procedure.

there's a problem with the ventilator, disconnect the patient from the ventilator and manually ventilate with 100% oxygen; use a handheld resuscitation bag connected to the ET or tracheostomy tube, troubleshoot the ventilator, and correct the problem. If you can't determine the cause, call for help and have the respiratory therapist evaluate the problem. (See *Understanding manual ventilation*.)

Oxygen therapy

In oxygen therapy, oxygen can be delivered by mask, nasal prongs, nasal catheter, or transtracheal catheter to prevent or reverse hypoxemia and reduce the work of breathing. Possible causes of hypoxemia include emphysema, pneumonia, Guillain-Barré syndrome, heart failure, and myocardial infarction. (See *Oxygen delivery systems*, pages 140 to 143.)

(Text continues on page 144.)

OXYGEN DELIVERY SYSTEMS

Patients may receive oxygen through one of several administration systems. Each has its own benefits, drawbacks, and indications for use. The advantages and disadvantages of each system are compared here.

Nasal cannula

Oxygen is delivered through plastic cannulas placed in the patient's nostrils.

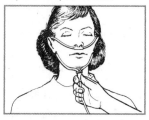

Advantages: Safe and simple, comfortable and easily tolerated, nasal prongs can be shaped to fit any face, effective for low oxygen concentrations, inexpensive and disposable, allows for movement, eating, and talking
Disadvantages: Can't deliver concentrations higher than 40%, can't be used in patients with complete nasal obstruction, may cause headaches or dry mucous membranes if flow rate exceeds 6 L/minute, can dislodge easily
Administration guidelines: Ensure patency of the patient's nostrils with a flashlight. If patent, hook the cannula tubing behind the patient's ears and under the chin. Slide the adjuster upward under the chin to secure the tubing. If using an elastic strap to secure the cannula, position it over the ears and around the back of the head. Avoid applying it too tightly, which can result in excess pressure on facial structures and cannula occlusion. With a nasal cannula, oral breathers achieve the same oxygen delivery as nasal breathers. Oxygen can be given without humidification at flow of less than or equal to 4 L/minute.

Simple mask

Oxygen flows through an entry port at the bottom of the mask and exits through large holes on the sides of the mask.

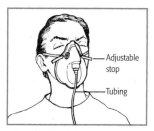

Adjustable stop

Tubing

Advantages: Can deliver concentrations of 35% to 50%
Disadvantages: Hot and confining, may irritate the patient's skin, interferes with eating and talking, impractical for long-term therapy because of imprecision, tight seal required for higher oxygen concentration may cause discomfort
Administration guidelines: Select the mask size that offers the best fit. Place the mask over the patient's nose, mouth, and chin, and mold the flexible metal edge to the bridge of the nose. Adjust the elastic band around the head to hold the mask firmly but comfortably over the cheeks, chin, and bridge of the nose. For an elderly or a cachectic patient with sunken cheeks, tape gauze pads to the mask over the cheek area to try to create an airtight seal. Without this seal, room air dilutes the oxygen, preventing delivery of the prescribed concentration. A minimum of 5 L/minute is required in all masks to flush expired carbon dioxide from the mask so that the patient doesn't rebreathe it.

Partial rebreather mask

The patient inspires oxygen from a reservoir bag along with atmospheric air and oxygen from the mask. The first third of exhaled tidal volume enters the bag; the rest exits the mask. Because air entering the reservoir bag comes from the trachea and bronchi, where no gas exchange occurs, the patient rebreathes the oxygenated air he just exhaled.

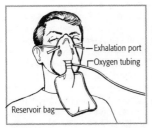

Exhalation port
Oxygen tubing
Reservoir bag

Advantages: Effectively delivers concentrations of 40% to 70%, openings in the mask allow the patient to inhale room air if oxygen source fails
Disadvantages: Hot and confining, tight seal required for accurate oxygen concentration may cause discomfort, interferes with eating and talking, may irritate skin, bag may twist or kink, impractical for long-term therapy
Administration guidelines: Follow the procedures listed for the simple mask. If the reservoir bag collapses more than slightly during inspiration, raise the flow rate until you see only a slight deflation. Marked or complete deflation indicates insufficient oxygen flow; carbon dioxide may accumulate in the mask and bag. Keep the reservoir bag from twisting or kinking. Ensure free expansion by making sure that the bag lies outside the patient's gown and bedcovers.

Nonrebreather mask

On inhalation, the one-way valve opens, directing oxygen from a reservoir bag into the mask. On exhalation, gas exits the mask through the one-way expiratory valve and enters the atmosphere. The patient only breathes air from the bag.

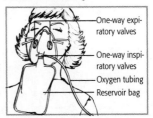

One-way expiratory valves
One-way inspiratory valves
Oxygen tubing
Reservoir bag

Advantages: Delivers the highest possible oxygen concentration (60% to 80%) short of intubation and mechanical ventilation, effective for short-term therapy, doesn't dry mucous membranes, can be converted to a partial rebreather mask, if necessary, by removing the one-way valve
Disadvantages: Requires a tight seal that may cause discomfort and be difficult to maintain, may irritate the patient's skin, interferes with talking and eating, impractical for long-term therapy
Administration guidelines: Follow procedures listed for the simple mask. Make sure that the mask fits very snugly and the one-way valves are secure and functioning. Because the mask excludes room air, valve malfunction can cause carbon dioxide buildup and suffocate an unconscious patient. If the reservoir bag collapses more than slightly during inspiration, raise the flow rate until you see only a slight deflation. Marked or complete deflation indicates an insufficient flow rate. Keep the reservoir bag from twisting or kinking. Ensure free expansion by making sure that the bag lies outside the patient's gown and bedcovers.

(continued)

OXYGEN DELIVERY SYSTEMS *(continued)*

CPAP mask
This system allows the spontaneously breathing patient to receive continuous positive airway pressure (CPAP) with or without an artificial airway.

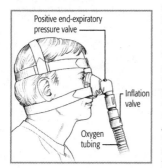

Positive end-expiratory pressure valve

Inflation valve

Oxygen tubing

Advantages: Noninvasively improves arterial oxygenation by increasing functional residual capacity, alleviates the need for intubation, allows the patient to talk and cough without interrupting positive pressure

Disadvantages: Requires a tight fit that may cause discomfort; interferes with eating and talking; heightened risk of aspiration if the patient vomits; increased risk of pneumothorax, diminished cardiac output, and gastric distention; contraindicated in patients with chronic obstructive pulmonary disease, bullous lung disease, low cardiac output, or tension pneumothorax

Administration guidelines: Place one strap behind the patient's head and the other strap over his head to ensure a snug fit. Attach one latex strap to the connector prong on one side of the mask. Then, use one hand to position the mask on the patient's face while using the other hand to connect the strap to the other side of the mask. After the mask is applied, assess the patient's respiratory, circulatory, and GI function every hour. Watch for signs of pneumothorax, decreased cardiac output, a drop in blood pressure, and gastric distention.

Venturi mask

The mask is connected to a Venturi device, which mixes a specific volume of air and oxygen.

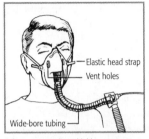

Elastic head strap
Vent holes
Wide-bore tubing

Advantages: Delivers highly accurate oxygen concentration despite the patient's respiratory pattern because the same amount of air is always entrained, has dilute jets that can be changed or a dial that changes oxygen concentration, doesn't dry mucous membranes, allows addition of humidity or aerosol

Disadvantages: Confining and may irritate skin, interferes with eating and talking, condensate possibly collecting and dripping on the patient if humidification is used, possible oxygen concentration alteration if mask fits loosely, tubing kinks, oxygen intake ports become blocked, flow is insufficient, or patient is hyperpneic

Administration guidelines: Make sure that the oxygen flow rate is set at the amount specified on each mask and the Venturi valve is set for the desired fraction of inspired oxygen.

Aerosols

A face mask, hood, tent, or tracheostomy tube or collar is connected to wide-bore tubing that receives aerosolized oxygen from a jet nebulizer. The jet nebulizer, which is attached near the oxygen source, adjusts air entrainment in a manner similar to the Venturi device.

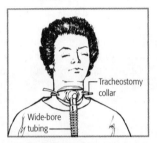

Tracheostomy collar
Wide-bore tubing

Advantages: Delivers high humidity, allows gas to be heated (when given through artificial airway) or cooled (when delivered through a tent)

Disadvantages: Condensate collected in the tracheostomy collar or T tube possibly draining into the tracheostomy, weight of the T tube possibly putting stress on the tracheostomy tube

Administration guidelines: Guidelines vary with the type of nebulizer used: the ultrasonic, large-volume, small-volume, or in-line. When using a high-output nebulizer, watch for signs of overhydration, pulmonary edema, crackles, and electrolyte imbalance.

The equipment used depends on the patient's age, condition, and the required fraction of inspired oxygen. High-flow systems, such as a Venturi mask and ventilators, deliver a precisely controlled air-oxygen mixture. Low-flow systems, such as nasal prongs, nasal catheter, simple mask, partial rebreather mask, and nonrebreather mask, allow variation in the oxygen percentage delivered, based on the patient's respiratory pattern.

Nasal prongs deliver oxygen at flow rates from 0.5 to 6 L/minute. Inexpensive and easy to use, the prongs permit talking, eating, and suctioning—interfering less with the patient's activities than other devices. Even so, the prongs may cause nasal drying and can't deliver high oxygen concentrations.

A nasal catheter can deliver low-flow oxygen at somewhat higher concentrations; however, it isn't commonly used because of discomfort and drying of the mucous membranes.

Masks deliver up to 100% oxygen concentrations but can't be used to deliver controlled oxygen concentrations. In addition, they may fit poorly, causing discomfort, and must be removed to eat. Children and infants don't tolerate masks. (See *Oxygen delivery to children.*)

Transtracheal oxygen catheters, used for patients requiring long-term oxygen therapy, permit highly efficient oxygen delivery and increased mobility with portable oxygen systems and avoid the adverse effects of nasal delivery systems. Even so, they may become a source of infection and require close monitoring and follow-up after insertion as well as daily maintenance care.

PATIENT PREPARATION

- Instruct the patient, his roommates, and visitors not to use improperly grounded radios, televisions, electric razors, or other equipment. Place an "OXYGEN PRECAUTIONS" sign on the outside of the patient's door.
- Perform a cardiopulmonary assessment, and check that baseline ABG or oximetry values have been obtained.
- Check the patency of the patient's nostrils (he may need a mask if they're blocked). Consult the physician if a change in administration route is necessary.
- Assemble the equipment, check the connections, and turn on the oxygen source. Make sure the humidifier bubbles and oxygen flows through the prongs, catheter, or mask.

AGE AWARE

OXYGEN DELIVERY TO CHILDREN

Oxygen delivery to children can be accomplished using an oxygen hood, nasal cannula or prongs, or a mist tent.

Oxygen hood

Oxygen delivery to an infant is best tolerated by giving it through an oxygen hood, as shown at right.

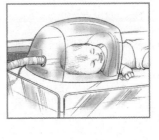

High and low concentrations of oxygen can be delivered by an oxygen hood. Remember to not allow the oxygen to flow directly on the infant's face. This cold stimulation can trigger the diving reflex, which results in bradycardia and shunting of blood to the central circulation. Older infants and children can also use a nasal cannula or nasal prongs.

Mist tent

For children beyond infancy, an oxygen tent or mist tent, shown at right, is another option. The drawback is that the concentration of the oxygen within the tent is very hard to control.

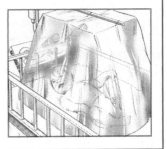

Remember to remove all toys that may produce a spark, including those that are battery operated. Oxygen supports combustion, and the smallest spark can cause a fire.

- Set the flow rate as ordered. If necessary, have the respiratory care practitioner check the flowmeter for accuracy.

MONITORING AND AFTERCARE

- Periodically perform a cardiopulmonary assessment on the patient receiving any form of oxygen therapy.
- If the patient is on bed rest, change his position frequently (at least every 2 hours) to ensure adequate ventilation and circulation.

- Provide good skin care to prevent irritation and breakdown caused by the tubing, prongs, or mask.
- Be sure to humidify oxygen flow exceeding 3 L/minute to help prevent drying of mucous membranes. However, humidity isn't added with Venturi masks because water can block the Venturi jets.
- Assess for signs of hypoxia, including decreased LOC, tachycardia, arrhythmias, diaphoresis, restlessness, altered blood pressure or respiratory rate, clammy skin, and cyanosis. If these occur, notify the physician, obtain a pulse oximetry reading, and check the oxygen delivery equipment to see if it's malfunctioning. Be especially alert for changes in respiratory status when you change or stop oxygen therapy.
- If your patient is using a nonrebreather mask, periodically check the valves to see if they're functioning properly. If the valves stick closed, the patient is reinhaling carbon dioxide and not receiving adequate oxygen. Replace the mask if necessary.
- If the patient receives oxygen concentrations exceeding 50% for more than 24 hours, ask about symptoms of oxygen toxicity, such as burning, substernal chest pain, dyspnea, and dry cough. Atelectasis and pulmonary edema may also occur.
- Encourage coughing and deep breathing to help prevent atelectasis. Monitor ABG levels frequently and reduce oxygen concentrations as soon as ABG values indicate this is feasible.
- Use a low flow rate if your patient has chronic pulmonary disease. However, don't use a simple face mask because low flow rates won't flush carbon dioxide from the mask, and the patient will rebreathe carbon dioxide. Watch for alterations in LOC, heart rate and rhythm, and respiratory rate and rhythm.
- If the patient needs oxygen at home, the physician will order the flow rate, the number of hours per day to be used, and the conditions of use. Several types of delivery systems are available, including a tank, concentrator, and liquid oxygen system. The chosen system depends on the patient's needs and the availability and cost of each system. Make sure the patient can use the prescribed system safely and effectively. He'll need regular follow-up care to evaluate his response to therapy. (See *Home ventilator therapy.*)

DISCHARGE TEACHING

HOME VENTILATOR THERAPY

If the patient requires a ventilator at home, conduct thorough patient teaching with him and a family member. Be sure to include these points:

● Show him how to check the device and its settings for accuracy and the nebulizer and oxygen equipment for proper functioning. Tell him to do so at least once per day.
● Tell him to be sure to refill his humidifier as necessary.
● Explain that his arterial blood gas levels will be measured periodically to evaluate his therapy.
● Demonstrate how to count his pulse rate, and tell him to report changes in rate or rhythm as well as chest pain, fever, dyspnea, or swollen extremities.
● Tell him to bring his ventilator with him if he needs to be treated for an acute problem because it may be possible to stabilize him without hospitalization. However, be sure to explain that, if hospitalization is required, he may not be able to use his own ventilator.
● Tell him to call his physician or respiratory therapist if he has questions or problems.

Weaning

The patient's body quickly comes to depend on artificial ventilation and must gradually be reintroduced to normal breathing.

Successful weaning depends on a strong spontaneous respiratory effort, a stable cardiovascular system, and sufficient respiratory muscle strength and LOC to sustain spontaneous breathing. Certain criteria must be met before weaning can begin. (See *Criteria for weaning*, pages 148 and 149.)

Several weaning methods are used:

■ In intermittent mandatory ventilation (IMV), the number of breaths produced by the ventilator is gradually reduced, allowing the patient to breathe independently. Decreasing the number of breaths allows the patient to gradually increase his respiratory muscle strength and endurance.

■ Pressure support ventilation may be used alone or as an adjunct to IMV in the weaning process. In this procedure, a set burst of pressure is applied during inspiration with the patient's normal breathing pattern, allowing the patient to build respiratory muscle strength.

CRITERIA FOR WEANING

Successful weaning from the ventilator depends on the patient's ability to breathe on his own. This means that he must have a spontaneous respiratory effort that can keep him ventilated, a stable cardiovascular system, and sufficient respiratory muscle strength and level of consciousness to sustain spontaneous breathing. The patient should meet some or all the following criteria.

Readiness criteria

● Arterial oxygen saturation (SaO_2) greater than 92% on fraction of inspired oxygen less than or equal to 40%, positive end-expiratory pressure (PEEP) less than or equal to 5 cm H_2O
● Hemodynamically stable, adequately resuscitated and doesn't require vasoactive support
● Serum electrolyte levels and pH within normal range
● Hematocrit greater than 25%
● Core body temperature greater than 96.8° F (36° C) and less than 102.2° F (39° C)
● Pain adequately managed
● Successful withdrawal of a neuromuscular blocker
● Arterial blood gas values within normal limits or at patient's baseline

Weaning intervention (long term—more than 72 hours)

● Transfer to pressure-support ventilation (PSV) mode and adjust support level to maintain patient's respiratory rate at less than 35 breaths/minute.
● Observe for 30 minutes for signs of early failure, such as:
   – sustained respiratory rate greater than 35 breaths/minute
   – SaO_2 less than 89%
   – tidal volume less than or equal to 5 ml/kg
   – sustained minute ventilation greater than 200 ml/kg/minute

▩ Spontaneous breathing trials are another step to weaning. In this procedure, a T-piece is attached to the end of the ET tube or a tracheostomy collar is attached to the tracheostomy tube. The ventilator is then disconnected, and the patient is allowed to breathe on his own through the ET or tracheostomy tube. The amount of time spent off the ventilator is initially short, 1 to 2 minutes, and then gradually increased as the patient can tolerate it.

NURSING CONSIDERATIONS
▩ When weaning the patient, continue to observe for signs of respiratory distress, fatigue, hypoxemia, and cardiac arrhythmias.

– evidence of respiratory or hemodynamic distress: labored respiratory pattern, increased diaphoresis or anxiety, sustained heart rate greater than 20% higher or lower than baseline, systolic blood pressure greater than 180 mm Hg or less than 90 mm Hg diastolic.

● If tolerated, continue trial for 2 hours, then return patient to "rest" settings by adding ventilator breaths or increasing PSV to achieve a total respiratory rate of less than 20 breaths/minute.

● After 2 hours of rest, repeat trial for 2 to 4 hours at same PSV level as previous trial. If the patient exceeds the tolerance criteria, stop the trial and return to "rest" settings. In this case, the next trial should be performed at a higher support level than the failed trial.

● Record the results after each weaning episode, including specific parameters and the time frame if failure was observed.

● The goal is to increase trial lengths and reduce the PSV level needed in increments.

● With each successful trial, the PSV level may be decreased by 2 to 4 cm H_2O or the time interval may be increased by 1 to 2 hours (or both), while keeping the patient within tolerable parameters.

● Ensure nocturnal ventilation at "rest" settings (with a respiratory rate of less than 20 breaths/minute) for at least 6 hours each night until the patient's weaning trials demonstrate readiness to stop support.

▨ Schedule weaning to comfortably and realistically fit into the patient's daily regimen. Avoid weaning during meals, baths, and lengthy therapeutic procedures.

▨ Document the length of the weaning trial and the patient's tolerance of the procedure.

▨ After the patient is successfully weaned and extubated, administer the appropriate oxygen therapy.

SURGERY

If drugs or other therapeutic approaches fail to maintain airway patency and protect healthy tissues from disease, surgical intervention may be necessary. Respiratory surgeries include chest tube insertion, lung transplantation, lung volume reduction surgery, thoracotomy, and tracheotomy.

Chest tube insertion

A chest tube may be required to help treat pneumothorax, hemothorax, empyema, pleural effusion, or chylothorax. Inserted into the pleural space, the tube allows blood, fluid, pus, or air to drain and allows the lung to reinflate. In pneumothorax, the tube restores negative pressure to the pleural space through an underwater-seal drainage system. The water in the system prevents air from being sucked back into the pleural space during inspiration. If a leak occurs through the bronchi and can't be sealed, suction applied to the underwater-seal system removes air from the pleural space faster than it can collect.

PATIENT PREPARATION

■ If time permits, the physician will obtain informed consent after explaining the procedure. Reassure the patient that chest tube insertion will help him breathe more easily.

■ Obtain baseline vital signs and give a sedative, as ordered.

■ Collect necessary equipment, including a thoracotomy tray and an underwater-seal drainage system. Prepare lidocaine (Xylocaine) for local anesthesia, as directed. The physician will clean the insertion site with povidone-iodine solution. Set up the underwater-seal drainage system according to the manufacturer's instructions and place it at the bedside, below the patient's chest level. Stabilize the unit to avoid knocking it over. (See *Closed chest-drainage system.*)

MONITORING AND AFTERCARE

■ When the patient's chest tube is stabilized, instruct him to take several deep breaths to inflate his lungs fully and help push pleural air out through the tube.

■ Obtain vital signs immediately after tube insertion and every 15 minutes thereafter, according to facility policy (usually for 1 hour).

■ Routinely assess chest tube function. Describe and record the amount of drainage on the intake and output sheet.

CLOSED CHEST-DRAINAGE SYSTEM

One-piece, disposable plastic drainage systems, such as the Pleur-evac (shown below), contain three chambers. The drainage chamber is on the right and has three calibrated columns that display the amount of drainage collected. When the first column fills, drainage carries over into the second and, when that fills, into the third. The water-seal chamber is located in the center. The suction-control chamber on the left is filled with water to achieve various suction levels. Rubber diaphragms are provided at the rear of the device to change the water level or remove samples of drainage. A positive-pressure relief valve at the top of the water-seal chamber vents excess pressure into the atmosphere, preventing pressure buildup.

PLEUR-EVAC

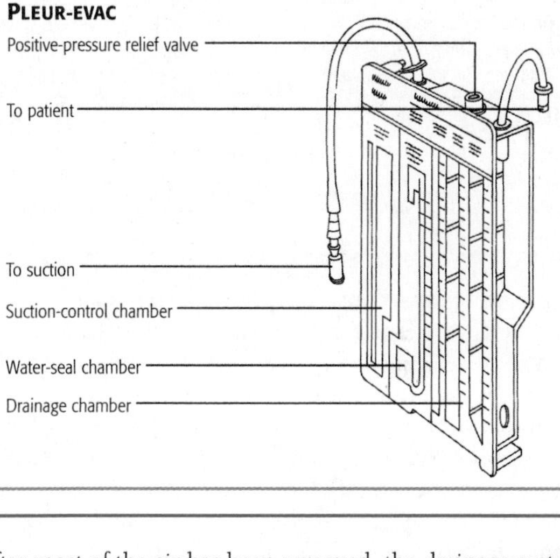

Positive-pressure relief valve

To patient

To suction

Suction-control chamber

Water-seal chamber

Drainage chamber

- After most of the air has been removed, the drainage system should bubble only during forced expiration unless the patient has a bronchopleural fistula. Constant bubbling in the system may indicate that a connection is loose or that the tube has advanced slightly out of the patient's chest. Promptly correct any loose connections to prevent complications.
- Change the dressing daily (or per facility policy) to clean the site and remove drainage.

COMBATING TENSION PNEUMOTHORAX

Tension pneumothorax—the entrapment of air within the pleural space—can be fatal without prompt treatment.

What causes it?
An obstructed or dislodged chest tube is a common cause of tension pneumothorax. Other causes include blunt chest trauma or high-pressure mechanical ventilation. In such cases, increased positive pressure within the patient's chest cavity compresses the affected lung and the mediastinum, shifting them toward the opposite lung. This impairs venous return and cardiac output and may cause the lung to collapse.

Telltale signs
Suspect tension pneumothorax if the patient develops dyspnea, chest pain, an irritating cough, vertigo, syncope, or anxiety after blunt chest trauma or if he has a chest tube in place. Is his skin cold, pale, and clammy? Are his respiratory and pulse rates unusually rapid? Does he have unequal bilateral chest expansion?

If you note these signs and symptoms, palpate the patient's neck, face, and chest wall for subcutaneous emphysema and palpate his trachea for deviation from midline. Auscultate the lungs for decreased or absent breath sounds on one side. Then percuss them for hyperresonance. If you suspect tension pneumothorax, immediately notify the physician and help identify the cause.

■ If the chest tube becomes dislodged, cover the opening immediately with petroleum gauze and apply pressure to prevent negative inspiratory pressure from sucking air into the chest. Call the physician and have an assistant collect equipment for tube reinsertion while you keep the opening closed. Reassure the patient and monitor him closely for signs of tension pneumothorax. (See *Combating tension pneumothorax*.)

■ The physician will remove the patient's chest tube after the lung is fully reexpanded. As soon as the tube is removed, apply an airtight, sterile petroleum dressing.

■ Typically, a patient is discharged with a chest tube only if it's used to drain a loculated empyema, which doesn't require an underwater-seal drainage system.

Lung transplantation
Lung transplantation involves the replacement of one or both lungs with a donor organ. Cystic fibrosis is the most common underlying disease that necessitates lung transplantation; others

include bronchopulmonary dysplasia, pulmonary hypertension, and pulmonary fibrosis.

In some cases, only one lobe may be involved in transplantation. Single-lung transplantation is considered for patients with end-stage chronic obstructive pulmonary disease. Typically, the patient has a life expectancy of less than 2 years. One-year survival rates after transplantation range from 75% to 85%, decreasing to 50% after 5 years.

To be a candidate for lung transplantation, a patient must:
- have a forced vital capacity of less than 40%
- have a forced expiratory volume of less than 30% of the predicted value
- have a partial pressure of arterial oxygen of less than 60 mm Hg on room air at rest
- exhibit evidence of major pulmonary complications
- demonstrate an increased antibiotic resistance.

Lung transplantation is contraindicated in cases of:
- active malignancy
- hepatitis C with positive biopsy for liver damage
- human immunodeficiency virus infection
- major organ dysfunction, especially involving the renal or cardiovascular system
- progressive neuromuscular disease.

Lung transplantation is performed under general anesthesia. Cardiopulmonary bypass is commonly used during the transplantation procedure. Bilateral anterior thoracotomy incisions and a transverse sternotomy provide access to the thoracic cavity. After removal of the patient's lungs, the donor lungs are implanted with anastomoses to the same areas as for single-lung transplantation.

The major complication after lung transplantation is organ rejection, which occurs because the recipient's body responds to the implanted tissue as a foreign body and triggers an immune response. This leads to fibrosis and scar formation. Another major complication after lung transplantation is infection due to immunosuppressive therapy. Other possible complications include hemorrhage and reperfusion edema.

Long-term complications (typically occurring after 3 years) include obliterative bronchiolitis and posttransplant lymphoproliferative disorder. Either may be fatal.

PATIENT PREPARATION

■ Provide care before and after transplant surgery.

■ Answer all questions about the transplant procedure and what the patient can expect. Explain postoperative care (intubation, for example), equipment used in the acute postoperative phase, and pain management.

■ Administer medications and obtain laboratory testing, as ordered.

MONITORING AND AFTERCARE

■ Assess cardiopulmonary status every 5 to 15 minutes in the immediate postoperative period, until the patient is stabilized. Be alert for a cardiac index of less than 2.2, hypotension, fever higher than 99.5° F (37.5° C), crackles or rhonchi, or decreased arterial oxygen saturation (SaO_2).

■ Assess respiratory status (breath sounds, effort, end-tidal carbon dioxide, and SaO_2) and ventilatory equipment frequently, and suction secretions as necessary. Expect frequent arterial blood gas (ABG) analyses and daily chest X-rays to evaluate the patient's readiness to wean from the ventilator.

■ Assess chest tube drainage for amount, color, and characteristics. Check for bleeding. Notify the physician according to the facility's and surgeon's parameters for abnormal drainage.

■ Closely monitor fluid intake and output. If the patient becomes hemodynamically unstable, administer fluids and vasoactive and inotropic drugs, as ordered, and titrate the dose to achieve the desired hemodynamic response.

■ After extubation, assess the patient often for shortness of breath, tachypnea, dyspnea, malaise, and increased sputum production; these symptoms suggest acute rejection.

■ After a single-lung transplantation, the newly implanted lung is denervated, but the patient's original lung continues to send messages to the brain indicating poor oxygenation. The patient may complain of shortness of breath and dyspnea even with SaO_2 levels of greater than 90%.

■ Maintain strict infection control precautions such as meticulous hand washing.

■ Inspect surgical dressings for bleeding in the early postoperative phase. Inspect the surgical incisions later for redness, swelling, and other signs of infection.

Lung volume reduction surgery

Lung volume reduction surgery is removal of the diseased portion of the lung to increase chest cavity space. The procedure can alter a flattened diaphragm to assume a normal shape, making the diaphragm function better. It results in improved shortness of breath, greater exercise tolerance, and better quality of life.

Lung volume reduction surgery can be performed through a unilateral or bilateral thoracoscopy, which is a minimally invasive technique that uses a videoscope placed through one of the incisions. A stapler and grasper are placed in the other incisions, and the diseased portions of the lungs are removed.

This procedure can also be performed using a bilateral sternotomy approach, in which an incision is made through the breast bone to expose the lungs. The lungs are then reduced at the same time. This is the most invasive technique and is only used when thoracoscopy isn't appropriate.

PATIENT PREPARATION

- Review with the patient the technique to be used and explain preprocedure and postprocedure nursing care.
- Verify that an appropriate consent form has been signed.
- Note and document patient allergies.
- Instruct the patient to fast for 6 to 12 hours before the procedure.
- Obtain vital signs and results of preprocedure studies; report abnormal findings.

MONITORING AND AFTERCARE

- Monitor the patient's vital signs, pulse oximetry, breath sounds, and intake and output.
- Maintain a patent airway and adequate oxygenation.
- Monitor patency and function of chest tubes, assess respiratory status and characteristics of sputum, measure drainage, and auscultate for crepitus and decreased breath sounds.
- Position the patient to promote chest expansion postoperatively.
- Observe the patient for bleeding.

■ Provide pulmonary rehabilitation, as ordered: suctioning, deep breathing, percussion, incentive spirometry, and respiratory treatments.

■ Check the follow-up chest X-ray for pneumothorax.

RED FLAG Immediately report subcutaneous crepitus around the patient's face, neck, or chest because it may indicate tracheal or bronchial perforation or pneumothorax.

Thoracotomy

A thoracotomy is the surgical removal of all or part of a lung. Its primary aim is to spare healthy lung tissue from disease. Lung excision may involve a pneumonectomy, lobectomy, segmental resection, or wedge resection.

A pneumonectomy is the excision of an entire lung; it's usually performed to treat bronchogenic carcinoma but may also be used to treat tuberculosis (TB), bronchiectasis, or a lung abscess. It's used only when a less radical approach can't remove all diseased tissue. Chest cavity pressures stabilize after a pneumonectomy and, over time, fluid enters the cavity where lung tissue was removed, preventing significant mediastinal shift.

A lobectomy is the removal of one of the five lung lobes; it's used to treat bronchogenic carcinoma, TB, a lung abscess, emphysematous blebs or bullae, benign tumors, or localized fungal infections. After a lobectomy, the remaining lobes expand to fill the entire pleural cavity.

A segmental resection is the removal of one or more lung segments; it preserves more functional tissue than lobectomy and is commonly used to treat bronchiectasis. A wedge resection is the removal of a small portion of the lung without regard to segments; it preserves the most functional tissue of all the surgeries but can treat only a small, well-circumscribed lesion. Remaining lung tissue must be reexpanded after both types of resection.

PATIENT PREPARATION

■ Explain the anticipated surgery to the patient and inform him that he'll receive a general anesthetic.

■ Inform the patient that postoperatively he may have chest tubes in place and may receive oxygen.

POST-THORACOTOMY HOME CARE

● Tell the patient to continue his coughing and deep-breathing exercises to prevent complications. Advise him to report changes in sputum characteristics to his physician.

● Instruct the patient to continue performing range-of-motion exercises to maintain mobility of his shoulder and chest wall.

● Tell the patient to avoid contact with people who have upper respiratory tract infections and to refrain from smoking.

● Provide instructions for wound care and dressing changes, as necessary.

▨ Teach him deep-breathing techniques, and explain that he'll perform these after surgery to help with lung reexpansion. Also teach him to use an incentive spirometer; record the volumes he achieves to provide a baseline.

MONITORING AND AFTERCARE

▨ After a pneumonectomy, the patient should lie only on the operative side or on his back until stabilized. This prevents fluid from draining into the unaffected lung if the sutured bronchus opens.

▨ Make sure the chest tube is functioning, if present, and observe for signs of tension pneumothorax.

▨ Provide pain management.

▨ Have the patient begin coughing and deep-breathing exercises as soon as his condition is stable. Auscultate his lungs, place him in semi-Fowler's position, and have him splint his incision to facilitate coughing and deep breathing.

▨ Perform passive range-of-motion (ROM) exercises the evening of surgery and two or three times daily thereafter. Progress to active ROM exercises.

▨ Provide discharge instructions for the patient going home after a thoracotomy. (See *Post-thoracotomy home care*.)

Tracheotomy

A tracheotomy provides an airway for an intubated patient who needs prolonged mechanical ventilation and facilitates removal of lower tracheobronchial secretions in a patient who can't clear

COMPARING TRACHEOSTOMY TUBES

Tracheostomy tubes are made of plastic or metal and come in uncuffed, cuffed, or fenestrated varieties. Tube selection depends on the patient's condition and the physician's preference. Make sure you're familiar with the advantages and disadvantages of these commonly used tracheostomy tubes.

Uncuffed
(plastic or metal)

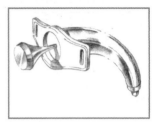

Advantages
● Free flow of air around tube and through larynx
● Reduced risk of tracheal damage
● Mechanical ventilation possible in patient with neuromuscular disease

Disadvantages
● Increased risk of aspiration in adults owing to lack of cuff
● Adapter possibly needed for ventilation

Plastic cuffed
(low pressure and high volume)

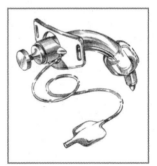

Advantages
● Disposable
● Cuff bonded to tube (won't detach accidentally inside trachea)
● Low cuff pressure that's evenly distributed against tracheal wall (no need to deflate periodically to lower pressure)
● Reduced risk of tracheal damage

Disadvantages
● Possibly more expensive than other tubes

COMPARING TRACHEOSTOMY TUBES *(continued)*

Fenestrated

Advantages
● Speech possible through upper airway when external opening is capped and cuff is deflated
● Breathing by mechanical ventilation possible with inner cannula in place and cuff inflated
● Easy removal of inner cannula for cleaning

Disadvantages
● Possible occlusion of fenestration
● Possible dislodgment of inner cannula
● Cap removal necessary before inflating cuff

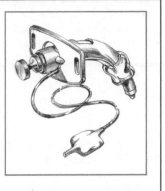

them. It's also performed in emergencies when endotracheal intubation isn't possible, to prevent an unconscious or paralyzed patient from aspirating food or secretions, and to bypass upper airway obstruction resulting from trauma, burns, epiglottiditis, or a tumor.

After the physician creates the surgical opening, he inserts a tracheostomy tube to permit access to the airway. He may select from several tube styles, depending on the patient's condition and needs. (See *Comparing tracheostomy tubes*.)

PATIENT PREPARATION

■ For an emergency tracheotomy, briefly explain the procedure to the patient as time permits and quickly obtain supplies or a tracheotomy tray.

■ For a scheduled tracheotomy, explain the procedure and the need for general anesthesia to the patient and his family. If possible, mention whether the tracheostomy will be temporary or permanent.

- Set up a communication system with the patient (letter board or flash cards), and practice it with him to make sure he'll be able to communicate comfortably while his speech is limited.
- Introduce a patient requiring a long-term or permanent tracheostomy to someone who has experienced the procedure and has adjusted well to tracheostomy care.
- Make sure that samples for ABG analysis and other diagnostic tests have been collected and that the patient or a responsible family member has signed a consent form.

MONITORING AND AFTERCARE

- Auscultate breath sounds every 2 hours after the procedure. Note crackles, rhonchi, or diminished breath sounds.
- Turn the patient every 2 hours to avoid pooling of tracheal secretions. As ordered, provide chest physiotherapy to help mobilize secretions, and note their quantity, consistency, color, and odor.
- Replace humidity lost in bypassing the nose, mouth, and upper airway mucosa to reduce the drying effects of oxygen on mucous membranes. Humidification will also help to thin secretions. Oxygen given through a T-piece or tracheostomy mask should be connected to a nebulizer or heated cascade humidifier.
- Monitor ABG results and compare them with baseline values to check adequacy of oxygenation and carbon dioxide removal. Also monitor the patient's oximetry values, as ordered.
- Suction the tracheostomy using sterile technique to remove excess secretions when necessary. Avoid suctioning a patient for longer than 10 seconds at a time to prevent hypoxia or trauma. Discontinue the procedure if the patient develops respiratory distress.
- Make sure the tracheostomy ties are secure but not too tight. To prevent accidental tube dislodgment or expulsion, avoid changing the ties until the stoma track is stable. Report any tube pulsation to the physician; this may indicate the tube is close to the innominate artery, which predisposes the patient to hemorrhage.
- Change the tracheostomy dressing when soiled or once per shift, using aseptic technique, and check the color, odor,

amount, and type of drainage. Also check for swelling, crepitus, erythema, and bleeding at the site and report excessive bleeding or unusual drainage immediately. Wear goggles, gloves, and mask when changing tracheostomy tubes.

■ Keep a sterile tracheostomy tube (with obturator) at the patient's bedside and be prepared to replace an expelled or contaminated tube. Also keep available a sterile tracheostomy tube (with obturator) that's one size smaller than the tube currently being used. The smaller tube may be necessary if the trachea begins to close after tube expulsion, making insertion of the same size tube difficult.

MISCELLANEOUS TREATMENTS

Other miscellaneous treatments include chest physiotherapy, mucus-clearing devices, extracorporeal membrane oxygenation (ECMO), and prone positioning.

Chest physiotherapy

Chest physiotherapy is usually performed with other treatments, such as suctioning, incentive spirometry, and administration of such medications as small-volume nebulizer aerosol treatments and expectorants. (See *Postural drainage positions,* pages 162 to 164.) Recent studies indicate that percussion vibration isn't an effective treatment of most diseases; exceptions include cystic fibrosis and bronchiectasis. Improved breath sounds, increased partial pressure of arterial oxygen (PaO_2), sputum production, and improved airflow suggest successful treatment.

PATIENT PREPARATION

■ If the patient is in pain or is preoperative, administer pain medication before the treatment, as ordered, and teach the patient to splint his incision.

■ Auscultate the lungs to determine baseline status, and check the physician's order to determine which lung areas require treatment.

■ Obtain pillows and a tilt board if necessary.

(Text continues on page 165.)

POSTURAL DRAINAGE POSITIONS

The following illustrations show the various postural drainage positions and the areas of the lungs affected by each.

Lower lobes: Posterior basal segments

Elevate the foot of the bed 30 degrees. Have the patient lie prone with his head lowered. Position pillows under his chest and abdomen. Percuss his lower ribs on both sides of his spine.

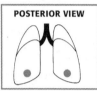

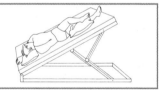

Lower lobes: Lateral basal segments

Elevate the foot of the bed 30 degrees. Instruct the patient to lie on his abdomen with his head lowered and his upper leg flexed over a pillow for support. Then have him rotate a quarter turn upward. Percuss his lower ribs on the uppermost portion of his lateral chest wall.

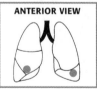

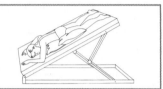

Lower lobes: Anterior basal segments

Elevate the foot of the bed 30 degrees. Instruct the patient to lie on his side with his head lowered. Then place pillows as shown. Percuss with a slightly cupped hand over his lower ribs just beneath the axilla. If an acutely ill patient has trouble breathing in this position, adjust the bed to an angle he can tolerate. Then begin percussion.

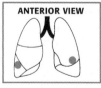

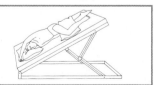

POSTURAL DRAINAGE POSITIONS *(continued)*

Lower lobes: Superior segments

With the bed flat, have the patient lie on his abdomen. Place two pillows under his hips. Percuss on both sides of his spine at the lower tips of his scapulae.

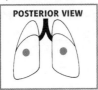
POSTERIOR VIEW

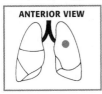

Right middle lobe: Medial and lateral segments

Elevate the foot of the bed 15 degrees. Have the patient lie on his left side with his head down and his knees flexed. Then have him rotate a quarter turn backward. Place a pillow beneath him. Percuss with your hand moderately cupped over the right nipple. For a woman, cup your hand so that its heel is under the armpit and your fingers extend forward beneath the breast.

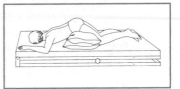
ANTERIOR VIEW

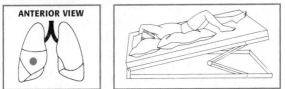

Left upper lobe: Superior and inferior segments, lingular portion

Elevate the foot of the bed 15 degrees. Have the patient lie on his right side with his head down and knees flexed. Then have him rotate a quarter turn backward. Place a pillow behind him, from shoulders to hips. Percuss with your hand moderately cupped over his left nipple. For a woman, cup your hand so that its heel is beneath the armpit and your fingers extend forward beneath the breast.

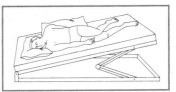
ANTERIOR VIEW

(continued)

POSTURAL DRAINAGE POSITIONS *(continued)*

Upper lobes: Anterior segments

Make sure that the bed is flat. Have the patient lie on his back with a pillow folded under his knees. Then have him rotate slightly away from the side being drained. Percuss between his clavicle and nipple.

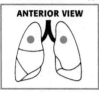
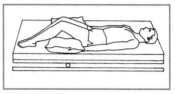

Upper lobes: Apical segments

Keep the bed flat. Have the patient lean back at a 30-degree angle against you and a pillow. Percuss with a cupped hand between his clavicles and the top of each scapula.

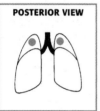
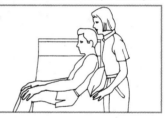

Upper lobes: Posterior segments

Keep the bed flat. Have the patient lean over a pillow at a 30-degree angle. Percuss and clap his upper back on each side.

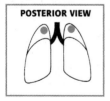
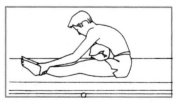

- Don't schedule therapy immediately after a meal; wait 2 to 3 hours to reduce the risk of nausea and vomiting.
- Make sure the patient is adequately hydrated to facilitate removal of secretions.
- If ordered, give bronchodilator and mist therapies before the treatment.
- Provide tissues, an emesis basin, and a cup for sputum.
- Set up suction equipment if the patient doesn't have an adequate cough to clear secretions.
- If he needs oxygen therapy or is borderline hypoxemic without it, provide adequate flow rates of oxygen during therapy. (See *Performing percussion and vibration,* page 166.)

MONITORING AND AFTERCARE
- Evaluate the patient's tolerance of the therapy and make adjustments as needed. Watch for fatigue and remember that the patient's ability to cough and breathe deeply lessens as he tires.
- Assess for difficulty expectorating secretions. Use suction if the patient has an ineffective cough or a diminished gag reflex.
- Provide oral hygiene after therapy; secretions may taste foul or have an unpleasant odor.
- Be aware that postural drainage positions can cause nausea, dizziness, dyspnea, and hypoxemia.
- The patient with chronic bronchitis, bronchiectasis, or cystic fibrosis may need chest physiotherapy at home.

Mucus-clearing devices

Patients with chronic respiratory disorders, such as cystic fibrosis, bronchitis, and bronchiectasis, require therapy to mobilize and remove mucus secretions from the lungs. A handheld mucus clearance device, also known as *the flutter,* can help such patients cough up secretions more easily. This device is basically a ball valve that vibrates as the patient exhales vigorously through it. The vibrations propagate throughout the airways during expiration, thereby loosening mucus. As the patient repeats this process, mucus progressively moves up the airways until it can be coughed out easily. A licensed practitioner should determine

PERFORMING PERCUSSION AND VIBRATION

To perform percussion, instruct the patient to breathe slowly and deeply, using the diaphragm, to promote relaxation. Cup your hands, with fingers flexed and thumbs pressed tightly against your index fingers. Percuss each segment for 1 to 2 minutes by alternating your hands against the patient in a rhythmic manner. Listen for a hollow sound on percussion to verify correct performance of the technique.

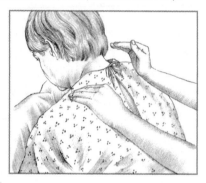

To perform vibration, ask the patient to inhale deeply and then exhale slowly through pursed lips. During exhalation, firmly press your fingers and the palms of your hands against the chest wall. Tense the muscles of your arms and shoulders in an isometric contraction to send fine vibrations through the chest wall. Vibrate during five exhalations over each chest segment.

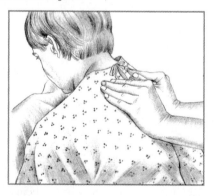

FLUTTER VALVE DEVICE

When the patient exhales through the flutter valve device, positive expiratory pressure and high-frequency oscillations help move mucus.

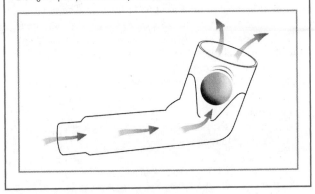

the frequency and duration with which this device can be used. (See *Flutter valve device*.)

PATIENT PREPARATION

- Explain the procedure to the patient. Tell him that this device will help move mucus through his airways so that he can eventually expectorate it.
- Tell the patient to hold the device so that the stem is parallel to the floor.
- Tell the patient to keep his cheeks as flat and hard as possible while exhaling. Suggest that he hold his cheeks lightly with his other hand.

MONITORING AND AFTERCARE

- To help the patient achieve the best fluttering effect, you may need to place one hand on his back and the other on his chest as he exhales through the device. If he's achieving the maximum effect, you'll feel the vibrations in his lungs as he exhales. If results are unsatisfactory at first, tell the patient to adjust the angle at which he's holding the device until optimal fluttering occurs.

- If the patient's final cough doesn't seem to work, he can try repeated, controlled, short, rapid exhalations ("huffing"), as though he were trying to cough a bread crumb out of his throat, to aid mucus removal.
- Make sure the patient cleans the device after each use to remove mucus from the internal components. Instruct him to clean it more thoroughly every 2 days. All parts should be washed in a solution of mild soap or detergent. Tell him not to use bleach or other chlorine-containing products. After thorough cleaning, all parts should be rinsed under a stream of hot tap water, wiped with a clean towel, and reassembled and stored in a clean, dry place.
- Auscultate for the patient's breath sounds to determine the effectiveness of his coughing.

Extracorporeal membrane oxygenation

ECMO, one of a group of supportive therapies called *extracorporeal life support,* involves the oxygenation of blood outside the body. It exposes a patient's lungs to low pressures as well as providing a means for oxygen delivery and carbon dioxide removal. When ECMO is used, lower fraction of inspired oxygen (FIO_2) concentrations and volumes can be delivered via mechanical ventilation, thereby reducing the risk of oxygen toxicity and barotrauma; however, it doesn't cure the underlying disease. Historically, ECMO was used to treat neonates who experienced severe respiratory distress. Today, ECMO is used to treat severe acute respiratory failure in neonates and adults. (See *ECMO in neonates.*)

Although the primary indication for using ECMO is severe respiratory failure, it may also be indicated in other situations, such as:

- acute respiratory distress syndrome (ARDS)
- a bridge to transplantation
- perioperative cardiac failure
- primary myocardial failure.

There are two basic types of ECMO: veno-arterial ECMO (VA-ECMO) and veno-venous ECMO (VV-ECMO).

AGE AWARE

ECMO IN NEONATES

In neonates, extracorporeal membrane oxygenation (ECMO) is considered the standard treatment for severe respiratory distress. However, in adults, ECMO is used only after other modes of ventilation have been used without success. These modes include:

● low tidal volume ventilation and high-level, positive end-expiratory pressure to facilitate mechanical ventilation

● pharmacologic therapy, such as neuromuscular blocking agents, sedatives, and opioids, to minimize oxygen consumption.

VA-ECMO, the standard type used for neonates, involves the insertion of a catheter into the internal jugular or femoral vein for blood removal. Blood is returned to the patient and arterial circulation via the carotid or femoral artery. This type of ECMO provides partial to complete cardiopulmonary bypass and is used most commonly when the patient has severe cardiac failure in addition to pulmonary failure. Unfortunately, this type of ECMO increases the risk of air being directly introduced into the arterial circulation, causing emboli. In addition, neurologic complications can occur with ligation of the carotid artery when therapy is stopped.

VV-ECMO involves the insertion of a catheter to remove and return blood to the right atrium via the right internal jugular or femoral vein. Usually, a double-lumen catheter is used. This type of ECMO is used for patients requiring only respiratory support such as for ARDS. It doesn't provide cardiac support to assist systemic circulation. Pulmonary blood flow is maintained, and the lungs are perfused with oxygenated blood.

As blood leaves the patient's body, it's pumped through a membrane oxygenator, which acts as an artificial lung, supplying oxygen to the blood. (See *ECMO setup*, page 170.)

The circuit also has numerous safety and pressure monitors located throughout. A roller pump regulates the blood flow to the oxygenator, turning off whenever the pump flow is greater than blood return to the patient. In this way, excessive pressure on the right atrium or major vessels is averted. The pump automatically restarts when the flow rate balances.

ECMO SETUP

Extracorporeal membrane oxygenation (ECMO) is managed by either a critical care nurse or respiratory therapist with special training in its operation. Illustrated below and described here is a typical ECMO setup:

● The *arterial filter* removes air bubbles and clots from the blood as it travels through the ECMO circuit.

● The *cannula* is a catheter through which blood travels to and from the patient.

● The *control desk module* continuously monitors pressure throughout the circuit and regulates blood flow as needed in response to changing pressures in the system.

● The *heater* generates heat needed to keep blood at a constant temperature.

● The *heat exchanger* uses heat generated by a heater to maintain the temperature of the blood as it's oxygenated.

● The *hemochron* monitors blood clotting.

● The *I.V. pump* allows injection of medications, such as antibiotics, into the cannula of the ECMO circuit.

● The *membrane oxygenator* serves as the artificial lung supplying oxygen to the blood.

● The *transonic blood flowmeter* measures the amount of blood flowing through the cannula at various places along the ECMO circuit.

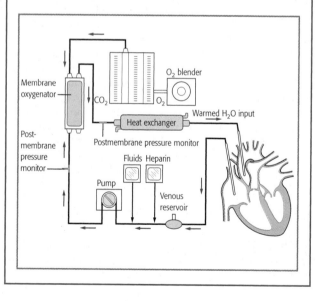

PATIENT PREPARATION

■ Instruct the patient and his family about the procedure and the rationale for treatment.

■ Also discuss the use of other equipment, such as continuous cardiac monitoring, nasogastric tube, indwelling urinary catheter and, possibly, a pulmonary artery catheter.

MONITORING AND AFTERCARE

■ Assess cardiopulmonary and hemodynamic status closely, including central venous pressure, pulmonary artery pressure, and cardiac output, at least every 15 minutes in the hour immediately after the procedure and then hourly or more frequently as indicated by the patient's condition or facility's policy.

■ Assess the endotracheal (ET) tube and mechanical ventilation.

■ Monitor oxygen saturation levels and arterial blood gas (ABG) values as ordered. Suction as necessary.

■ After ECMO is initiated and the patient's gas exchange shows signs of improvement, expect to lower ventilator settings.

■ Be alert to changes in tidal volume, which should increase as the lungs improve.

■ Perform chest physiotherapy, as needed.

■ Change the patient's position frequently. Anticipate placing the patient with ARDS in the prone position, which helps to improve oxygenation.

■ Administer sedatives and analgesia, as ordered, to ease the patient's tolerance of the procedure, maximize oxygen delivery, provide for patient comfort, and decrease the risk of catheter dislodgment. If necessary, apply soft restraints, as ordered, to reduce the risk of the patient touching the catheter.

■ Monitor intake and output at least hourly and assess daily weight.

■ Monitor blood urea nitrogen and serum creatinine levels closely for renal dysfunction (a complication of ECMO).

■ Assess for signs and symptoms of acute renal failure.

■ Monitor clotting times, as indicated, and assist with adjustments to heparin infusion.

■ Obtain hemoglobin level, hematocrit, and platelet count every 4 hours and as needed. Expect to give blood transfusions.

- Inspect ECMO catheter insertion sites for oozing or hematoma. Observe ECMO catheter insertion sites hourly; change dressings as needed to keep the site clean and dry. If needed, weigh saturated dressings to determine fluid volume loss.
- Assess the patient's neurologic status frequently, at least every 2 hours.
- Assess the affected extremity distal to the ECMO catheter insertion site for pulses, color, and temperature at least every 2 hours to prevent ischemia.
- Throughout the patient's care, explain all procedures and treatments, even if he's sedated. Offer emotional support to the patient's family; encourage them to visit and interact with the patient.

Prone positioning

Prone positioning is a therapeutic maneuver to improve oxygenation and pulmonary mechanics in patients with acute lung injury or ARDS. Also known as *proning,* prone positioning involves physically turning a patient face down from his back (supine position). This positioning improves oxygenation by shifting blood flow to regions of the lung that are less severely injured and better aerated.

The criteria for prone positioning frequently include:
- acute onset of respiratory signs and symptoms
- hypoxemia; specifically, a PaO_2/FIO_2 ratio of 300 or less for acute lung injury and a PaO_2/FIO_2 ratio of 200 or less for ARDS
- no evidence of left atrial hypertension
- radiologic evidence of diffuse bilateral pulmonary infiltrates.

With the appropriate equipment, prone positioning may also facilitate better movement of the diaphragm by allowing the abdomen to expand more fully. It's usually performed for 6 or more hours per day, for as long as 10 days, until the requirement for a high concentration of inspired oxygen resolves. Patients who respond to prone positioning by an increase in the PaO_2/FIO_2 ratio of more than 20 or PaO_2 greater than 20% within 2 hours of being turned from supine to prone are classified as responders to prone positioning.

Prone positioning is indicated to support mechanically ventilated patients with ARDS who require high concentrations of inspired oxygen. It also corrects severe hypoxemia and maintains adequate oxygenation (PaO_2 greater than 60%) in patients with acute lung injury, while avoiding ventilator-induced lung injury.

Prone positioning is contraindicated in patients whose heads can't be supported in a face-down position or those who can't tolerate a head-down position. Hemodynamically unstable patients (systolic blood pressure less than 90 mm Hg) despite aggressive fluid resuscitation and vasopressors shouldn't be placed in the prone position. It's also contraindicated in patients who are extremely obese (typically, more than 300 lb [136 kg]); in patients with cerebral hypertension unresponsive to therapy, unstable bone fractures, or left-sided heart failure (nonpulmonary respiratory failure); and in patients with an active intra-abdominal process.

PATIENT PREPARATION

- Assess the patient's hemodynamic status to determine if he can tolerate the prone position.
- Assess the patient's mental status before prone positioning. Although agitation isn't a contraindication for prone positioning, it must be effectively managed.
- Determine whether the patient's size and weight will allow turning him on a generally narrow critical care bed.
- Explain the purpose and procedure of prone positioning to the patient and his family.
- Remove anterior chest wall electrocardiogram monitoring leads, but make sure the patient's cardiac rate and rhythm can be monitored. These leads are repositioned onto the patient's back after he's prone.
- Provide eye care, if indicated, including lubrication and horizontal taping of eyelids.
- Make sure that the patient's tongue stays inside his mouth; if the tongue is edematous or protruding, insert a bite block.
- Secure the patient's ET or tracheostomy tube to prevent dislodgment.

▓ Make sure that the brake of the bed is engaged. Attach the surface of the prone positioner to the bed frame, as recommended by the manufacturer.

▓ Position staff appropriately while positioning the patient; a minimum of three people is required: one on either side of the bed and one at the head of the bed.

▓ Adjust all patient tubing and invasive monitoring lines to prevent dislodgement, kinking, disconnection, or contact with the patient's body during the turning procedure and while the patient remains in the prone pelvic piece of the device so that it rests ½″ (1.3 cm) above the iliac crest.

MONITORING AND AFTERCARE

▓ Monitor the patient's response to prone positioning through his vital signs, pulse oximetry, and mixed venous oxygen saturation. During the initial prone positioning, obtain ABG analysis within ½ hour of the procedure and within ½ hour before returning the patient to the supine position.

▓ Reposition the patient's head hourly while he's prone to prevent facial breakdown. As one person lifts the patient's head, the second person moves the headpieces to provide head support in a different position.

▓ Provide range-of-motion exercises to the patient's arms and legs every 2 hours.

▓ Prone positioning should be stopped when the patient no longer demonstrates improved oxygenation with the position change.

Infection and inflammation

Infectious and inflammatory disorders of the respiratory tract include bronchiectasis, croup, epiglottiditis, pharyngitis, pleural effusion and empyema, pleurisy, pneumonia, severe acute respiratory syndrome, sinusitis, tonsillitis, and tuberculosis.

BRONCHIECTASIS

Bronchiectasis is characterized by chronic abnormal dilation of the bronchi and destruction of the bronchial walls. It can occur throughout the tracheobronchial tree or be confined to one segment or lobe. It's usually bilateral and involves the basilar segments of the lower lobes.

The disease has three forms: cylindrical (fusiform), varicose, and saccular (cystic). It affects people of both sexes and all ages. With antibiotics available to treat acute respiratory tract infections, the incidence of bronchiectasis has dramatically decreased during the past 20 years. Its incidence is highest among Inuit populations in the Northern Hemisphere and the Maoris of New Zealand. Bronchiectasis is irreversible. (See *Forms of bronchiectasis,* page 176.)

Pathophysiology

Bronchiectasis results from conditions associated with repeated damage to bronchial walls and with abnormal mucociliary clearance, which causes a breakdown of supporting tissue adjacent to the airways. Such conditions include:

- complications of measles, pneumonia, pertussis, or influenza

FORMS OF BRONCHIECTASIS

The different forms of bronchiectasis may occur separately or simultaneously:
● In *cylindrical bronchiectasis,* the bronchi expand unevenly, with little change in diameter, and end suddenly in a squared-off fashion.
● In *varicose bronchiectasis,* abnormal, irregular dilation and narrowing of the bronchi give the appearance of varicose veins.
● In *saccular bronchiectasis,* many large dilations end in sacs. These sacs balloon into pus-filled cavities as they approach the periphery and are then called *saccules.*

- congenital anomalies (rare), such as bronchomalacia, congenital bronchiectasis, and Kartagener's syndrome (bronchiectasis, sinusitis, and dextrocardia), and various rare disorders such as immotile cilia syndrome
- immune disorders (agammaglobulinemia, for example)
- inhalation of corrosive gas or repeated aspiration of gastric juices
- cystic fibrosis
- obstruction (by a foreign body, tumor, or stenosis) with recurrent infection
- recurrent, inadequately treated bacterial respiratory tract infections such as tuberculosis.

In bronchiectasis, hyperplastic squamous epithelia denuded of cilia replace ulcerated columnar epithelia. Abscess formation occurs, involving all layers of the bronchial walls. This produces inflammatory cells and fibrous tissues. The result is both dilation and narrowing of the airways. Sputum stagnates in the dilated bronchi and leads to secondary infection, characterized by inflammation and leukocytic accumulations. Additional debris collects in and occludes the bronchi. Building pressure from the retained secretions induces mucosal injury. Extensive vascular proliferation of bronchial circulation occurs and produces frequent hemoptysis.

Complications
- Amyloidosis
- Chronic malnutrition

- Cor pulmonale
- Right-sided heart failure

Assessment findings

- The patient may complain of frequent bouts of pneumonia; a history of coughing up blood or blood-tinged sputum; a chronic cough that produces copious, foul-smelling, mucopurulent secretions (up to several cups daily); dyspnea; weight loss; and malaise.
- Inspection of the patient's sputum may show a cloudy top layer, a central layer of clear saliva, and a heavy, thick, purulent bottom layer.
- In advanced disease, the patient may have clubbed fingers and toes and cyanotic nail beds.
- If the patient also has a complicating condition, such as pneumonia or atelectasis, percussion may detect dullness over lung fields.
- Auscultation may reveal coarse crackles during inspiration over involved lobes or segments and, occasionally, wheezes.
- With complicating atelectasis or pneumonia, you may hear diminished breath sounds during auscultation.

Diagnostic test results

- Bronchography identifies the location and extent of disease.
- Bronchoscopy helps to identify the source of secretions or the bleeding site in hemoptysis.
- Chest X-rays show peribronchial thickening, atelectatic areas, and scattered cystic changes that suggest bronchiectasis.
- Complete blood count can reveal anemia and leukocytosis.
- Computed tomography scan reveals anatomic changes.
- Pulmonary function tests detect decreased vital capacity, expiratory flow, and hypoxemia; these tests also help evaluate disease severity, therapeutic effectiveness, and the patient's suitability for surgery.
- Sputum culture and Gram stain identify predominant pathogens.
- Sweat electrolyte tests may reveal cystic fibrosis.

Treatment

Antibiotic therapy (oral or I.V.) for 7 to 10 days—or until sputum production decreases—is the principal treatment. Bronchodilators and postural drainage and chest percussion help remove secretions if the patient has bronchospasm and thick, tenacious sputum. Occasionally, bronchoscopy may be used to remove secretions. Oxygen therapy may be used for hypoxia. Segmental resection, bronchial artery embolization, or lobectomy may be necessary if pulmonary function is poor.

The only cure for bronchiectasis is surgical removal of the affected lung portion. However, the patient with bronchiectasis affecting both lungs probably won't benefit from surgery.

Nursing interventions

- Provide supportive care, and help the patient adjust to the lifestyle changes that irreversible lung damage causes.
- Give antibiotics, as ordered, and record the patient's response.
- Give oxygen, as needed, and assess gas exchange by monitoring arterial blood gas values, as ordered.
- Perform chest physiotherapy, including postural drainage and chest percussion for involved lobes, several times per day, especially in the early morning and before bedtime.
- Provide a warm, quiet, comfortable environment. Also, help the patient to alternate rest and activity periods.
- Provide well-balanced, high-calorie meals for the patient. Offer small, frequent meals to prevent fatigue.
- Make sure the patient receives adequate hydration to help thin secretions and promote easier removal.
- Give frequent mouth care to remove foul-smelling sputum. Provide the patient with tissues and a waxed bag for disposal of the contaminated tissues.
- Watch for developing complications, such as right-sided heart failure and cor pulmonale.
- After surgery, give meticulous postoperative care. Monitor vital signs, encourage deep breathing and position changes every 2 hours, and provide chest tube care. (See *Bronchiectasis teaching topics.*)

BRONCHIECTASIS TEACHING TOPICS

● Show family members how to perform postural drainage and percussion. Also, teach the patient coughing and deep-breathing exercises to promote good ventilation and assist in secretion removal. Instruct him to maintain each postural drainage position for 10 minutes. Then direct the caregiver in performing percussion and instructing the patient to cough.

● Advise the patient to stop smoking because it stimulates secretions and irritates the airways. Refer the patient to a local smoking-cessation group.

● Instruct the patient to avoid air pollutants and people with known upper respiratory tract infections.

● Direct the patient to take medications (especially antibiotics) exactly as ordered. Make sure he knows the adverse effects associated with his medications. Instruct him to notify the physician if any of these effects occur.

● Teach the patient to dispose of all secretions properly to avoid spreading the infection to others. Advise him to wash his hands thoroughly after disposing of contaminated tissues.

● Urge the patient to keep up-to-date in his immunization schedule to prevent childhood diseases.

● Encourage the patient to rest as much as possible.

● Discuss dietary measures. Encourage the patient to follow a balanced, high-protein diet. Suggest that he eat small, frequent meals. Explain that milk products may increase the viscosity of secretions.

● Encourage the patient to drink plenty of fluids to thin secretions and aid expectoration.

● If the patient needs surgery, offer complete preoperative and postoperative instructions. Forewarn him if he is to have an I.V. line and chest tubes. Explain the reason for these procedures.

● Tell the patient to seek prompt attention for respiratory infections.

● Tell the patient to avoid air pollutants and people with upper respiratory tract infections. Instruct him to take medications (especially antibiotics) exactly as prescribed.

CROUP

Croup is a severe inflammation and obstruction of the upper airway. This childhood disease affects boys more than girls. The barking cough of croup results from soft tissue collapsing in the airway and then being forced open. Older children develop rings of cartilage that prevent the collapse.

Croup usually occurs in the winter as acute laryngotracheobronchitis (the most common form), laryngitis, or acute spasmodic laryngitis. It must be distinguished from epiglottiditis.

Usually mild and self-limiting, acute laryngotracheobronchitis appears mostly in children ages 3 months to 3 years. Acute spasmodic laryngitis affects children ages 1 to 3, particularly those with allergies and a family history of croup. Overall, up to 15% of patients have a family history of croup. Recovery is usually complete.

Pathophysiology
Croup usually results from a viral infection. Parainfluenza viruses cause about two-thirds of such infections; adenoviruses, respiratory syncytial virus (RSV), influenza viruses, measles viruses, and bacteria (pertussis and diphtheria) account for the rest.

Complications
- Airway obstruction
- Dehydration
- Ear infection
- Pneumonia
- Respiratory failure

Assessment findings
- Typically, the child or his parents report a recent upper respiratory tract infection preceding croup.
- On inspection, you may observe the use of accessory muscles with nasal flaring during breathing.
- You typically hear the child's sharp, barklike cough and hoarse or muffled vocal sounds.
- As croup progresses, the patient may display further upper airway obstruction with severely compromised ventilation. (See *How croup affects the upper airway.*)
- Auscultation may disclose inspiratory stridor and diminished breath sounds. These signs and symptoms may last for only a few hours, or they may persist for 1 to 2 days.

LARYNGOTRACHEOBRONCHITIS
- The patient may complain of fever and breathing problems that occur more often at night. Typically, the child becomes frightened because he can't exhale (because inflammation causes edema in the bronchi and bronchioles).

HOW CROUP AFFECTS THE UPPER AIRWAY

In croup, inflammatory swelling and spasms constrict the larynx, thereby reducing airflow. This cross-sectional drawing (from chin to chest) shows the upper airway changes caused by croup. Inflammatory changes almost completely obstruct the larynx (which includes the epiglottis) and significantly narrow the trachea.

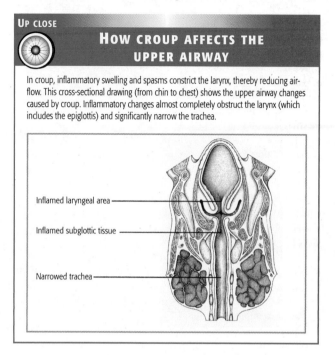

Inflamed laryngeal area

Inflamed subglottic tissue

Narrowed trachea

- During auscultation, you may hear diffusely decreased breath sounds, expiratory rhonchi, and scattered crackles.

LARYNGITIS
- The patient usually reports mild signs and symptoms and no respiratory distress. If the patient is an infant, however, some respiratory distress may occur.
- In children, the history may include such signs and symptoms as a sore throat and cough that, rarely, may progress to marked hoarseness.
- Inspection may disclose suprasternal and intercostal retractions, inspiratory stridor, dyspnea, diminished breath sounds, restlessness and, in later stages, severe dyspnea and exhaustion.

ACUTE SPASMODIC LARYNGITIS

■ The patient history may reveal mild to moderate hoarseness and nasal discharge, followed by the characteristic cough and noisy inspiration that typically awaken the child at night.

■ The child may become anxious, which leads to increasing dyspnea and transient cyanosis.

■ Inspection may disclose labored breathing with retractions and clammy skin.

■ Palpation may reveal a rapid pulse rate. These severe signs diminish after several hours but reappear in a milder form on the next one or two nights.

Diagnostic test results

■ Blood cultures can distinguish bacterial from viral infections.

■ Laryngoscopy may reveal inflammation and obstruction in epiglottal and laryngeal areas.

■ Throat cultures can rule out diphtheria.

■ Throat cultures can also identify infecting organisms and their sensitivity to antibiotics when bacterial infection is the cause.

■ X-rays of the neck may show upper airway narrowing and edema in subglottic folds.

Treatment

For most children with croup, home care with rest, cool humidification during sleep, and antipyretic drugs such as acetaminophen (Tylenol) relieve signs and symptoms. However, respiratory distress that interferes with oral hydration usually requires hospitalization and parenteral fluid replacement to prevent dehydration. If the patient has croup from a bacterial infection, he needs antibiotic therapy. Oxygen therapy may also be required.

For moderately severe croup, aerosolized racemic epinephrine may temporarily reduce airway swelling. Intubation is performed only if other means of preventing respiratory failure are unsuccessful.

Corticosteroids reduce subglottic edema and inflammation. Dexamethasone (Decadron) given in a single dose early in the course of croup allows a shorter hospital stay and reduces cough, dyspnea and, commonly, the need for intubation.

Nursing interventions

- Monitor cough and breath sounds, hoarseness, severity of retractions, inspiratory stridor, cyanosis, respiratory rate and character (especially prolonged and labored respirations), restlessness, fever, and heart rate.

- Keep the child as quiet as possible but avoid sedation, which may depress respiration. If the patient is an infant, position him in an infant seat or prop him up with a pillow; place an older child in Fowler's position. If an older child requires a cool-mist tent to help him breathe, describe it to him and his parents and explain why it's needed.

- Change bed linens as necessary to keep the patient dry.

- Control the patient's energy output and oxygen demand by providing age-appropriate diversional activities to keep him quietly occupied.

- If possible, isolate patients suspected of having RSV and parainfluenza infections. Wash your hands carefully before leaving the room to avoid transmitting germs to other patients, particularly infants.

- Control fever with sponge baths and antipyretics. Keep a hypothermia blanket on hand if the patient's temperature rises above 102° F (38.9° C). Watch for seizures in infants and young children with high fevers. Give I.V. antibiotics as ordered.

- Relieve sore throat with soothing, water-based ices, such as fruit sherbet and ice pops. Avoid thicker, milk-based fluids if the patient has thick mucus or swallowing difficulties. Apply petroleum jelly or another ointment around the nose and lips to decrease irritation from nasal discharge and mouth breathing.

- Institute measures to prevent the patient's crying, which increases respiratory distress. As necessary, adapt treatment to conserve the patient's energy and to include parents, who can provide reassurance.

- Reassure the parents that they made the right decision by bringing their child to the emergency department, especially at night when the night air may improve the child's breathing significantly, leaving the parents wondering if they overreacted.

CROUP TEACHING TOPICS

Because this disease primarily affects young children, patient teaching usually centers on the parents.

● Warn parents that ear infections and pneumonia may complicate croup. These disorders may follow croup about 5 days after recovery. Urge the parents to seek immediate medical attention if the patient has an earache, productive cough, high fever, or increased shortness of breath.

● Teach the parents effective home care. Suggest the use of a cool humidifier (vaporizer). To relieve croupy spells, tell parents to carry the child into the bathroom, shut the door, and turn on the hot water. Breathing in warm, moist air quickly eases an acute spell of croup.

■ Watch for signs of complete airway obstruction, such as increased heart and respiratory rates, use of respiratory accessory muscles in breathing, nasal flaring, and increased restlessness. (See *Croup teaching topics*.)

EPIGLOTTIDITIS

Epiglottiditis, an acute inflammation of the epiglottis and surrounding area, is a life-threatening emergency that rapidly causes edema and induration. If untreated, epiglottiditis results in complete airway obstruction. Epiglottiditis can occur from infancy to adulthood in any season. It's fatal in 8% to 12% of patients, typically children ages 2 to 8.

Pathophysiology

Epiglottiditis usually results from infection with *Haemophilus influenzae* type B and, occasionally, pneumococci or group A streptococci. Epiglottiditis is becoming more rare.

Complications

■ Airway obstruction
■ Death

AIRWAY CRISIS

Epiglottiditis can progress to complete airway obstruction within minutes. To prepare for this medical emergency, keep these tips in mind.

● Watch for increasing restlessness, tachycardia, fever, dyspnea, and intercostal and substernal retractions. These are warning signs of total airway obstruction and the need for an emergency tracheotomy.

● Keep the following equipment available at the patient's bedside in case of sudden, complete airway obstruction: a tracheotomy tray, endotracheal tubes, a manual resuscitation bag, oxygen equipment, and a laryngoscope with blades of various sizes.

● Remember that using a tongue blade or throat culture swab can initiate sudden, complete airway obstruction.

● Before examining the patient's throat, arrange for trained personnel (such as an anesthesiologist) to be present in case the patient requires insertion of an emergency airway.

Assessment findings

■ The patient or his parents may report an earlier upper respiratory tract infection.

■ Additional complaints include sore throat, dysphagia, and the sudden onset of a high fever.

■ On inspection, the patient may be febrile, drooling, pale or cyanotic, restless, apprehensive, and irritable.

■ You may also observe nasal flaring.

■ The patient may sit in a tripod position: upright, leaning forward with the chin thrust out, mouth open, and tongue protruding. This position helps relieve severe respiratory distress.

■ The patient's voice usually sounds thick and muffled.

■ Because manipulation may trigger sudden airway obstruction, attempt throat inspection only when immediate intubation is needed and can be performed. (See *Airway crisis.*)

■ The patient's throat appears red and inflamed.

■ Auscultation of the lung fields may reveal rhonchi and diminished breath sounds, usually transmitted from the upper airway.

Diagnostic test results

- Direct laryngoscopy reveals the hallmark of acute epiglottiditis: a swollen, beefy-red epiglottis. The throat examination should follow X-rays and, in most cases, shouldn't be performed if significant obstruction is suspected or if immediate intubation isn't possible.
- Lateral neck X-rays show an enlarged epiglottis and distended hypopharynx.
- Additional X-rays of the chest and cervical trachea help to confirm the diagnosis.

Treatment

A patient with acute epiglottiditis and airway obstruction requires emergency hospitalization. Place the patient in a cool-mist tent with added oxygen. If complete or near-complete airway obstruction occurs, he may also need emergency endotracheal intubation or a tracheotomy. Arterial blood gas (ABG) analysis or pulse oximetry may be used to assess his progress.

Treatment may also include parenteral fluids to prevent dehydration when the disease interferes with swallowing and a 10-day course of parenteral antibiotics—usually ampicillin (Principen). If the patient is allergic to penicillin or could have ampicillin-resistant endemic *H. influenzae*, chloramphenicol (Chloromycetin) or another antibiotic may be prescribed.

Corticosteroids may be prescribed to reduce edema during early treatment. Oxygen therapy also may be used.

Keep in mind that preventive measures should be taken. In the late 1980s, the American Academy of Pediatrics recommended that all children receive the *Haemophilus* b conjugate (Hib) vaccine, and it remains on the recommended schedule of immunizations today. Begin Hib vaccine immunization at age 2 months and continue for three or four doses, depending on the manufacturer. Since the introduction of the Hib vaccine, the incidence of epiglottiditis has declined dramatically.

Nursing interventions

- Place the patient in a sitting position to ease his respiratory difficulty unless he finds another, more comfortable position.
- Monitor pulse oximetry.

EPIGLOTTIDITIS TEACHING TOPICS

● Inform the patient and his family that epiglottal swelling usually subsides after 24 hours of antibiotic therapy. The epiglottis usually returns to normal size within 72 hours.

● If the patient's home care regimen includes oral antibiotic therapy, emphasize the need for completing the entire prescription. Explain proper administration. Discuss drug storage, dosage, adverse effects, and whether the medication can be taken with food or milk.

● If the patient should require the *Haemophilus* b conjugate vaccine, discuss the rationale for immunization, and help the family obtain the vaccine.

▧ Place the patient in a cool-mist tent. Change the sheets frequently because they quickly become saturated.

▧ Encourage the parents to remain with their child. Offer reassurance and support to relieve family members' anxiety and fear.

▧ Monitor the patient's temperature, vital signs, and respiratory rate and pattern frequently. Also monitor ABG (to detect hypoxia and hypercapnia) and pulse oximetry values (to detect decreasing oxygen saturation). Report changes.

▧ Observe the patient continuously for signs of impending airway closure, which may develop at any time.

▧ Calm the patient during X-rays of his chest and cervical trachea.

▧ Minimize external stimuli.

▧ Start an I.V. line for antibiotic therapy and fluid replacement if the patient can't maintain adequate fluid intake. Draw blood for laboratory analysis, as ordered.

▧ Keep tracheostomy equipment at the bedside.

▧ Record intake and output precisely to monitor and prevent dehydration.

▧ If the patient has a tracheostomy, anticipate his needs because he can't cry or call out. Provide emotional support. Reassure him and his family that a tracheostomy is a short-term intervention (usually 4 to 7 days). Monitor the patient for signs of secondary infection, including increasing temperature, increasing pulse rate, and hypotension. (See *Epiglottiditis teaching topics.*)

PHARYNGITIS

Pharyngitis, the most common throat disorder, is an acute or chronic inflammation of the pharynx. It's widespread among adults who live or work in dusty or dry environments, use their voices excessively, habitually use tobacco or alcohol, or suffer from chronic sinusitis, persistent coughs, or allergies. Uncomplicated pharyngitis usually subsides in 3 to 10 days.

Beta-hemolytic streptococci, which cause 15% to 20% of the cases of acute pharyngitis, may precede the common cold or other communicable diseases. Chronic pharyngitis is usually an extension of nasopharyngeal obstruction or inflammation.

Viral pharyngitis accounts for about 70% of acute pharyngitis cases.

Pathophysiology

Pharyngitis may occur as a result of a virus, such as rhinovirus, coronavirus, adenovirus, influenza, and parainfluenza. Mononucleosis can also cause pharyngitis. In children, streptococcal bacteria commonly cause pharyngitis. Fungal pharyngitis can develop with prolonged use of an antibiotic in an immunosuppressed patient, such as one with human immunodeficiency virus. Gonococcal pharyngitis is caused by release of a toxin produced by *Corynebacterium diphtheriae*.

Complications

- Otitis media
- Sinusitis
- Mastoiditis
- Rheumatic fever
- Nephritis

Assessment findings

- Typically, the patient complains of a sore throat and slight difficulty swallowing; swallowing saliva hurts more than swallowing food.
- The patient may also complain of a sensation of a lump in the throat, a constant and aggravating urge to swallow, a head-

ache, and muscle and joint pain (especially in bacterial pharyngitis).
▧ Assessment of vital signs may reveal mild fever.
▧ On inspection, the posterior pharyngeal wall appears fiery red, with swollen, exudate-flecked tonsils and lymphoid follicles.
▧ If the patient has bacterial pharyngitis, the throat is acutely inflamed, with patches of white and yellow follicles.
▧ The tongue may be strawberry red in color.
▧ Neck palpation may reveal enlarged, tender cervical lymph nodes.

AGE AWARE Over 90% of cases of sore throat and fever in children are viral. Associated symptoms usually include a runny nose and a nonproductive cough.

Diagnostic test results
▧ Computed tomography scan is helpful in identifying the location of abscesses.
▧ Rapid strep tests generally detect group A streptococcal infections, but they miss the fairly common streptococcal groups C and G.
▧ Throat culture may be used to identify the bacterial organisms causing the inflammation, but it may not detect other causative organisms.
▧ White blood cell (WBC) count is used to determine atypical lymphocytes; total WBC count is elevated.

Treatment
Based on the patient's symptoms, treatment for acute viral pharyngitis consists mainly of rest, warm saline gargles, throat lozenges containing a mild anesthetic, plenty of fluids, and an analgesic, as needed. If the patient can't swallow fluids, he may need hospitalization for I.V. hydration.

Bacterial pharyngitis requires rigorous treatment with penicillin (or another broad-spectrum antibiotic if the patient is allergic to penicillin) because streptococcus is the chief infecting organism. Continue antibiotic therapy for 48 hours after visible signs of infection have disappeared or for at least 7 to 10 days.

DISCHARGE TEACHING

PHARYNGITIS TEACHING TOPICS

● If the patient has acute bacterial pharyngitis, emphasize the importance of completing the full course of antibiotic therapy. Tell him to call the physician if he experiences an adverse reaction.

● Teach the patient with chronic pharyngitis how to minimize sources of throat irritation in the environment—by using a bedside humidifier, for example. Refer him to a self-help group to stop smoking, if appropriate.

● Inform the patient and his family that in the case of a positive streptococcal infection, the family should undergo throat cultures, regardless of the presence or absence of symptoms. Those with positive cultures require penicillin therapy.

● Teach the patient to avoid using irritants, such as alcohol, which may worsen symptoms.

An antifungal is used to treat fungal pharyngitis. An equine antitoxin is given for diphtheria pharyngitis.

Chronic pharyngitis requires the same supportive measures as acute pharyngitis, but with greater emphasis on eliminating the underlying cause such as an allergen.

Preventive measures include humidifying the air and avoiding excessive exposure to air conditioning. In addition, urge patients who smoke to stop.

Nursing interventions

- Give an analgesic and warm saline gargles, as ordered and as appropriate.
- Encourage the patient to drink fluids (up to 2½ qt [2.5 L] per day). Monitor intake and output scrupulously, and watch for signs of dehydration (cracked lips, dry mucous membranes, low urine output, poor skin turgor). Provide meticulous mouth care to prevent dry lips and oral pyoderma.
- Obtain throat cultures, and give an antibiotic, as ordered.
- Maintain a restful environment, especially if the patient is febrile, to conserve energy.
- Advise a soft, light diet with plenty of liquids to combat the commonly experienced anorexia. An antiemetic can be given before eating, if ordered.

- Examine the skin twice per day for possible drug sensitivity rashes or for rashes indicating a communicable disease.
- Give an antitussive, as ordered, if the patient has a cough.
- Give an analgesic, as ordered. (See *Pharyngitis teaching topics.*)

PLEURAL EFFUSION AND EMPYEMA

The pleural space normally contains a small amount (about 20 ml) of extracellular fluid that lubricates the pleural surfaces. If fluid accumulates as a result of increased production or inadequate removal, pleural effusion occurs. Empyema is a type of pleural effusion in which pus and necrotic tissue accumulate in the pleural space. Blood (hemothorax) and chyle (chylothorax) may also collect in this space.

The incidence of pleural effusion increases with heart failure (the most common cause), parapneumonia, cancer, and pulmonary embolism.

Pathophysiology

A transudative pleural effusion—an ultrafiltrate of plasma containing a low concentration of protein—may result from heart failure, hepatic disease with ascites, peritoneal dialysis, hypoalbuminemia, and disorders that increase intravascular volume.

The effusion stems from an imbalance of osmotic and hydrostatic pressures. Normally, the balance of these pressures in parietal pleural capillaries causes fluid to move into the pleural space; balanced pressure in visceral pleural capillaries promotes reabsorption of this fluid. However, when excessive hydrostatic pressure or decreased osmotic pressure causes excessive fluid to pass across intact capillaries, a transudative pleural effusion results.

Exudative pleural effusions can result from tuberculosis (TB), subphrenic abscess, pancreatitis, bacterial or fungal pneumonitis or empyema, cancer, parapneumonia, pulmonary embolism (with or without infarction), collagen disease (lupus erythematosus and rheumatoid arthritis), myxedema, intra-abdominal abscess, esophageal perforation, and chest trauma.

Such an effusion occurs when capillary permeability increases, with or without changes in hydrostatic and colloid osmotic pressures, allowing protein-rich fluid to leak into the pleural space.

Empyema usually stems from an infection in the pleural space. The infection may be idiopathic or may be related to pneumonitis, carcinoma, perforation, penetrating chest trauma, or esophageal rupture.

Complications
- Atelectasis
- Hypoxemia, respiratory acidosis, or thoracic shift (in large pleural effusions)
- Infection

Assessment findings
- The patient's history characteristically shows underlying pulmonary disease.
- If he has a large amount of effusion, he typically complains of dyspnea.
- If he has pleurisy, he may report pleuritic chest pain.
- If he has empyema, he may also complain of a general feeling of malaise and he may have a fever.
- Inspection may indicate that the trachea has deviated away from the affected side.
- On palpation, you may note decreased tactile fremitus with a large amount of effusion.
- Percussion may disclose dullness over the effused area that doesn't change with respiration.
- When you auscultate the chest, you may hear diminished or absent breath sounds over the effusion and a pleural friction rub during inspiration and expiration. (This pleural friction rub is transitory, however, and disappears as fluid accumulates in the pleural space.)
- You may also hear bronchial breath sounds, sometimes with the patient's pronunciation of the letter "e" sounding like the letter "a."

Diagnostic test results

■ Chest X-rays show radiopaque fluid-independent regions (usually with fluid accumulation of more than 250 ml).
■ Thoracentesis allows analysis of aspirated fluid and may show:
  – transudative effusion that usually has a specific gravity of less than 1.015 and contains less than 3 g/dl of protein
  – exudative effusion with a ratio of protein in fluid to protein in serum of greater than or equal to 0.5, pleural fluid lactate dehydrogenase (LD) of greater than or equal to 200 IU, and a ratio of LD in pleural fluid to LD in serum of greater than or equal to 0.6
  – aspirated fluid in empyema containing acute inflammatory white blood cells and microorganisms and showing leukocytosis
  – fluid in empyema and rheumatoid arthritis, which can be the cause of an exudative pleural effusion, showing an extremely decreased pleural fluid glucose level
  – pleural effusion from esophageal rupture or pancreatitis, usually with fluid amylase levels higher than serum amylase levels
  – test results of aspirated fluid for lupus erythematosus cells, antinuclear antibodies, and neoplastic cells; color and consistency; acid-fast bacillus, fungal, and bacterial cultures; and triglycerides (in chylothorax).
■ Other diagnostic tests may be ordered. A negative tuberculin skin test helps to rule out TB as a cause. If thoracentesis doesn't provide a definitive diagnosis in exudative pleural effusion, a pleural biopsy can help confirm TB or cancer.

Treatment

Depending on the amount of fluid present, symptom producing effusion may require thoracentesis to remove fluid or careful monitoring of the patient's own reabsorption of the fluid. Chemical pleurodesis—the instillation of a sclerosing agent, such as tetracycline (Achromycin), bleomycin (Blenoxane), or nitrogen mustard through the chest tube to create adhesions between the two pleurae—may prevent recurrent effusions.

The patient with empyema needs one or more chest tubes inserted after thoracentesis. These tubes allow purulent material to drain. The patient may also need decortication (surgical removal of the thick coating over the lung) or rib resection to allow open drainage and lung expansion. He also requires parenteral antibiotics and, if he has hypoxia, oxygen administration.

Hemothorax requires drainage to prevent fibrothorax formation.

Nursing interventions

- During thoracentesis, remind the patient to breathe normally and avoid sudden movements, such as coughing or sighing. Monitor his vital signs, and watch for syncope. Also be alert for bradycardia, hypotension, pain, pulmonary edema, and cardiac arrest, which indicate that fluid is being removed too quickly. Reassure the patient throughout the procedure.
- After thoracentesis, watch for respiratory distress and signs of pneumothorax (sudden onset of dyspnea and cyanosis).
- Provide oxygen and, in empyema, antibiotics, as ordered. Record the patient's response to these care measures.

DISCHARGE TEACHING

PLEURAL EFFUSION AND EMPYEMA TEACHING TOPICS

- If the patient developed pleural effusion because of pneumonia or influenza, tell him to seek medical attention promptly whenever he gets a chest cold.
- Teach the patient the signs and symptoms of respiratory distress. If any of these develop, tell him to notify his physician.
- Fully explain the drug regimen, including adverse effects. Emphasize the importance of completing the prescribed regimen.
- If the patient smokes, urge him to stop, and refer him to a support group. Request smoking cessation aids, such as nicotine patches (Nicoderm) or bupropion (Wellbutrin), for use during hospitalization.

- Use an incentive spirometer to promote deep breathing, and encourage the patient to perform deep-breathing exercises to promote lung expansion.
- Provide meticulous chest tube care, and use aseptic technique for changing dressings around the tube insertion site in the patient with empyema. Be aware of signs and symptoms of problems with the chest drainage unit in use.
- Follow your facility's policy for milking the tube. Keep petroleum gauze at the bedside in case of chest tube dislodgment.
- Don't clamp the chest tube; this may cause tension pneumothorax.
- If the patient has open drainage through a rib resection or intercostal tube, use precautions. The patient usually needs weeks of such drainage to obliterate the space, so make home health nurse referrals if he's to be discharged with the tube in place.
- Throughout therapy, listen to the patient's fears and concerns and remain with him during periods of extreme stress and anxiety. Encourage him to identify care measures and actions that make him comfortable and relaxed. Perform these measures, and encourage the patient to do so as well. (See *Pleural effusion and empyema teaching topics*.)

PLEURISY

Also called *pleuritis,* pleurisy is an inflammation of the visceral and parietal pleurae that line the inside of the thoracic cage and envelop the lungs. The disorder causes the pleurae to become swollen and congested, hampering pleural fluid transport and increasing friction between the pleural surfaces.

Pathophysiology

Pleurisy can result from pneumonia, tuberculosis, viruses, systemic lupus erythematosus, rheumatoid arthritis, uremia, Dressler's syndrome, cancer, pulmonary infarction, and chest trauma.

Complications
- Permanent adhesions that can restrict lung expansion

Assessment findings
- The patient may report a sudden, sharp, stabbing pain that worsens on inspiration, the result of inflammation or irritation of sensory nerve endings in the parietal pleura that rub against one another during respiration.
- Severe pain may cause shallow, rapid breathing and may limit the patient's movement on the affected side during breathing.
- He may also have dyspnea.
- Other symptoms vary depending on the underlying pathologic process.
- When you auscultate the chest, you may hear a characteristic pleural friction rub—a coarse, creaky sound heard during late inspiration and early expiration—directly over the area of pleural inflammation.
- Palpation over the affected area may reveal coarse vibration.

Diagnostic test results
- Chest X-rays can identify pneumonia.
- Electrocardiography rules out coronary artery disease as the source of the patient's pain.

Treatment
Symptomatic treatment includes anti-inflammatory agents, analgesics, and bed rest. Severe pain may require an intercostal nerve block of two or three intercostal nerves. Pleurisy with pleural effusion calls for thoracentesis as both a diagnostic and therapeutic measure.

Nursing interventions
- Assess the patient for pain every 2 to 4 hours, and give antitussives and pain medication. Make sure you don't overmedicate. Pain relief allows for maximum chest expansion.
- Encourage the patient to take deep breaths and to cough. To minimize pain, apply firm pressure at the site of the pain while the patient coughs (splinting).

- Encourage the use of incentive spirometry every hour, and instruct the patient on proper use.
- Place the patient in high Fowler's position to help lung expansion. Positioning him on the affected side may aid in splinting.
- Assess the patient's respiratory status at least every 4 hours to detect early signs of compromise. Monitor the patient for such complications as fever, increased dyspnea, and changes in breath sounds.
- Plan your care to allow the patient as much uninterrupted rest as possible.
- Pain can impair the patient's mobility, so help him perform active and passive range-of-motion exercises to prevent contractures and promote muscle strength. Encourage the patient to walk, as tolerated.
- If the patient needs thoracentesis, remind him to breathe normally and avoid sudden movements, such as coughing or sighing, during the procedure. (See *Pleurisy teaching topics.*) Monitor his vital signs, and watch for syncope. Also watch for indications that fluid is being removed too quickly: bradycardia, hypotension, pain, pulmonary edema, and cardiac arrest. Reassure the patient throughout the procedure.

RED FLAG After thoracentesis, watch for respiratory distress and signs of pneumothorax (sudden onset of dyspnea and cyanosis).

- Throughout therapy, listen to the patient's fears and concerns, and answer his questions. Remain with him during periods of extreme stress and anxiety. Encourage him to identify actions and care measures that help make him comfortable and re-laxed. Perform these measures, and encourage the patient to do so as well.
- Whenever possible, include the patient in care decisions, and include family members in all phases of the patient's care.

PNEUMONIA

Pneumonia is an acute infection of the lung parenchyma that commonly impairs gas exchange. Pneumonia can be classified in several ways. Based on microbiological etiology, it may be viral, bacterial, fungal, protozoal, mycobacterial, mycoplasmal, or rickettsial in origin.

Based on location, pneumonia may be classified as bron-chopneumonia, lobular pneumonia, or lobar pneumonia. Bron-chopneumonia involves distal airways and alveoli; lobular pneu-monia, part of a lobe; and lobar pneumonia, an entire lobe.

The infection is also classified as one of three types: primary, secondary, or aspiration pneumonia. Primary pneumonia results directly from inhalation or aspiration of a pathogen, such as bac-teria or a virus; it includes pneumococcal and viral pneumonia. Secondary pneumonia may follow initial lung damage from a noxious chemical or other insult (superinfection), or may result from hematogenous spread of bacteria from a distant area. Aspi-ration pneumonia results from inhalation of foreign matter, such as vomitus or food particles, into the bronchi. It's more likely to occur in elderly or debilitated patients, those receiving nasogas-tric (NG) tube feedings, and those with an impaired gag reflex, poor oral hygiene, or a decreased level of consciousness.

Pneumonia occurs in both sexes and at all ages. More than 3 million cases of pneumonia occur annually in the United

States. The infection carries a good prognosis for patients with normal lungs and adequate immune systems. In debilitated patients, however, bacterial pneumonia ranks as the leading cause of death. Pneumonia is also the leading cause of death from infectious disease in the United States.

Pathophysiology

In bacterial pneumonia, which can occur in any part of the lungs, an infection initially triggers alveolar inflammation and edema. Capillaries become engorged with blood, causing stasis. As the alveolocapillary membrane breaks down, alveoli fill with blood and exudate, resulting in atelectasis. In severe bacterial infections, the lungs assume a heavy, liverlike appearance, as in acute respiratory distress syndrome (ARDS).

Viral infection, which typically causes diffuse pneumonia, first attacks bronchiolar epithelial cells, causing interstitial inflammation and desquamation. It then spreads to the alveoli, which fill with blood and fluid. In advanced infection, a hyaline membrane may form. As with bacterial infection, severe viral infection may clinically resemble ARDS.

In aspiration pneumonia, aspiration of gastric juices or hydrocarbons triggers similar inflammatory changes and inactivates surfactant over a large area. Decreased surfactant leads to alveolar collapse. Acidic gastric juices may directly damage the airways and alveoli. Particles with the aspirated gastric juices may obstruct the airways and reduce airflow, which leads to secondary bacterial pneumonia.

Certain predisposing factors increase the risk of pneumonia. For bacterial and viral pneumonia, these include chronic illness and debilitation, cancer (particularly lung cancer), abdominal and thoracic surgery, atelectasis, common colds or other viral respiratory infections, chronic respiratory disease (chronic obstructive pulmonary disease, asthma, bronchiectasis, cystic fibrosis), influenza, smoking, malnutrition, alcoholism, sickle cell disease, tracheostomy, exposure to noxious gases, aspiration, and immunosuppressive therapy. (See *Causes of pneumonia,* pages 200 to 205.)

(*Text continues on page 204.*)

CAUSES OF PNEUMONIA

CHARACTERISTICS

VIRAL PNEUMONIAS

INFLUENZA
- Prognosis poor even with treatment
- 50% mortality from cardiopulmonary collapse
- Signs and symptoms: cough (initially nonproductive; later, purulent sputum), marked cyanosis, dyspnea, high fever, chills, substernal pain and discomfort, moist crackles, frontal headache, myalgia

ADENOVIRUS
- Insidious onset
- Generally affects young adults
- Good prognosis; usually clears without residual effects
- Signs and symptoms: sore throat, fever, cough, chills, malaise, small amounts of mucoid sputum, retrosternal chest pain, anorexia, rhinitis, adenopathy, scattered crackles, rhonchi

RESPIRATORY SYNCYTIAL VIRUS
- Most prevalent in infants and children
- Complete recovery in 1 to 3 weeks
- Signs and symptoms: listlessness, irritability, tachypnea with retraction of intercostal muscles, slight sputum production, fine moist crackles, fever, severe malaise, possibly cough or croup

MEASLES (RUBEOLA)
- Signs and symptoms: fever, dyspnea, cough, small amounts of sputum, coryza, rash, cervical adenopathy

CHICKENPOX (VARICELLA)
- Uncommon in children but present in 30% of adults with varicella
- Signs and symptoms: characteristic rash, cough, dyspnea, cyanosis, tachypnea, pleuritic chest pain, hemoptysis and rhonchi 1 to 6 days after onset of rash

DIAGNOSTIC TESTS	TREATMENT
● Chest X-ray: diffuse bilateral broncho-pneumonia radiating from hilus ● White blood cell (WBC) count: normal to slightly elevated ● Sputum smears: no specific organisms	● Supportive treatment for respiratory failure includes endotracheal intubation and ventilator assistance; for fever, hypothermia blanket or antipyretics; for influenza A, amantadine (Symmetrel) or rimantadine (Flumadine).
● Chest X-ray: patchy distribution of pneumonia, more severe than indicated by physical examination ● WBC count: normal to slightly elevated	● Treatment goal is to relieve symptoms.
● Chest X-ray: patchy bilateral consolidation ● WBC count: normal to slightly elevated	● Supportive treatment includes humidified air, oxygen, antimicrobials (typically given until viral cause is confirmed), and aerosolized ribavirin (Virazole).
● Chest X-ray: reticular infiltrates, sometimes with hilar lymph node enlargement ● Lung tissue specimen: characteristic giant cells	● Supportive treatment includes bed rest, adequate hydration, antimicrobials and, if necessary, assisted ventilation.
● Chest X-ray: more extensive pneumonia than indicated by examination; bilateral, patchy, diffuse, nodular infiltrates ● Sputum analysis: predominant mononuclear cells and characteristic intranuclear inclusion bodies	● Supportive treatment includes adequate hydration and, in critically ill patients, oxygen therapy. ● Patients who are immunocompromised also receive I.V. acyclovir (Zovirax).

(continued)

CAUSES OF PNEUMONIA *(continued)*

CHARACTERISTICS

VIRAL PNEUMONIAS (continued)

CYTOMEGALOVIRUS
● Difficult to distinguish from other nonbacterial pneumonias. In adults with healthy lung tissue, resembles mononucleosis and is generally benign; in neonates, occurs as devastating multisystemic infection; in immunocompromised hosts, varies from clinically inapparent to fatal infection
● Signs and symptoms: fever, cough, shaking chills, dyspnea, cyanosis, weakness, diffuse crackles

PROTOZOAN PNEUMONIA

PNEUMOCYSTIS CARINII
● Occurs in immunocompromised patients
● Symptoms: dyspnea, nonproductive cough, anorexia, weight loss, fatigue, low-grade fever

BACTERIAL PNEUMONIAS

STREPTOCOCCUS
● Caused by *Streptococcus pneumoniae*
● Signs and symptoms: sudden onset of a single, shaking chill and sustained temperature of 102° to 104° F (38.9° to 40° C); commonly preceded by upper respiratory tract infection

KLEBSIELLA
● More likely in patients with chronic alcoholism, pulmonary disease, and diabetes
● Signs and symptoms: fever and recurrent chills; cough producing rusty, bloody, viscous sputum (currant jelly); cyanosis of lips and nail beds from hypoxemia; shallow, grunting respirations

DIAGNOSTIC TESTS	TREATMENT
● Chest X-ray: in early stages, variable patchy infiltrates; later, bilateral, nodular, and more predominant in lower lobes ● Percutaneous aspiration of lung tissue, transbronchial biopsy or open lung biopsy: typical intranuclear and cytoplasmic inclusions on microscopic examination (the virus can be cultured from lung tissue)	● Supportive treatment includes adequate hydration and nutrition, oxygen therapy, and bed rest. ● Disease is more severe in patients who are immunocompromised, warranting ganciclovir (Cytovene) or foscarnet. (Foscavir)
● Fiber-optic bronchoscopy: obtains specimen for histology studies ● Chest X-ray: for specific infiltrations, nodular lesions, or spontaneous pneumothorax	● Antimicrobial therapy consists of co-trimoxazole (Bactrim, Septra) or pentamidine therapy. ● Supportive treatment includes oxygen, improved nutrition, and mechanical ventilation.
● Chest X-ray: areas of consolidation, commonly lobar ● WBC count: elevated ● Sputum culture: possibly gram-positive *S. pneumoniae*	● Antimicrobial therapy consists of penicillin G or, if the patient is allergic to penicillin, erythromycin (E-mycin); therapy is begun after obtaining culture specimen, but without waiting for results, and continues for 7 to 10 days.
● Chest X-ray: typically, but not always, consolidation in the upper lobe that causes bulging of fissures ● WBC count: elevated ● Sputum culture and Gram stain: possibly gram-negative cocci *Klebsiella*	● Antimicrobial therapy consists of an aminoglycoside and, in serious infections, a cephalosporin.

(continued)

CAUSES OF PNEUMONIA *(continued)*

CHARACTERISTICS

BACTERIAL PNEUMONIAS (continued)

STAPHYLOCOCCUS
● Commonly occurs in patients with viral illness, such as influenza or measles, and in those with cystic fibrosis
● Signs and symptoms: temperature of 102° to 104° F, recurrent shaking chills, bloody sputum, dyspnea, tachypnea, hypoxemia

ASPIRATION PNEUMONIA

● Results from vomiting and aspiration of gastric or oropharyngeal contents into trachea and lungs or from ineffective swallowing muscles
● Noncardiogenic pulmonary edema possible with damage to respiratory epithelium from contact with gastric acid
● Subacute pneumonia possible with cavity formation
● Lung abscess possible if foreign body present
● Signs and symptoms: crackles, dyspnea, cyanosis, hypotension, tachycardia

Complications
▨ Septic shock
▨ Hypoxemia
▨ Respiratory failure
▨ Empyema
▨ Lung abscess (see *Understanding lung abscess,* page 206)
▨ Bacteremia
▨ Endocarditis
▨ Pericarditis
▨ Meningitis

Assessment findings
▨ In bacterial pneumonia, the patient may report pleuritic chest pain, a cough, excessive sputum production, and chills.
▨ On assessment, you may note that the patient has a fever.
▨ During inspection, you may observe that the patient is shaking and coughs up sputum.

DIAGNOSTIC TESTS	TREATMENT
● Chest X-ray: multiple abscesses and infiltrates; frequently empyema ● WBC count: elevated ● Sputum culture and Gram stain: possibly gram-positive staphylococci	● Antimicrobial therapy consists of nafcillin or oxacillin (Bactocill) for 14 days if staphylococci are producing penicillinase. ● A chest tube drains empyema.
● Chest X-ray: location of areas of infiltrates (suggests diagnosis)	● Antimicrobial therapy consists of penicillin G or clindamycin (Cleocin). ● Supportive therapy includes oxygen therapy, suctioning, coughing, deep breathing, adequate hydration, and I.V. corticosteroids.

- Creamy yellow sputum suggests staphylococcal pneumonia, green sputum denotes pneumonia caused by *Pseudomonas* organisms, and sputum that looks like currant jelly indicates pneumonia caused by *Klebsiella*. (Clear sputum means that the patient doesn't have an infective process.)
- In advanced cases of all types of pneumonia, you'll hear dullness when you percuss.
- Auscultation may disclose crackles, wheezing, or rhonchi over the affected lung area as well as decreased breath sounds and decreased vocal fremitus.

Diagnostic test results
- Arterial blood gas (ABG) levels vary depending on the severity of pneumonia and the underlying lung state.
- Blood cultures reflect bacteremia and help to determine the causative organism.

UNDERSTANDING LUNG ABSCESS

In lung abscess, a localized bacterial infection causes purulence and tissue destruction. Bacteria may spread and cause multiple abscesses throughout the lungs.

Lung abscess may be secondary to localized pneumonia or necrosis from a neoplasm that can't drain. Other causes include necrotizing infections or cysts, cavitary infarctions or cancers, and necrotic lesions from pneumoconiosis.

The patient history includes coughing, sometimes with bloody or purulent sputum, and pleuritic chest pain and dyspnea. Headache, anorexia, malaise, diaphoresis, chills, fever, and clubbing of the fingers may occur. You may detect dullness over affected lung tissue, crackles, and decreased and cavernous breath sounds.

Chest X-rays show a solid mass or localized infiltrate with clear spaces that contain air and fluid. Causative organisms are identified through blood and sputum cultures and Gram stain. White blood cell count is elevated. Computed tomography scan helps to differentiate the type of lesion. Bronchoscopy may be necessary later to collect specimens and identify obstruction.

Treatment includes extensive antibiotic therapy and, possibly, postural drainage and oxygen therapy. Massive hemoptysis, cancer, or bronchiectasis may require lesion or lobe resection. All patients require rigorous follow-up and serial chest X-rays.

- Bronchoscopy or transtracheal aspiration allows the collection of material for culture.
- Chest X-rays show infiltrates, confirming the diagnosis.
- Sputum specimen for Gram stain and culture and sensitivity tests shows acute inflammatory cells.
- Pleural fluid culture may also be obtained.
- Pulse oximetry may show a reduced level of arterial oxygen saturation.
- White blood cell count indicates leukocytosis in bacterial pneumonia and a normal or low count in viral or mycoplasmal pneumonia.

Treatment

The patient needs antimicrobial treatment based on the causative agent. Therapy should be reevaluated early in the course of treatment.

Supportive measures include humidified oxygen therapy for hypoxia, bronchodilator therapy, antitussives, mechanical venti-

lation for respiratory failure, a high-calorie diet and adequate
fluid intake, bed rest, and an analgesic to relieve pleuritic chest
pain. A patient with severe pneumonia on mechanical ventilation may need positive end-expiratory pressure to maintain adequate oxygenation.

Nursing interventions

- Maintain a patent airway and adequate oxygenation. Measure
  the patient's ABG levels, especially if he's hypoxic. Provide
  supplemental oxygen if his partial pressure of arterial oxygen
  falls below 55 mm Hg. If he has an underlying chronic lung
  disease, give oxygen cautiously.

- In severe pneumonia that requires endotracheal (ET) intubation or a tracheostomy with or without mechanical ventilation, provide thorough respiratory care and suction often using sterile technique to remove secretions.

- Obtain sputum specimens as needed. Use suction if the patient can't produce a specimen. Collect the specimens in a
  sterile container and deliver them promptly to the laboratory.

- Give antibiotics, as ordered, and pain medication as needed.
  Provide I.V. fluids and electrolyte replacement, if needed, for
  fever and dehydration.

- Provide a high-calorie, high-protein diet of soft foods to offset
  the calories the patient uses to fight the infection. If necessary,
  supplement oral feedings with NG tube feedings or parenteral
  nutrition.

- To prevent aspiration during NG tube feedings, elevate the
  patient's head, check the tube position, and give the feeding
  slowly. Don't give large volumes at one time because this can
  cause vomiting.

- If the patient has an ET tube, inflate the tube cuff before feeding. Keep his head elevated for at least 30 minutes after feeding.

- Monitor the patient's fluid intake and output.

- To control the spread of infection, dispose of secretions properly. Tell the patient to sneeze and cough into a disposable tissue, and tape a waxed bag to the side of the bed for used tissues.

DISCHARGE TEACHING

PNEUMONIA TEACHING TOPICS

● Emphasize the importance of adequate rest to promote full recovery and prevent a relapse. Explain that the practitioner will advise the patient when he can resume full activity and return to work.

● Review the patient's medication. Stress the need to take the entire course of medication, even if he feels better, to prevent a relapse.

● Teach the patient procedures to clear lung secretions, such as deep-breathing and coughing exercises, as well as home oxygen therapy. Explain deep breathing and pursed-lip breathing.

● Urge the patient to drink 2 to 3 qt (2 to 3 L) of fluid per day to maintain adequate hydration and keep mucus secretions thin for easier removal.

● Teach the patient and his family about chest physiotherapy. Explain that postural drainage, percussion, and vibration help to mobilize and remove mucus from the lungs.

● Urge the patient to avoid irritants that stimulate secretions, such as cigarette smoke, dust, and significant environmental pollution. If necessary, refer him to community programs or agencies that can help him stop smoking.

■ Provide a quiet, calm environment, with frequent rest periods. Make sure the patient has diversionary activities appropriate to his age.

■ Listen to the patient's fears and concerns, and remain with him during periods of severe stress and anxiety. Encourage him to identify actions and care measures that promote comfort and relaxation.

■ When possible, include the patient in care decisions.

■ Include family members in all phases of the patient's care, and encourage them to visit. (See *Pneumonia teaching topics*.)

SEVERE ACUTE RESPIRATORY SYNDROME

Severe acute respiratory syndrome (SARS) is a viral respiratory infection that can progress to pneumonia and, eventually, death. The disease was first recognized in 2003 with outbreaks in China, Canada, Singapore, Taiwan, and Vietnam, with other countries, including the United States, reporting smaller numbers of cases.

Pathophysiology

SARS is caused by the SARS-associated coronavirus (SARS-CoV). Coronaviruses are a common cause of mild respiratory illnesses in humans, but researchers believe that a virus may have mutated, allowing it to cause this potentially life-threatening disease.

Close contact with a person who's infected with SARS, including contact with infectious aerosolized droplets or body secretions, is the method of transmission. Most people who contracted the disease during the 2003 outbreak did so while traveling to endemic areas. However, the virus can live on hands, tissues, and other surfaces for up to 6 hours in its droplet form and it can live in the stool of people with SARS for up to 4 days. The virus may survive for months or years in below-freezing temperatures.

Complications

- Respiratory failure
- Liver failure
- Heart failure
- Myelodysplastic syndromes
- Death

Assessment findings

- The incubation period for SARS is typically 3 to 5 days but may last as long as 14 days.
- Initial signs and symptoms include fever, shortness of breath and other minor respiratory symptoms, general discomfort, headache, rigors, chills, myalgia, sore throat, and dry cough.
- Some people may develop diarrhea or a rash.

Diagnostic test results

- Diagnosis of severe respiratory illness is made when the patient has a fever higher than 100.4° F (38° C) or signs and symptoms of lower respiratory illness and a chest X-ray showing pneumonia or acute respiratory distress syndrome.
- Laboratory validation for the virus includes cell culture of SARS-CoV, detection of SARS-CoV ribonucleic acid by the reverse transcription polymerase chain reaction (RT-PCR) test, or detection of serum antibodies to SARS-CoV. Detectable lev-

DISCHARGE TEACHING

SARS TEACHING TOPICS

● Provide patient and family teaching, including the importance of frequent hand washing, covering the mouth and nose when coughing or sneezing, and avoiding close personal contact while infected or potentially infected. Instruct the patient and his family not to share such items as eating utensils, towels, and bedding until they have been washed with soap and hot water, and to use disposable gloves and household disinfectant to clean any surface that may have been exposed to the patient's body fluids.

● Emphasize to the patient the importance of not going to work, school, or other public places, as recommended by the physician.

els of antibodies may not be present until 21 days after the onset of illness, but some individuals develop antibodies within 14 days. A negative PCR, antibody test, or cell culture doesn't rule out the diagnosis.

Treatment

Treatment is symptomatic and supportive and includes maintenance of a patent airway and adequate nutrition. Other treatment measures include supplemental oxygen, chest physiotherapy, or mechanical ventilation. In addition to standard precautions, contact precautions requiring gowns and gloves for all patient contacts and airborne precautions utilizing a negative-pressure isolation room and properly fitted N-95 respirators are recommended for patients who are hospitalized. Quarantine may be used to prevent the spread of infection.

Antibiotics may be given to treat bacterial causes of atypical pneumonia. Antiviral medications also have been used. High doses of corticosteroids have been used to reduce lung inflammation. In some serious cases, serum from individuals who have already recovered from SARS (convalescent serum) has been given. The general benefit of these treatments hasn't been determined conclusively.

Nursing interventions

■ Report suspected cases of SARS to local and national health organizations.

- Frequently monitor the patient's vital signs and respiratory status.
- Maintain isolation as recommended. The patient will need emotional support to deal with anxiety and fear related to the diagnosis of SARS and as a result of isolation. (See *SARS teaching topics.*)

SINUSITIS

Infection and inflammation of the paranasal sinuses may be acute, subacute, chronic, allergic, or hyperplastic. Acute sinusitis usually results from the common cold; in about 10% of patients, it lingers in subacute form. Chronic sinusitis follows persistent bacterial infection, generally occurring when a cold spreads to the sinuses.

Allergic sinusitis accompanies allergic rhinitis. Hyperplastic sinusitis is a combination of purulent acute sinusitis and allergic sinusitis or rhinitis. For all types, the prognosis is good.

Pathophysiology

Sinusitis usually results from a bacterial infection (*Haemophilus influenzae,* anaerobes) or, less frequently, from a viral infection. Viral sinusitis usually follows an upper respiratory tract infection in which the virus penetrates the normal mucous membrane, decreasing ciliary transport.

Fungal sinusitis is uncommon and is typically found in immunosuppressed patients. The most common types are aspergillosis, mucomycosis, candidiasis, histoplasmosis, and coccidiomycosis. The spores causing them are usually found in soil and enter through the respiratory tract.

Acute sinusitis is most commonly caused by *H. influenzae, Staphylococcus aureus, Streptococcus pneumoniae,* and *S. pyogenes.* Predisposing factors include any condition that interferes with sinus drainage and ventilation, such as chronic nasal edema, a deviated septum, and viscous mucus. Bacterial invasion may also result from swimming in contaminated water. Generalized debilitating conditions, including chemotherapy, malnutrition, diabetes, blood dyscrasias, long-term steroids, and immunodeficiency, may predispose an individual to sinusitis.

UNDERSTANDING BRAIN ABSCESS

Brain (intracranial) abscess is free or encapsulated purulence, typically in the frontal, parietal, temporal, or occipital lobes or, less commonly, in the cerebellum or basal ganglia. It can occur at any age (mostly ages 10 to 35) and is rare in elderly people.

Brain abscess is usually secondary to another infection, most commonly mastoid or ear infection. Untreated brain abscess is usually fatal; with treatment, the prognosis is only fair.

Typically, the patient reports recent or recurrent infection or a history of congenital heart disease. Nausea, vomiting, and a constant, intractable headache may occur along with changes in level of consciousness, confusion or disorientation, and signs of a focal neurologic disorder. Signs of increased intracranial pressure

(ICP) may be apparent, including abnormal pupillary response and depressed respirations.

EEG, computed tomography scan and, occasionally, arteriography can help identify the abscess site. Cerebrospinal fluid analysis can help confirm infection, but is risky because the process can provoke cerebral herniation. Other tests include culture and sensitivity tests, skull X-rays, and radioisotope scans.

Therapy consists of an antibiotic and surgical aspiration, drainage, or removal of the abscess (after it becomes encapsulated). Other treatments may include mechanical ventilation, I.V. fluid and diuretic administration, and a glucocorticoid to combat increased ICP and cerebral edema. An anticonvulsant can help prevent seizures.

AGE AWARE The incidence of acute and chronic sinusitis increases in later childhood. Sinusitis may be more prevalent in children who have had tonsils and adenoids removed.

Complications
- Meningitis
- Cavernous sinus thrombosis syndrome
- Bacteremia
- Septicemia
- Brain abscess (see *Understanding brain abscess*)
- Frontal lobe abscess
- Osteomyelitis
- Mucocele
- Orbital cellulitis or abscess

LOCATING THE PARANASAL SINUSES

The location of a patient's sinusitis pain indicates the affected sinus. For example, an infected maxillary sinus can cause tooth pain. (*Note:* The sphenoid sinus, which lies under the eye and above the soft palate, isn't shown here.)

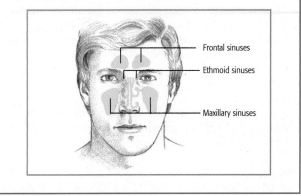

Frontal sinuses
Ethmoid sinuses
Maxillary sinuses

Assessment findings

- A patient with acute sinusitis typically complains of nasal congestion that preceded a gradual buildup of pressure in the affected sinus.
- He may state that for 24 to 48 hours after onset, a nasal discharge was present and later became purulent.
- He may also list a sore throat, a localized headache, and a general feeling of malaise.
- The patient may point to pain specific to the affected sinus: in the cheeks and upper teeth (maxillary sinusitis); over the eyes (ethmoid sinusitis); over the eyebrows (frontal sinusitis); or behind the eyes, over the occiput, or at the top of the head (sphenoid sinusitis, a rare condition). (See *Locating the paranasal sinuses.*)
- The patient also may report purulent nasal drainage that continues longer than 3 weeks after an acute infection subsides, which usually suggests subacute sinusitis.

- The patient with chronic sinusitis may report continuous and mucopurulent discharge. In the acute form, the patient may complain of a stuffy nose, vague facial discomfort, edema, edematous nasal mucosa, fatigue, and a nonproductive cough.
- Assessment of vital signs may reveal a low-grade fever of 99° to 99.5° F (37.2° to 37.5° C).
- The areas over the sinuses may appear swollen (caused by bacterial growth on diseased tissue in hyperplastic sinusitis).
- Inspection also may reveal enlarged turbinates and thickening of the mucosal lining and mucosal polyps (hyperplastic sinusitis).
- Palpation may cause pain and pressure over the affected sinus areas.
- Transillumination may expose diminished areas of light, which indicate areas of purulent drainage that prevent the passage of light.

Diagnostic test results

- Antral puncture promotes drainage and removal of purulent material. It also may be used to collect a specimen for culture and sensitivity identification of the infecting organism, but this test is rarely performed.
- Sinus endoscopy indicates purulent nasal drainage, nasal edema, and obstruction of ostia.
- Sinus X-rays reveal cloudiness in the affected sinus, air-fluid levels, or a thickened mucosal lining; ultrasonography and computed tomography scan may uncover suspected complications, recurrent or chronic sinusitis, or unresolved and serious sinusitis.

Treatment

ACUTE SINUSITIS

Administration of antibiotics—usually amoxicillin (Amoxil) or ampicillin (Principen)—is the primary treatment to combat persistent sinus infection. An analgesic may be prescribed to relieve pain. Other appropriate measures include a vasoconstrictor, such as epinephrine (Adrenalin) and phenylephrine (Neo-Synephrine), to decrease nasal secretions. Steam inhalation also promotes vasoconstriction and encourages drainage. Local heat application may help to relieve pain and congestion.

SUBACUTE SINUSITIS

As with acute sinusitis, antibiotic therapy is the treatment of choice, along with a vasoconstrictor to help reduce nasal secretions.

ALLERGIC SINUSITIS

Treatment of allergic sinusitis must include treatment of allergic rhinitis—administration of an antihistamine, identification of allergens by skin testing, and desensitization by immunotherapy. Severe allergic symptoms may require treatment with a corticosteroid and epinephrine.

CHRONIC OR HYPERPLASTIC SINUSITIS

For patients with these types of sinusitis, an antibiotic and a steroid nasal spray may relieve pain and congestion. An antihistamine may be judiciously prescribed for symptomatic relief but should be given cautiously because it may thicken nasal secretions and prevent effective sinus drainage.

OTHER TREATMENTS

If a subacute infection persists, the maxillary sinus may be irrigated. The ethmoid and sphenoid sinuses can be drained indirectly with the Proetz displacement method—a technique that uses gravity to displace thick, purulent material with thin irrigating fluid. If these irrigating techniques fail to relieve symptoms, one or more sinuses may require surgery. (See *Surgery for chronic and hyperplastic sinusitis,* page 216.) Functional endoscopic surgery may be an option because all sinuses are accessible by this method (however, frontal sinus access is limited). This procedure is performed under local or general anesthesia with direct visualization through the nose using specialized endoscopes and forceps.

Nursing interventions

- Encourage the patient to drink plenty of fluids to promote drainage.

SURGERY FOR CHRONIC AND HYPERPLASTIC SINUSITIS

When drug therapy and irrigation fail to relieve infection, surgery may be needed to correct chronic and hyperplastic sinusitis. The following procedures are common:

For maxillary sinusitis
● Nasal window procedure creates an opening in the sinus, allowing secretions and pus to drain through the nose.
● Caldwell-Luc procedure removes diseased mucosa in the maxillary sinus through an incision under the upper lip.

For chronic ethmoid sinusitis
● Ethmoidectomy removes all infected tissue through an external or intranasal incision into the ethmoid sinus.

● External ethmoidectomy removes infected ethmoid sinus tissue through a crescent-shaped incision, beginning under the inner eyebrow and extending along the side of the nose.

For chronic frontal sinusitis
● Fronto-ethmoidectomy removes infected frontal sinus tissue through an extended external ethmoidectomy.
● Osteoplastic flap drains the sinuses through an incision across the skull, behind the hairline.

■ Encourage the patient to express his concerns, and answer his questions. Include the patient and his family in planning and implementing the patient's care.

■ To relieve pain and promote drainage, apply warm compresses continuously or four times daily at 2-hour intervals. Give an analgesic, a vasoconstrictor, a nasal spray, an antibiotic, an antifungal, and an antihistamine, as ordered and as needed, monitoring the patient's response. Humidifiers and saline dressings are also helpful.

■ Watch for and report vomiting, chills, fever, edema of the forehead or eyelids, blurred or double vision, and personality changes, which could indicate complications.

AFTER SURGERY
■ Monitor the patient for excessive drainage or bleeding.

■ To prevent edema and promote drainage, place the patient in semi-Fowler's position. To relieve edema and pain and minimize bleeding, apply ice compresses or a rubber glove filled with ice chips over the nose and iced saline gauze over the eyes. Continue these measures for 24 hours.

■ Frequently change the mustache dressing or drip pad, recording the consistency, amount, and color of drainage (expect scant, bright-red drainage with some clots).

■ Because the patient is breathing through the mouth, provide meticulous and frequent mouth care. (See *Sinusitis teaching topics*.)

TONSILLITIS

Inflammation of the tonsils can be acute or chronic. Uncomplicated acute tonsillitis usually lasts 4 to 6 days and commonly affects children ages 5 to 10. Tonsils tend to hypertrophy during childhood and atrophy after puberty.

UNDERSTANDING THROAT ABSCESSES

Throat abscesses may be peritonsillar or retropharyngeal. Peritonsillar abscess, usually unilateral, is most common in adolescents and young adults. Acute retropharyngeal abscess commonly affects children younger than age 2. Chronic retropharyngeal abscess can occur at any age.

Peritonsillar abscess follows acute tonsillitis, usually from streptococcal or staphylococcal infection. Acute retropharyngeal abscess commonly follows upper respiratory tract infection. Chronic retropharyngeal abscess results from tuberculosis of the cervical spine.

Peritonsillar abscess causes severe throat pain and, possibly, ear pain, gland tenderness, swallowing difficulty, chills and fever, malaise, rancid breath, nausea and, sometimes, spasm of the jaw muscles and muffled speech. Retropharyngeal abscess may cause pain, dysphagia, fever, nasal or laryngeal obstruction, neck hyperextension and, in children, drooling and muffled crying. The soft palate and posterior pharyngeal wall may be red and swollen, displacing the tonsils or uvula.

X-rays may show a displaced larynx. Throat culture and sensitivity testing isolates the causative organism. A computed tomography scan can enable viewing of abscesses.

Early peritonsillar abscess necessitates large doses of an antibiotic. Late-stage abscess with cellulitis usually requires incision and drainage, followed by I.V. antibiotic therapy. Chronic recurrence may necessitate tonsillectomy. Retropharyngeal abscess may require drainage by incision or needle aspiration, followed by an analgesic and an I.V. antibiotic.

Pathophysiology

Tonsillitis usually results from infection with beta-hemolytic streptococci but may also result from other bacteria or viruses.

Complications

- Chronic upper airway obstruction
- Sleep apnea or sleep disturbances
- Cor pulmonale
- Failure to thrive
- Eating or swallowing disorders
- Speech abnormalities
- Febrile seizures
- Otitis media
- Cardiac valvular disease

- Abscesses
- Glomerulonephritis
- Subacute bacterial endocarditis
- Abscessed cervical lymph nodes (see *Understanding throat abscesses*)

Assessment findings

- The patient with acute tonsillitis may complain of mild to severe sore throat. In a child too young to complain about throat pain, the parents may report that the child has stopped eating.
- The patient or his parents also may report muscle and joint pain, chills, malaise, headache, and pain that's frequently referred to the ears.
- Because of excess secretions, the patient may complain of a constant urge to swallow and a constricted feeling in the back of the throat. Such discomfort usually subsides after 72 hours.
- Fever of 100° F (37.8° F) or higher may be present, and palpation may reveal swollen, tender lymph nodes in the submandibular area.
- Inspection of the throat may reveal generalized inflammation of the pharyngeal wall, with swollen tonsils that project from between the pillars of the fauces and exude white or yellow follicles.
- Purulent drainage becomes apparent when you apply pressure to the tonsillar pillars.
- The uvula may also be edematous and inflamed.
- Patients with chronic tonsillitis may report recurrent sore throats and attacks of acute tonsillitis. Inspection may expose purulent drainage in the tonsillar crypts.

Diagnostic test results

- Needle biopsy helps differentiate cellulitis from abscess.
- Throat culture may reveal the infecting organism and indicate appropriate antibiotic therapy.
- White blood cell count usually reveals leukocytosis.

Treatment

Management of acute tonsillitis stresses symptom relief and requires rest, adequate fluid intake, aspirin or acetaminophen (Tylenol) or ibuprofen (Advil) and, for bacterial infection, an antibiotic. For group A beta-hemolytic streptococcus, penicillin (Pen-Vee K) is the drug of choice. Erythromycin (Erythrocin) or another broad-spectrum antibiotic may be given if the patient is allergic to penicillin. To prevent complications, continue antibiotics for 10 days.

Chronic tonsillitis or complications may require tonsillectomy, but only after the patient has been free from tonsillar or respiratory tract infections for 3 to 4 weeks.

Nursing interventions

- Despite dysphagia, urge the patient to drink plenty of fluids, especially if fever is present. Offer a child ice cream and flavored drinks and ices. Assess hydration status. Increased humidification may provide comfort.
- Monitor the effect of pain medication.
- Suggest gargling to soothe the throat.
- Before surgery, assess the patient for bleeding abnormalities.
- Keep a tracheostomy tray at the bedside in case of emergency.

AFTER SURGERY
- Maintain a patent airway. To prevent aspiration, place the patient on his side. Keep suction equipment nearby.
- Monitor vital signs frequently and check for bleeding. Immediately report excessive bleeding, increased pulse rate, or decreased blood pressure.
- When the patient is fully alert and the gag reflex has returned, give him water. Later, encourage him to drink nonirritating fluids. Avoid milk products; they coat the throat, causing throat clearing and increased risk of bleeding.
- Provide an analgesic for pain relief. Because crying irritates the operative site, keep the child comfortable.
- Encourage deep-breathing exercises to prevent pulmonary complications. (See *Tonsillitis teaching topics.*)

TUBERCULOSIS

Tuberculosis (TB) is an acute or chronic infection characterized by pulmonary infiltrates and by the formation of granulomas with caseation, fibrosis, and cavitation. The incidence of TB has been increasing in the United States secondary to homelessness, drug abuse, and human immunodeficiency virus infection. Globally, TB is the leading infectious cause of morbidity and mortality, generating 8 to 10 million new cases each year.

The disease is twice as common in men as in women and four times as common in nonwhites as in whites. Incidence is highest in people who live in crowded, poorly ventilated, unsanitary conditions, such as prisons, tenement houses, and homeless shelters. The typical newly diagnosed patient with TB is a single, homeless, nonwhite man. With proper treatment, the prognosis is usually excellent. However, mortality is 50% in strains of TB resistant to two or more of the major antitubercular agents.

Pathophysiology
TB results from exposure to *Mycobacterium tuberculosis* and, sometimes, other strains of mycobacteria. Transmission occurs

UNDERSTANDING TUBERCULOSIS

When a person without immunity inhales droplets infected with *Mycobacterium tuberculosis*, the bacilli lodge in the alveoli, causing irritation. The immune system responds by sending leukocytes, lymphocytes, and macrophages to surround the bacilli, and the local lymph nodes swell and become inflamed.

If the encapsulated bacilli (tubercles) and the inflamed nodes rupture, the infection contaminates the surrounding tissue and may spread through the blood and lymphatic circulation to distant sites— a process called *hematogenous dissemination*. This same phagocytic cycle oc-

curs whenever the bacilli spread. Sites of extrapulmonary tuberculosis (TB) include the pleura, meninges, joints, lymph nodes, peritoneum, and GI tract.

After exposure to *M. tuberculosis*, roughly 5% of infected people develop active TB within 1 year. In the remainder, microorganisms cause a latent infection. The host's immunologic defense system usually destroys the bacillus or walls it up in a tubercle. However, the live, encapsulated bacilli may lie dormant within the tubercle for years, reactivating later to cause active infection. In this respect, the disease is an opportunistic infection.

when an infected person coughs or sneezes, spreading infected droplets. (See *Understanding tuberculosis*.)

These at-risk populations have a high incidence of TB:
- Black and Hispanic men, ages 25 to 44
- drug abusers and alcoholics
- gastrectomy patients
- homeless persons
- nursing home residents (10 times more likely to contract TB than anyone in the general population)
- patients in mental health facilities
- patients receiving immunosuppressant or corticosteroid treatment
- patients with silicosis, diabetes, malnutrition, cancer, Hodgkin's disease, or leukemia
- people in close contact with a newly diagnosed patient with TB
- people who have had TB before
- people with multiple sexual partners
- people with weak immune systems or diseases that affect the immune system, especially those with acquired immunodeficiency syndrome (AIDS)

- prisoners
- recent immigrants to the United States.

Complications
- Massive pulmonary tissue damage
- Inflammation and tissue necrosis
- Respiratory failure
- Bronchopleural fistulas
- Pneumothorax
- Hemorrhage
- Pleural effusion
- Pneumonia
- Liver involvement from drug therapy

Assessment findings
- The patient with a primary infection after an incubation period of 4 to 8 weeks is usually asymptomatic but may complain of weakness and fatigue, anorexia and weight loss, low-grade fever, and night sweats.
- The patient with reactivated TB may report chest pain and a cough that produces blood or mucopurulent or blood-tinged sputum.
- The patient with reactivated TB may also have a low-grade fever.
- On percussion, you may note dullness over the affected area, a sign of consolidation or the presence of pleural fluid.
- On auscultation, you may hear crepitant crackles, bronchial breath sounds, wheezes, and whispered pectoriloquy.

   AGE AWARE Fever and night sweats, the typical hallmarks of TB, may not be present in elderly patients, who instead may exhibit a change in activity or weight. Assess older patients carefully.

Diagnostic test results
- Several of these tests may be necessary to distinguish TB from other diseases that may mimic it, such as lung carcinoma, lung abscess, pneumoconiosis, and bronchiectasis.
  - Bronchoscopy may be performed if the patient can't produce an adequate sputum specimen.

  – Chest X-rays show nodular lesions, patchy infiltrates
    (mainly in upper lobes), cavity formation, scar tissue, and
    calcium deposits. They may not help distinguish active
    from inactive TB.
  – Computed tomography scans or magnetic resonance imag-
    ing allow the evaluation of lung damage or confirm a diffi-
    cult diagnosis.
  – Stains and cultures of sputum, cerebrospinal fluid, urine,
    drainage from abscess, or pleural fluid show heat-sensitive,
    nonmotile, aerobic, acid-fast bacilli.
  – A tuberculin skin test reveals that the patient has been in-
    fected with TB at some point, but it doesn't indicate active
    disease. In this test, intermediate-strength purified protein
    derivative or 5 tuberculin units (0.1 ml) are injected intra-
    dermally on the forearm and read in 48 to 72 hours. A
    positive reaction (greater than or equal to a 10-mm indura-
    tion) develops within 2 to 10 weeks after infection with the
    tubercle bacillus in active and inactive TB. However, a se-
    verely immunosuppressed patient may not have a positive
    reaction.
▪ Because many immigrants have received the bacille Calmette-
  Guérin (BCG) vaccine, skin tests won't be effective screening
  tools for these people. Chest X-rays are needed for screening
  people who have previously been vaccinated against TB with
  BCG.

Treatment

Antitubercular therapy with daily oral doses of isoniazid (Laniazid), rifampin (Rifadin), and pyrazinamide (Tebrazid; with
ethambutol [Myambutol] added in some cases) for at least 6
months usually cures TB. After 2 to 4 weeks, the disease is no
longer infectious and the patient can resume normal activities
while continuing to take medication. A longer course of treatment may be necessary if the patient is slow to respond to treatment; patients with AIDS may also require extended treatment.
    The patient with atypical mycobacterial disease or drug-
resistant TB may require second-line drugs, such as capreomy-

cin (Capastat), streptomycin, para-aminosalicylic acid, cycloser-ine (Seromycin), amikacin (Amikin), and quinolone drugs.

Nursing interventions

- Give ordered antibiotics and antitubercular agents.
- Isolate the infectious patient in a quiet, properly ventilated room, as per guidelines from the Centers for Disease Control and Prevention, and maintain TB precautions such as a negative-pressure room. Provide diversional activities and check on him frequently. Make sure the call button is nearby.
- Place a covered trash can nearby, or tape a waxed bag to the bedside for used tissues. Tell the patient to wear a mask when outside his room. Tell visitors and health care personnel to take proper precautions, such as wearing a mask while in the room and following strict hand-washing precautions when leaving the room.
- Make sure the patient gets plenty of rest. Provide for periods of rest and activity to promote health as well as conserve energy and reduce oxygen demand.
- Provide the patient with well-balanced, high-calorie foods, preferably in small, frequent meals to conserve energy and to encourage the anorexic patient to eat more. Record the patient's weight weekly. If he needs oral supplements, consult with the dietitian.
- Watch for adverse reactions to the medications.
- Give isoniazid with food. This drug can cause hepatitis or peripheral neuritis, so monitor levels of aspartate aminotransferase and alanine aminotransferase. To prevent or treat peripheral neuritis, give pyridoxine (vitamin B_6), as ordered.
- If the patient receives ethambutol, watch for signs of optic neuritis; report them to the physician, who's likely to stop the drug. Check the patient's vision monthly, and give this medication with food.
- If the patient receives rifampin, watch for signs of hepatitis, purpura, and a flulike syndrome as well as other complications such as hemoptysis. Monitor liver and kidney function tests throughout therapy.

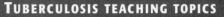

TUBERCULOSIS TEACHING TOPICS

● Show the patient and his family how to perform postural drainage and chest percussion. Also teach the patient coughing and deep-breathing exercises. Instruct him to maintain each position for 10 minutes and then to perform percussion and cough.

● Teach the patient the adverse effects of his medication, and tell him to report them immediately. Emphasize the importance of regular follow-up examinations, and instruct him and his family members about the signs and symptoms of recurring tuberculosis. Stress the importance of faithfully following long-term treatment.

● Advise anyone exposed to an infected patient to receive tuberculin tests and, if a positive reaction occurs, to obtain chest X-rays and prophylactic isoniazid (Laniazid).

● Warn the patient taking rifampin (Rifadin) that the drug temporarily makes body secretions, such as urine, appear orange; reassure him that this effect is harmless. Caution the female patient taking hormonal contraceptives that these may be less effective while she's taking rifampin, so it's important to use other methods of birth control such as condoms with spermicide foam.

● Teach the patient the signs and symptoms that require medical assessment: increased cough, hemoptysis, unexplained weight loss, fever, and night sweats.

● Stress the importance of eating high-calorie, high-protein, balanced meals.

● Emphasize the importance of scheduling and keeping follow-up appointments.

● Refer the patient to such support groups as the American Lung Association.

■ Perform chest physiotherapy, including postural drainage and chest percussion, several times per day.

■ Give the patient supportive care, and help him adjust to the changes he may have to make during his illness. Include the patient in care decisions, and let the family take part in the patient's care whenever possible. (See *Tuberculosis teaching topics.*)

Obstructive disorders

Among chronic obstructive disorders of the lung, chronic obstructive pulmonary disease (COPD), also called *chronic obstructive lung disorder,* is the most common. It affects an estimated 30 million Americans and its numbers are rising.

Early COPD may not produce symptoms and may cause only minimal disability in many patients, but it tends to worsen with time.

Types of COPD include chronic bronchitis, cystic fibrosis, emphysema and, more commonly, a combination of these conditions (usually bronchitis and emphysema).

CHRONIC BRONCHITIS

Bronchitis is acute or chronic inflammation of the bronchi caused by irritants or infection. The distinguishing characteristic of bronchitis is obstruction of airflow. In chronic bronchitis, a form of chronic obstructive pulmonary disease, hypersecretion of mucus and chronic productive cough are present during 3 months of the year for at least 2 consecutive years.

AGE AWARE Children of parents who smoke are at higher risk for respiratory tract infection, which can lead to chronic bronchitis.

Pathophysiology
Chronic bronchitis develops when irritants are inhaled for a prolonged period. The irritants inflame the tracheobronchial tree, leading to increased mucus production and a narrowed or

MUCUS BUILDUP IN CHRONIC BRONCHITIS

In chronic bronchitis, excessive production of mucus obstructs the small airways resulting in even more reduced oxygenation.

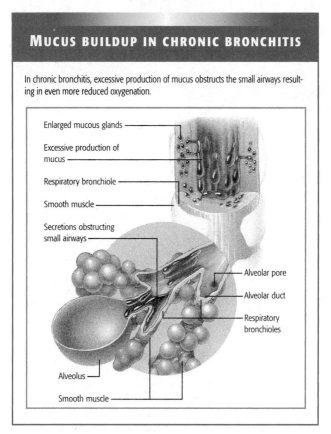

blocked airway. As the inflammation continues, changes in the cells lining the respiratory tract increase resistance in the small airways, and severe imbalance in the ventilation-perfusion ($\dot{V}/\dot{Q}$) ratio decreases arterial oxygenation.

Chronic bronchitis causes hypertrophy of airway smooth muscle and hyperplasia of the mucus glands, increased number of goblet cells, ciliary damage, squamous metaplasia of the columnar epithelium, and chronic leukocytic and lymphocytic infiltration of bronchial walls. Hypersecretion of the goblet cells blocks the free movement of the cilia, which normally sweep dust, irritants, and mucus away from the airways. Accumulating mucus and debris impair the defenses and increase the likelihood of respiratory tract infections. (See *Mucus buildup in chronic bronchitis.*)

Additional effects include narrowing and widespread inflammation within the airways. Bronchial walls become inflamed and thickened from edema and accumulation of inflammatory cells, and smooth-muscle bronchospasm further narrows the lumen. Initially, only large bronchi are involved, but eventually all airways are affected. Airways become obstructed and close, especially on expiration, trapping the gas in the distal portion of the lung. Consequent hypoventilation leads to a $\dot{V}/\dot{Q}$ mismatch and resultant hypoxemia and hypercapnia.

Complications
■ Recurrent respiratory tract infection
■ Cor pulmonale
■ Polycythemia

Assessment findings
The clinical effects of chronic bronchitis may include:
■ insidious onset with progressive cough and exertional dyspnea
■ upper respiratory infections associated with increased sputum production and worsening dyspnea, which takes progressively longer to resolve; copious gray, white, or yellow sputum
■ weight gain due to edema
■ cyanosis
■ tachypnea
■ prolonged expiratory time and use of accessory muscles of respiration.

Diagnostic test results
■ Arterial blood gas (ABG) analysis may show decreased partial pressure of arterial oxygen and normal or increased partial pressure of arterial carbon dioxide.
■ Chest X-ray may show hyperinflation and increased bronchovascular markings.

- Electrocardiogram may show atrial arrhythmias; peaked P waves in leads II, III, and aV_F; and, occasionally, right ventricular hypertrophy.
- Pulmonary function tests show increased residual volume, decreased vital capacity and forced expiratory volumes, and normal static compliance and diffusing capacity.

Treatment

Antibiotics are given to treat infections. Avoidance of smoking and air pollutants is strongly recommended. Bronchodilators are given to relieve bronchospasm and facilitate mucociliary clearance. The patient will require adequate fluid intake and chest physiotherapy to move secretions. Ultrasonic or mechanical nebulizer treatments may be needed to loosen secretions and aid in mobilization. The patient may occasionally require corticosteroids. Diuretics may be given for edema. Oxygen will be given to the patient with hypoxemia or cor pulmonale.

Nursing interventions

- Answer the patient's questions, and encourage him and his family to express their concerns about the illness. Include the patient and his family in care decisions. Refer them to other support services, as appropriate.
- Assess for changes in baseline respiratory function. Evaluate sputum quality and quantity, restlessness, increased tachypnea, and altered breath sounds. Report changes immediately.
- As needed, perform chest physiotherapy, including postural drainage and chest percussion and vibration for involved lobes, several times daily.
- Weigh the patient three times per week, and assess for edema.
- Provide the patient with a high-calorie, protein-rich diet. Offer small, frequent meals to conserve the patient's energy and prevent fatigue.
- Make sure the patient receives adequate fluids (at least 3 qt [3 L]/day) to loosen secretions.
- Schedule respiratory therapy at least 1 hour before or after meals. Provide mouth care after bronchodilator inhalation therapy.

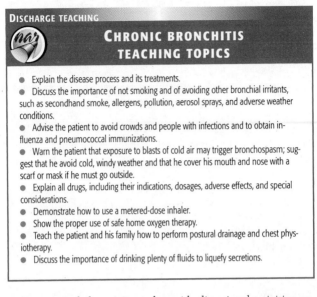

DISCHARGE TEACHING

CHRONIC BRONCHITIS TEACHING TOPICS

- Explain the disease process and its treatments.
- Discuss the importance of not smoking and of avoiding other bronchial irritants, such as secondhand smoke, allergens, pollution, aerosol sprays, and adverse weather conditions.
- Advise the patient to avoid crowds and people with infections and to obtain influenza and pneumococcal immunizations.
- Warn the patient that exposure to blasts of cold air may trigger bronchospasm; suggest that he avoid cold, windy weather and that he cover his mouth and nose with a scarf or mask if he must go outside.
- Explain all drugs, including their indications, dosages, adverse effects, and special considerations.
- Demonstrate how to use a metered-dose inhaler.
- Show the proper use of safe home oxygen therapy.
- Teach the patient and his family how to perform postural drainage and chest physiotherapy.
- Discuss the importance of drinking plenty of fluids to liquefy secretions.

▦ Encourage daily activity, and provide diversional activities, as appropriate. To conserve the patient's energy and prevent fatigue, help him to alternate periods of rest and activity.

▦ Give medications as ordered, and note the patient's response to them. (See *Chronic bronchitis teaching topics*.)

CYSTIC FIBROSIS

Cystic fibrosis is a chronic, progressive, inherited disease that affects the exocrine (mucus-secreting) glands. The disease is transmitted as an autosomal recessive trait and is the most common fatal genetic disease of white children. When both parents are carriers of the recessive gene, they have a 25% chance of transmitting the disease with each pregnancy.

The incidence of cystic fibrosis is highest in people of northern European ancestry. The disease is less common in Blacks, Native Americans, and people of Asian ancestry. It occurs with equal frequency in both sexes.

Cystic fibrosis is incurable; however, medical research is underway to find better treatments. Life expectancy has greatly increased; it's now about 32 years.

Pathophysiology

The gene responsible for cystic fibrosis, located on chromosome 7, encodes a membrane-associated protein called the cystic fibrosis transmembrane conductance regulator protein. The exact function of this protein remains unknown, but it appears to help regulate chloride transport across epithelial membranes. The immediate causes of symptoms are increased viscosity of bronchial, pancreatic, and other mucous gland secretions and consequent destruction of glandular ducts. Cystic fibrosis accounts for almost all cases of pancreatic enzyme deficiency in children.

Complications

- Bronchiectasis
- Pneumonia
- Atelectasis
- Hemoptysis
- Dehydration
- Distal intestinal obstructive syndrome
- Malnutrition
- Fat-soluble vitamin deficiency
- Gastroesophageal reflux
- Nasal polyps
- Rectal prolapse
- Cor pulmonale
- Hepatic disease
- Diabetes
- Pneumothorax
- Arthritis
- Pancreatitis
- Cholecystitis
- Hypochloremia
- Hyponatremia
- Clotting problems
- Retarded bone growth
- Delayed sexual development

AGE AWARE

PEDIATRIC SYMPTOMS OF CF

Some children display symptoms of cystic fibrosis (CF) at birth, as in a meconium ileus. A meconium ileus occurs because of a missing enzyme; specifically, the enzyme that moistens and makes all body fluids free-flowing. This results in the production of thick, tenacious meconium. In other children, CF isn't diagnosed until weeks, months, or even years after birth. Some children may have a mild form of the disease, whereas others have extensive digestive and pulmonary involvement.

Children with CF commonly display a barrel chest, cyanosis, and clubbing of the fingers and toes. They suffer recurring bronchitis and pneumonia, with associated nasal polyps and sinusitis. Death typically results from pneumonia, emphysema, or atelectasis.

Assessment findings

The clinical effects of cystic fibrosis may become apparent soon after birth or may take years to develop. They include major aberrations in sweat gland, respiratory, and GI functions.

- Hyponatremia and hypochloremia
- Wheezing
- Dry, nonproductive, paroxysmal cough
- Dyspnea
- Tachypnea
- Barrel chest
- Cyanosis
- Clubbing of the fingers and toes
- Recurring bronchitis and pneumonia
- Nasal polyps and sinusitis
- Meconium ileus (abdominal distention, vomiting, constipation, dehydration, and electrolyte imbalance) (see *Pediatric symptoms of CF*)
- Frequent, bulky, foul-smelling, and pale stool with a high fat content
- Poor growth
- Poor weight gain
- Ravenous appetite
- Distended abdomen
- Thin extremities
- Sallow skin with poor turgor

- Deficiency of fat-soluble vitamins (A, D, E, and K)
- Clotting problems

Diagnostic test results

According to the Cystic Fibrosis Foundation, a definitive diagnosis requires:

- two clearly positive sweat tests using pilocarpine solution (a sweat inducer) and the presence of an obstructive pulmonary disease-confirmed pancreatic insufficiency or failure to thrive or a family history of cystic fibrosis
- chest X-rays that show early signs of lung obstruction
- stool specimen analysis that shows the absence of trypsin, suggesting pancreatic insufficiency.

These test results may support the diagnosis:

- Deoxyribonucleic acid testing can now locate the presence of the Delta F 508 deletion (found in about 70% of patients with cystic fibrosis, although the disease is caused by more than 800 different mutations). This test can also be used for carrier detection and prenatal diagnosis in families with a previously affected child.
- Liver enzyme tests may reveal hepatic insufficiency.
- If pulmonary exacerbation exists, pulmonary function tests can reveal decreased vital capacity, elevated residual volume due to air entrapments, and decreased forced expiratory volume in 1 second.
- Serum albumin levels help to assess nutritional status, and electrolyte analysis is used to assess for dehydration.
- Sputum cultures may reveal organisms that patients typically and chronically colonize, such as *Pseudomonas* and *Staphylococcus*.

Treatment

Because cystic fibrosis has no cure, the goal of treatment is to help the patient lead as normal a life as possible. Specific treatments depend on the organ systems involved.

To combat electrolyte loss through sweat, the patient should generously salt his food and, during hot weather, take salt supplements.

Taking oral pancreatic enzymes with meals and snacks offsets pancreatic enzyme deficiencies. Such supplements improve absorption and digestion and help satisfy hunger on a reasonable caloric intake. The patient should also follow a diet high in fat, protein, and calories and that includes vitamin A, D, E, and K supplements.

To manage pulmonary dysfunction, the patient should undergo chest physiotherapy, nebulization to loosen secretions followed by postural drainage, and breathing exercises several times daily to help remove lung secretions. However, he shouldn't receive antihistamines, which dry mucous membranes, making mucus expectoration difficult. Oxygen therapy is used as needed.

Dornase alfa (Pulmozyme), a pulmonary enzyme given by aerosol nebulizer, helps to thin airway mucus, improving lung function and reducing the risk of pulmonary infection.

A patient with pulmonary infection needs to loosen and remove mucopurulent secretions by using intermittent nebulizer and postural drainage to relieve obstruction. Broad-spectrum antibiotics are used to control infection. Lung transplantation may reduce the effects of the disease.

Nursing interventions

- Give drugs as ordered. Give pancreatic enzymes with meals and snacks.
- Perform chest physiotherapy, including postural drainage and chest percussion designed for all lobes, several times a day, as ordered.
- Give oxygen therapy, as ordered. Check arterial oxygen saturation levels using pulse oximetry.
- Provide a well-balanced, high-calorie, high-protein diet. Include plenty of fats, which, though difficult for the patient to digest, are nutritionally necessary. Give him enzyme capsules to help combat most of the effects of fat malabsorption. Include vitamin A, D, E, and K supplements if laboratory analysis indicates deficiencies.
- Make sure the patient receives plenty of liquids to prevent dehydration, especially in warm weather.
- Provide exercise and activity periods for the patient to promote health. Encourage him to perform breathing exercises to help improve his ventilation.

DISCHARGE TEACHING

CYSTIC FIBROSIS TEACHING TOPICS

- Inform the patient and his family about the disease, and thoroughly explain treatment measures. Make sure they know about tests that can determine if family members carry the cystic fibrosis gene.
- Teach the patient and his family about the medications the patient may be receiving. Explain possible adverse reactions, and urge them to notify the physician if these reactions occur.
- Instruct the patient and his family about aerosol therapy, including intermittent nebulizer treatments before postural drainage. Tell them that these treatments help to loosen secretions and dilate the bronchi.
- Instruct the patient's family about proper methods of chest physiotherapy.
- If the physician prescribes aerobic exercises, teach the patient how to do them, and review their importance in maintaining respiratory muscle and cardiopulmonary function and in improving activity tolerance.
- Teach the patient and his family signs of infection and sudden changes in the patient's condition that they should report to the physician. These include increased coughing, decreased appetite, sputum that thickens or contains blood, shortness of breath, and chest pain.
- Advise the parents of a child with the disease not to be overly protective. Instead, help them explore ways to enhance their child's quality of life and to foster responsibility and independence in him from an early age. Stress the importance of good communication so that the child may express his fears and concerns.
- Encourage participation in local groups, such as the Cystic Fibrosis Foundation, to help meet patient and family needs.

- Provide the young child with play periods, and enlist the help of the physical therapy department. Some pediatric facilities have play therapists who provide essential play time for young patients.
- Provide emotional support to the parents of children with cystic fibrosis. Because it's an inherited disease, the parents may feel enormous guilt. Encourage them to discuss their fears and concerns, and answer their questions as honestly as possible.
- Be flexible with care and visiting hours during hospitalization to allow the child to continue schoolwork and friendships.
- Include the family in all phases of the child's care. If the child is an adolescent, he may want to perform much of his own treatment protocol. Encourage him to do so. (See *Cystic fibrosis teaching topics*.)

EMPHYSEMA

Emphysema is one of several diseases labeled as chronic obstructive pulmonary disease. It's the most common cause of death from respiratory disease in the United States. Emphysema is more prevalent in men than in women; approximately 2 million Americans are affected with the disease. Postmortem findings reveal few adult lungs without some degree of emphysema.

Emphysema may be caused by a genetic deficiency of alpha$_1$-antitrypsin (AAT) and by cigarette smoking. Genetically, 1 in 3,000 neonates is found with the disease, and 1% to 3% of all cases of emphysema are the result of AAT deficiency. Cigarette smoking and exposure to secondhand smoke are primary causes of emphysema. Other causative factors include air pollution, genetic abnormalities, and occupational irritants.

Primary emphysema has been linked to an inherited deficiency of the enzyme AAT, a major component of alpha$_1$-globulin. AAT inhibits the activation of several proteolytic enzymes; deficiency of this enzyme is an autosomal recessive trait that predisposes an individual to develop emphysema because proteolysis in lung tissues isn't inhibited. Homozygous individuals have up to an 80% chance of developing lung disease; people who smoke have a greater chance of developing emphysema. Patients who develop emphysema before or during their early 40s and those who are nonsmokers are believed to have an AAT deficiency.

Pathophysiology

In emphysema, recurrent inflammation is associated with the release of proteolytic enzymes from lung cells. This causes irreversible enlargement of the air spaces distal to the terminal bronchioles. Enlargement of air spaces destroys the alveolar walls, which results in breakdown of elasticity and loss of fibrous and muscle tissue, thus making the lungs less compliant.

In normal breathing, the air moves into and out of the lungs to meet metabolic needs. A change in airway size compromises the lung's ability to circulate sufficient air. In patient's with emphysema, recurrent pulmonary inflammation damages and

AIR TRAPPING IN EMPHYSEMA

After alveolar walls are damaged or destroyed, they can't support the airways and keep them open. The alveolar walls then lose their elastic recoil capability. Collapse then occurs on expiration.

Normal expiration
Normal expiration, as shown here, involves normal recoil and an open bronchiole.

Impaired expiration
Impaired expiration, as shown here, involves decreased elastic recoil and a narrowed bronchiole.

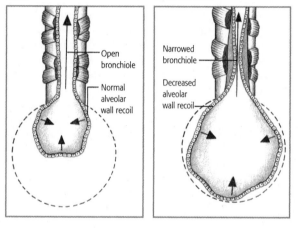

Open bronchiole

Normal alveolar wall recoil

Narrowed bronchiole

Decreased alveolar wall recoil

eventually destroys the alveolar walls, creating large air spaces. (See *Air trapping in emphysema*.)

The alveolar septa are initially destroyed, eliminating a portion of the capillary bed and increasing air volume in the acinus. This breakdown leaves the alveoli unable to recoil normally after expanding and results in bronchiolar collapse on expiration. The damaged or destroyed alveolar walls can't support the airways to keep them open.

The amount of air that can be expired is passively diminished, thus trapping air in the lungs and leading to overdistention. Hyperinflation of the alveoli produces bullae (air spaces) adjacent to pleura (blebs). Septal destruction also decreases airway calibration. Part of each inspiration is trapped because of increased residual volume and decreased calibration. Septal destruction may affect only the respiratory bronchioles and alveolar ducts, leaving alveolar sacs intact, or it can involve the entire acinus with damage more random and involving the lower lobes of the lungs.

Complications
- Recurrent respiratory tract infections
- Cor pulmonale
- Respiratory failure
- Spontaneous pneumothorax
- Pneumomediastinum

Assessment findings
- The patient's history may reveal that he's a long-time smoker.
- The patient may report shortness of breath and a chronic cough.
- The patient's history may also reveal anorexia with resultant weight loss and a general feeling of malaise.
- Inspection may show a barrel-chested patient who breathes through pursed lips and uses accessory muscles.
- You may notice peripheral cyanosis, clubbed fingers and toes, and tachypnea.
- Palpation may reveal decreased tactile fremitus and decreased chest expansion.
- Percussion may detect hyperresonance.
- On auscultation, you may hear decreased breath sounds, crackles, and wheezing during inspiration, a prolonged expiratory phase with grunting respirations, and distant heart sounds.

AGE AWARE Age-related changes in the respiratory system can worsen the symptoms of emphysema. Decreased peak airflow, gas exchange, and vital capacity can increase shortness of breath experienced by the patient as he ages. These changes can be complicated by smoking, which speeds up the process of aging in the lungs and further worsens symptoms. What's more, defense mechanisms in the lungs and immune system decrease, increasing the aging person's risk of pneumonia after bacterial or viral infection.

Diagnostic test results

- Arterial blood gas analysis usually shows reduced partial pressure of arterial oxygen and normal partial pressure of arterial carbon dioxide ($PaCO_2$) until late in the disease, when $PaCO_2$ increases significantly.
- Chest X-rays in advanced disease may show a flattened diaphragm, reduced vascular markings at the lung periphery, overaeration of the lungs, a vertical heart, an enlarged anteroposterior chest diameter, and a large retrosternal air space.
- Electrocardiography may reveal tall, symmetrical P waves in leads II, III, and aV_F; a vertical QRS axis; and signs of right ventricular hypertrophy late in the disease.
- Pulmonary function tests typically indicate increased residual volume and total lung capacity, reduced diffusing capacity, increased inspiratory flow, and decreased forced expiratory volume in 1 second and forced vital capacity.
- Red blood cell count usually demonstrates an increased hemoglobin level (polycythemia) late in the disease when the patient has persistent severe hypoxia.

Treatment

Emphysema management usually includes bronchodilators, such as aminophylline (Truphylline), to promote mucociliary clearance, antibiotics to treat respiratory tract infection, and immunizations to prevent influenza and pneumococcal pneumonia. Diuretics may be given for edema.

Other treatment measures include adequate hydration (in selected patients) and chest physiotherapy to mobilize secretions. Ultrasonic mechanical nebulizer treatments may be needed to loosen secretions and aid in mobilization.

Some patients may require oxygen therapy (at low settings) to correct hypoxia. They may also require transtracheal catheterization to receive oxygen at home. Counseling about avoiding smoking and air pollutants is necessary. Surgery may include bullectomy, lung volume reduction, or lung transplantation.

Nursing interventions

- Provide supportive care, and help the patient adjust to lifestyle changes resulting from a chronic illness.

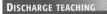

EMPHYSEMA TEACHING TOPICS

- Explain the disease process and treatments.
- Urge the patient to avoid inhaled irritants, such as automobile exhaust fumes, aerosol sprays, and industrial pollutants.
- Advise the patient to avoid crowds and people with infections and to obtain annual pneumonia and flu vaccines.
- Warn the patient that exposure to blasts of cold air may trigger bronchospasm; suggest that he avoid cold, windy weather and that he cover his mouth and nose with a scarf or mask if he must go outside in such conditions.
- Explain all drugs, including their indications, dosages, adverse effects, and special considerations.
- Inform the patient about signs and symptoms that suggest ruptured alveolar blebs and bullae, and urge him to seek immediate medical attention if they occur.
- Demonstrate how to use a metered-dose inhaler.
- Teach the safe use of home oxygen therapy.
- Teach the patient and his family how to perform postural drainage and chest physiotherapy.
- Discuss the importance of drinking plenty of fluids to liquefy secretions.
- For family members of a patient with familial emphysema, recommend a blood test for alpha$_1$-antitrypsin. If a deficiency is found, stress the importance of not smoking and avoiding areas where smoking is permitted.

- Answer the patient's questions about his illness as honestly as possible. Encourage him to express his fears and concerns about his illness. Remain with him during periods of extreme stress and anxiety. (See *Emphysema teaching topics.*)
- Include the patient and his family in care-related decisions. Refer the patient to appropriate support services as needed.
- If ordered, perform chest physiotherapy, including postural drainage and chest percussion and vibration, several times daily.
- Provide the patient with a high-calorie, protein-rich diet to promote health and healing. Give small, frequent meals to conserve energy and prevent fatigue.
- Schedule respiratory treatments at least 1 hour before or after meals. Provide mouth care after bronchodilator therapy.
- Make sure the patient receives adequate fluids (at least 3 qt [3 L]/day) to loosen secretions.

- Encourage daily activity, and provide diversionary activities, as appropriate. To conserve energy and prevent fatigue, have the patient alternate periods of rest and activity.
- Give medications, as ordered. Record the patient's response to these medications.
- Watch for complications, such as respiratory tract infections, cor pulmonale, spontaneous pneumothorax, respiratory failure, and peptic ulcer disease.

Restrictive disorders

Restrictive disorders affect the interstitium of the lungs (alveoli, blood vessels, and surrounding tissues). In restrictive disorders, a decrease in the lung capacity results from the inability of the lungs to expand and relax at the rate and completeness the diaphragm and intercostal muscles demand. With restrictive pulmonary disease, thickening of the lung tissues can occur and will result in a decrease in arterial oxygen levels.

Restrictive disorders reduce vital capacity and the functional residual capacity, but airflow remains normal. Conditions such as pulmonary fibrosis damage lung tissue and result in loss of elasticity. Typically, the onset of these disorders is slow and insidious, and dyspnea is the most common symptom.

Restrictive disorders include acute respiratory distress syndrome, acute respiratory failure, asbestosis, asthma, atelectasis, berylliosis, coal workers' pneumoconiosis, idiopathic pulmonary fibrosis, respiratory distress syndrome, sarcoidosis, and silicosis.

ACUTE RESPIRATORY DISTRESS SYNDROME

Acute respiratory distress syndrome (ARDS) is a form of pulmonary edema that can quickly lead to acute respiratory failure. It's also known as *shock, stiff, white, wet,* or *Da Nang lung.* It may follow direct or indirect lung injury.

Trauma is the most common cause of ARDS. Trauma-related factors, such as fat emboli, sepsis, shock, pulmonary contusions,

AGE AWARE

ARDS IN CHILDREN

Acute respiratory distress syndrome (ARDS) is a significant cause of mortality in children. Children at risk for ARDS include those with infections that cause fluid accumulation in the lungs. Children with any type of lung infection should receive prompt treatment to avoid this serious condition.

traumatic tissue injury, and multiple transfusions increase the likelihood of microemboli developing.

Other common causes of ARDS include anaphylaxis, aspiration of gastric contents, diffuse pneumonia (especially viral), drug overdose (for example, heroin, aspirin, and ethchlorvynol), idiosyncratic drug reaction (to ampicillin and hydrochlorothiazide [HydroDIURIL]), inhalation of noxious gases (such as nitrous oxide, ammonia, and chlorine), near-drowning, and ventilator-induced oxygen toxicity.

Less common causes of ARDS include coronary artery bypass grafting, hemodialysis, leukemia, acute miliary tuberculosis, pancreatitis, thrombotic thrombocytopenic purpura, uremia, and venous air embolism. (See *ARDS in children*.)

Pathophysiology

Increased permeability of the alveolocapillary membranes allows fluid to accumulate in the lung interstitium, alveolar spaces, and small airways, causing the lung to stiffen. This impairs ventilation, reducing oxygenation of pulmonary capillary blood. The disorder is difficult to recognize and can prove fatal within 48 hours of onset if not promptly diagnosed and treated. (See *What happens in ARDS*.)

This four-stage syndrome can progress to intractable and fatal hypoxemia; however, patients who recover may have little or no permanent lung damage.

In some patients, the syndrome may coexist with disseminated intravascular coagulation (DIC). It remains unclear whether ARDS stems from DIC or develops independently. Patients with three concurrent ARDS risk factors have an 85% probability of developing ARDS.

WHAT HAPPENS IN ARDS

These illustrations depict the process and progress of acute respiratory distress syndrome (ARDS).

1. The body responds to insult.

Injury reduces normal blood flow to the lungs, allowing platelets to aggregate. These platelets release such substances as serotonin (S), bradykinin (B) and, especially, histamine (H) that inflame and damage the alveolar membrane and later increase capillary permeability. At this early stage, signs and symptoms of ARDS are undetectable.

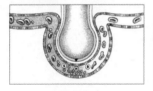

2. Fluid shift causes symptoms.

Increased capillary permeability allows fluid to shift into the interstitial space. As a result, the patient may experience tachypnea, dyspnea, and tachycardia.

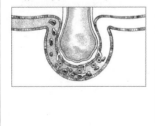

3. Pulmonary edema results.

As capillary permeability continues to increase, shifting of proteins and fluid increases interstitial osmotic pressure and causes pulmonary edema. At this stage, the patient may experience increased tachypnea, dyspnea, and cyanosis. Hypoxia (usually unresponsive to increased fraction of inspired oxygen), decreased pulmonary compliance, and crackles and rhonchi may also develop.

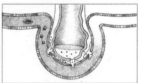

4. Alveoli collapse.

Fluid in the alveoli and decreased blood flow damage surfactant in the alveoli, reducing the cells' ability to produce more surfactant. Without surfactant, alveoli collapse, impairing gas exchange. Look for thick, frothy sputum and marked hypoxemia with increased respiratory distress.

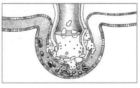

(continued)

WHAT HAPPENS IN **ARDS** *(continued)*

5. Gas exchange slows.

The patient breathes faster, but sufficient oxygen (O_2) can't cross the alveolocapillary membrane. Carbon dioxide (CO_2), however, crosses more easily and is lost with every exhalation. Both O_2 and CO_2 levels in the blood decrease. Look for increased tachypnea, hypoxemia, and hypocapnia.

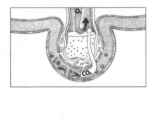

6. Metabolic acidosis occurs.

Pulmonary edema worsens. Meanwhile, inflammation leads to fibrosis, which further impedes gas exchange. The resulting hypoxemia leads to metabolic acidosis. At this stage, look for increased partial pressure of arterial carbon dioxide; decreased bicarbonate level, pH, and partial pressure of arterial oxygen; and mental confusion.

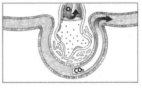

Complications
- Metabolic and respiratory acidosis
- Respiratory and cardiac arrest

Assessment findings
As you conduct your assessment, be alert for the patient's particular stage of ARDS. Each has its typical signs and symptoms.

STAGE I
- The patient may complain of dyspnea, especially on exertion.
- Respiratory and pulse rates are normal to high.
- Auscultation may reveal diminished breath sounds.

STAGE II
- Respiratory distress becomes more apparent.
- The patient may use accessory muscles to breathe and may appear pallid, anxious, and restless.

- He may have a dry cough with thick, frothy sputum and bloody, sticky secretions.
- Palpation may disclose cool, clammy skin.
- Tachycardia and tachypnea may accompany elevated blood pressure.
- He may have a change or decrease in mental status.
- Auscultation may reveal basilar crackles. (Stage II signs and symptoms may be incorrectly attributed to other causes such as multiple traumas.)
- The patient needs intubation and ventilation.

STAGE III

- The patient struggles to breathe.
- Vital signs reveal tachypnea (more than 30 breaths/minute), tachycardia with arrhythmias (usually premature ventricular contractions), and a labile blood pressure. Inspection may reveal a productive cough and pale, cyanotic skin.
- He may demonstrate a change or decrease in mental status. Auscultation may disclose crackles and rhonchi.

STAGE IV

- Acute respiratory failure with severe hypoxia occurs.
- The patient's mental status deteriorates, and he may become comatose.
- His skin appears pale and cyanotic.
- Spontaneous respirations aren't evident. Bradycardia with arrhythmias accompanies hypotension.
- Metabolic acidosis and respiratory acidosis develop.
- When ARDS reaches this stage, the patient is at high risk for fibrosis.
- Pulmonary damage becomes life-threatening.

Diagnostic test results

- Arterial blood gas (ABG) analysis (with the patient breathing room air) initially shows a reduced partial pressure of arterial oxygen (PaO_2) of less than 60 mm Hg and a decreased partial pressure of arterial carbon dioxide ($PaCO_2$) of less than 35 mm Hg. Hypoxemia despite increased supplemental oxygen is the hallmark of ARDS. The resulting blood pH usually reflects respiratory alkalosis. As ARDS worsens, ABG values show respiratory acidosis (increasing $PaCO_2$ [greater than 45 mm Hg]) and metabolic acidosis (decreasing bicarbonate levels [less than 22 mEq/L]) and declining PaO_2 despite oxygen therapy. The PaO_2 to fraction of inspired oxygen ratio is 200 mm Hg or less, regardless of the positive end-expiratory pressure (PEEP) level.

- Differential diagnosis must rule out cardiogenic pulmonary edema, pulmonary vasculitis, and diffuse pulmonary hemorrhage. Etiologic tests may involve sputum analyses (including Gram stain and culture and sensitivity), blood cultures (to identify infectious organisms), toxicology tests (to screen for drug ingestion), and various serum amylase tests (to rule out pancreatitis).
- Pulmonary artery catheterization helps to identify the cause of pulmonary edema by measuring pulmonary artery wedge pressure (PAWP). This procedure also allows the collection of samples of pulmonary artery and mixed venous blood that shows decreased oxygen saturation, reflecting tissue hypoxia. Normal PAWP values in ARDS are 12 mm Hg or less.
- Serial chest X-rays in early stages show bilateral infiltrates. In later stages, findings demonstrate lung fields with a ground-glass appearance and, eventually (with irreversible hypoxemia), "whiteouts" of both lung fields.

Treatment

Therapy focuses on correcting the cause of ARDS, if possible, and preventing the progression of life-threatening hypoxemia and respiratory acidosis. Supportive care consists of giving humidified oxygen through a tightly fitting mask, which facilitates the use of continuous positive airway pressure (CPAP). However, this therapy alone seldom fulfills the patient's ventilatory requirements. If the patient's hypoxemia doesn't subside with this treatment, he may require intubation, mechanical ventilation, and PEEP. Prevention of health care–related infections is also important. Other supportive measures include fluid restriction, diuretic therapy, and correction of electrolyte and acid-base imbalances.

When a patient with ARDS needs mechanical ventilation, sedatives, opioids, or neuromuscular blockers (such as vecuronium [Norcuron]) may be ordered to minimize restlessness (and thereby oxygen consumption and carbon dioxide production) and facilitate ventilation.

When ARDS results from fatty emboli or a chemical injury, a short course of high-dose corticosteroids may help if given early. Treatment with sodium bicarbonate may be necessary to reverse severe metabolic acidosis, and fluids and vasopressors may be needed to maintain blood pressure. Nonviral infections require treatment with antimicrobial drugs.

Nursing interventions

- Frequently assess the patient's respiratory status. Be alert for inspiratory retractions. Note respiratory rate, rhythm, and depth. Watch for dyspnea and accessory muscle use. Listen for adventitious or diminished breath sounds. Check for clear, frothy sputum (indicating pulmonary edema).
- Evaluate and document the patient's level of consciousness, noting confusion or mental sluggishness.
- Be alert for signs of treatment-induced complications, including arrhythmias, DIC, GI bleeding, infection, malnutrition, paralytic ileus, pneumothorax, pulmonary fibrosis, renal failure, thrombocytopenia, and tracheal stenosis.
- Maintain a patent airway by suctioning. Use sterile, nontraumatic technique. Ensure adequate humidification to help liquefy tenacious secretions.
- Closely monitor heart rate and blood pressure. Watch for arrhythmias that may result from hypoxemia, acid-base disturbances, or electrolyte imbalance.
- With pulmonary artery catheterization, know the desired PAWP level; check readings often, and watch for decreasing mixed venous oxygen saturation. Change dressings according to facility guidelines, using strict aseptic technique.
- Monitor serum electrolyte levels, and correct imbalances. Measure intake and output. Weigh the patient daily.
- Check ventilator settings frequently; drain condensation from the tubing promptly to ensure maximum oxygen delivery. Monitor ABG levels; document and report changes in arterial

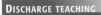
oxygen saturation as well as metabolic and respiratory acidosis and PaO_2 changes.

■ Be ready to provide CPAP to the patient with severe hypoxemia.

■ Give sedatives, as ordered, to reduce restlessness. Monitor and record the patient's response to medication.

RED FLAG Because PEEP may lower cardiac output, check for hypotension, tachycardia, and decreased urine output. To maintain PEEP, suction only as needed. High-frequency jet ventilation and pressure-controlled ventilation may also be required.

■ Reposition the patient often. Proning—maintaining the patient in a prone position for 6 or more hours per day—may be used to improve ventilation-perfusion mismatch.

■ Record an increase in secretions, temperature, or hypotension that may indicate a deteriorating condition.

■ Monitor the patient's nutritional intake, and record caloric intake. Give tube feedings and parenteral nutrition as ordered. Plan patient care to allow periods of uninterrupted sleep. To promote health and prevent fatigue, arrange for alternate periods of rest and activity.

■ Maintain joint mobility by performing passive range-of-motion (ROM) exercises. If possible, help the patient perform active ROM exercises.

■ Provide meticulous skin care. To prevent skin breakdown, reposition the endotracheal tube from side to side every 24 hours.

- Provide emotional support. Answer the patient's and family's questions as completely as possible to allay their fears and concerns.
- Watch for and immediately report all respiratory changes in the patient with injuries that may adversely affect the lungs—especially in the first few days after the injury when the patient's condition may appear to be improving.
- Provide alternative communication means for the patient on mechanical ventilation. (See *ARDS teaching topics.*)

ACUTE RESPIRATORY FAILURE

When the lungs can't adequately maintain arterial oxygenation or eliminate carbon dioxide, acute respiratory failure occurs. If not checked and treated, the condition leads to tissue hypoxia. In patients with essentially normal lung tissue, acute respiratory failure usually produces a partial pressure of arterial carbon dioxide ($PaCO_2$) greater than 50 mm Hg and a partial pressure of arterial oxygen (PaO_2) less than 50 mm Hg.

These limits, however, don't apply to patients with chronic obstructive pulmonary disease (COPD). These patients consistently have high $PaCO_2$ (hypercapnia) and low PaO_2 (hypoxemia) levels. For patients with COPD, only acute deterioration in arterial blood gas (ABG) values and corresponding clinical deterioration signal acute respiratory failure.

Pathophysiology

Respiratory failure results from impaired gas exchange. Conditions associated with alveolar hypoventilation, ventilation-perfusion mismatch, and intrapulmonary (right-to-left) shunting can cause acute respiratory failure if left untreated. Acute respiratory failure may develop in patients with COPD from any condition that increases the work of breathing and decreases the respiratory drive. These conditions can result from respiratory tract infection (such as bronchitis or pneumonia), bronchospasm, or accumulated secretions secondary to cough suppression. Other common causes are related to ventilatory failure, in which the brain fails to direct respiration, and gas exchange fail-

UP CLOSE

WHAT HAPPENS IN ACUTE RESPIRATORY FAILURE

Three major malfunctions account for impaired gas exchange and subsequent acute respiratory failure: alveolar hypoventilation, ventilation-perfusion ($\dot{V}/\dot{Q}$) mismatch, and intrapulmonary (right-to-left) shunting.

Alveolar hypoventilation

Decreased oxygen saturation may result when chronic airway obstruction reduces alveolar minute ventilation. In such cases, partial pressure of arterial oxygen (PaO_2) levels fall and partial pressure of arterial carbon dioxide levels rise, and hypoxia results.

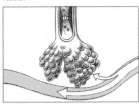

$\dot{V}/\dot{Q}$ mismatch

The most common cause of hypoxemia—imbalances in ventilation and perfusion—occur when conditions such as pulmonary embolism or acute respiratory distress syndrome interrupt normal gas exchange in a specific lung region. Either too little ventilation with normal blood flow or too little blood flow with normal ventilation may cause the imbalance. Whichever happens, the result is the same: PaO_2 levels fall.

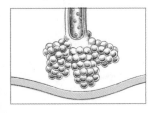

Right-to-left shunting

Untreated ventilation or perfusion imbalances can lead to right-to-left shunting, in which blood passes from the heart's right side to its left without being oxygenated.

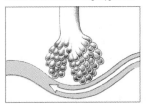

Implications

The hypoxemia and hypercapnia characteristic of respiratory failure stimulate strong compensatory responses by all body systems, including the respiratory, cardiovascular, and central nervous systems.

In response to hypoxemia, for example, the sympathetic nervous system triggers vasoconstriction, increases peripheral resistance, and boosts the heart rate.

The body responds to hypercapnia with cerebral depression, hypotension, circulatory failure, and an increased heartbeat and cardiac output. Hypoxemia or hypercapnia (or both) cause the brain's respiratory control center to first increase respiratory depth (tidal volume) and then increase the respiratory rate. As respiratory failure worsens, intercostal, supraclavicular, and suprasternal retractions may also occur.

CAUSES OF RESPIRATORY FAILURE

Problems with the brain, lungs, muscles and nerves, or pulmonary circulation can impair gas exchange and cause respiratory failure. Here's a list of conditions that can cause respiratory failure.

Brain
- Anesthesia
- Cerebral hemorrhage
- Cerebral tumor
- Drug overdose
- Head trauma
- Skull fracture

Lungs
- Acute respiratory distress syndrome
- Asthma
- Chronic obstructive pulmonary disease
- Cystic fibrosis
- Flail chest
- Massive bilateral pneumonia
- Sleep apnea
- Tracheal obstruction

Muscles and nerves
- Amyotrophic lateral sclerosis
- Guillain-Barré syndrome
- Multiple sclerosis
- Muscular dystrophy
- Myasthenia gravis
- Polio
- Spinal cord trauma

Pulmonary circulation
- Heart failure
- Pulmonary edema
- Pulmonary embolism

ure, in which respiratory structures fail to function properly. (See *What happens in acute respiratory failure*.)

Other causes of acute respiratory failure include:
- airway irritants, such as smoke or fumes
- cardiovascular disorders (myocardial infarction, heart failure, or pulmonary emboli)
- central nervous system depression owing to head trauma or injudicious use of sedatives, opioids, tranquilizers, or oxygen
- endocrine or metabolic disorders, such as myxedema or metabolic acidosis
- thoracic abnormalities, such as chest trauma, pneumothorax, or thoracic or abdominal surgery
- noncompliance with prescribed bronchodilator or corticosteroid therapy. (See *Causes of respiratory failure*.)

Complications

- Tissue hypoxia
- Metabolic acidosis
- Respiratory and cardiac arrest

Assessment findings

Because acute respiratory failure in COPD is life-threatening, you probably don't have time to conduct an in-depth patient interview. Instead, rely on family members or the patient's medical records to discover the precipitating incident.

- On inspection, note cyanosis of the oral mucosa, lips, and nail beds; nasal flaring; and ashen skin.
- You may observe the patient yawning and using accessory muscles to breathe.
- He may appear restless, anxious, depressed, lethargic, agitated, confused, or combative.
- The patient usually exhibits tachypnea, which signals impending respiratory failure.
- Palpation may reveal cold, clammy skin and asymmetrical chest movement, which suggests pneumothorax.
- If tactile fremitus is present, notice that it decreases over an obstructed bronchi or pleural effusion and increases over consolidated lung tissue.
- Percussion—especially in patients with COPD—reveals hyperresonance.
- If acute respiratory failure results from atelectasis or pneumonia, percussion usually produces a dull or flat sound.
- Auscultation typically reveals diminished breath sounds.
- In patients with pneumothorax, breath sounds may be absent. In other cases of respiratory failure, you may hear such adventitious breath sounds as wheezes (in asthma) and rhonchi (in bronchitis).
- If you hear crackles, suspect pulmonary edema as the cause of respiratory failure. (See *Identifying respiratory failure*.)

Diagnostic test results

- ABG analysis is the key to the diagnosis (and subsequent treatment) of acute respiratory failure. Progressively deteriorating ABG values and pH compared with the patient's nor-

IDENTIFYING RESPIRATORY FAILURE

Use the following measurements to identify respiratory failure:
- Vital capacity less than 15 ml/kg
- Tidal volume less than 3 ml/kg
- Negative inspiratory force less than −25 cm H_2O
- Respiratory rate more than twice the normal rate
- Diminished partial pressure of arterial oxygen despite increased fraction of inspired oxygen
- Elevated partial pressure of arterial carbon dioxide with pH less than 7.25

mal values strongly suggest acute respiratory failure. In the patient with essentially normal lung tissue, a pH of less than 7.35 usually indicates acute respiratory failure. In the patient with COPD, the pH deviation from the normal value is even lower.

- Blood tests such as white blood cell count are used to detect underlying causes. Abnormally low hematocrit and decreased hemoglobin level signal blood loss, which indicates decreased oxygen-carrying capacity.
- Chest X-rays are used to identify underlying pulmonary diseases or conditions, such as emphysema, atelectasis, lesions, pneumothorax, infiltrates, and effusions.
- Electrocardiography can demonstrate arrhythmias. Common electrocardiographic patterns point to cor pulmonale and myocardial hypoxia.
- Pulmonary artery catheterization helps to distinguish pulmonary and cardiovascular causes of acute respiratory failure and is used to monitor hemodynamic pressures.
- Pulse oximetry reveals decreasing arterial oxygen saturation but isn't as reliable as ABG analysis.
- Serum electrolyte findings vary. Hypokalemia may result from compensatory hyperventilation, the body's attempt to correct alkalosis; hypochloremia usually occurs in metabolic alkalosis.
- Additional tests, such as blood culture, Gram stain, and sputum culture, may be used to identify the pathogen.

Treatment

Acute respiratory failure in the patient with COPD is an emergency. The patient needs cautious oxygen therapy (nasal prongs or a Venturi mask) to increase his PaO_2. If significant respiratory acidosis persists, mechanical ventilation with an endotracheal (ET) or tracheostomy tube may be needed. High-frequency ventilation may be initiated if the patient doesn't respond to conventional mechanical ventilation. Treatment routinely includes antibiotics (for infection), bronchodilators and, possibly, corticosteroids.

If the patient also has cor pulmonale and decreased cardiac output, fluid restrictions and administration of positive inotropic agents, vasopressors, and diuretics may be ordered.

Nursing interventions

- Orient the patient and his family to the treatment unit. Most patients with acute respiratory failure receive intensive care. Helping the patient understand procedures, sounds, and sights may ease his anxiety.
- To reverse hypoxemia, give oxygen at appropriate concentrations to maintain PaO_2 at a minimum pressure range of 50 to 60 mm Hg. The patient with COPD usually needs only small amounts of supplemental oxygen. Watch for a positive response, such as improved breathing, color, and ABG values.
- Maintain a patent airway. If your patient retains carbon dioxide, encourage him to cough and breathe deeply with pursed lips. If he's alert, have him use an incentive spirometer.
- If he's intubated and lethargic, reposition him every 1 to 2 hours. Use postural drainage and chest physiotherapy to help clear secretions.
- Observe the patient closely for respiratory arrest. Auscultate chest sounds. Monitor ABG values and vital signs, and report changes immediately. Notify the physician of deterioration in oxygen saturation levels detected by pulse oximetry.
- Watch for treatment complications, especially oxygen toxicity and acute respiratory distress syndrome.
- Frequently monitor vital signs. Note and report an increasing pulse rate, increasing or decreasing respiratory rate, declining blood pressure, or febrile state.

- Monitor and record serum electrolyte levels carefully. Take steps to correct imbalances. Monitor fluid balance by recording the patient's intake and output and daily weight.
- Check the cardiac monitor for arrhythmias.
- Perform oral hygiene measures frequently.
- Apply soft wrist restraints for the confused patient, if needed. This prevents him from disconnecting the oxygen setup. However, remember that these restraints can increase anxiety, fear, and agitation.
- Position the patient for comfort and optimal gas exchange. Place the call button within his reach.
- Keep the patient in a normothermic state to reduce the body's demand for oxygen.
- Pace and group patient care activities to maximize the patient's energy level and provide needed rest.

  If the patient requires mechanical ventilation:

- Check ventilator settings, cuff pressures, and ABG values often to ensure correct fraction of inspired oxygen (FIO_2) settings, which are determined by ABG levels. Draw blood samples for ABG analysis 20 to 30 minutes after every change in the FIO_2 setting or as ordered.
- Suction the trachea as needed. Observe for a change in sputum quality, consistency, and color. Provide humidification to liquefy secretions.
- Watch for complications of mechanical ventilation, such as reduced cardiac output, pneumothorax or other barotrauma, increased pulmonary vascular resistance, diminished urine output, increased intracranial pressure, and GI bleeding.
- Routinely assess ET tube position and patency. Make sure the tube is placed properly and taped securely. Immediately after intubation, check for accidental intubation of the esophagus or the mainstem bronchus, which may have occurred during ET tube insertion. Also be alert for transtracheal or laryngeal perforation, aspiration, broken teeth, nosebleeds, arrhythmias, hypertension, and vagal reflexes such as bradycardia.
- After tube placement, watch for complications, such as tube displacement, herniation of the tube's cuff, respiratory infection, and tracheal malacia and stenosis.

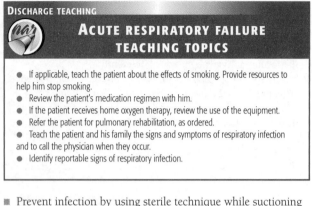

DISCHARGE TEACHING

ACUTE RESPIRATORY FAILURE TEACHING TOPICS

● If applicable, teach the patient about the effects of smoking. Provide resources to help him stop smoking.
● Review the patient's medication regimen with him.
● If the patient receives home oxygen therapy, review the use of the equipment.
● Refer the patient for pulmonary rehabilitation, as ordered.
● Teach the patient and his family the signs and symptoms of respiratory infection and to call the physician when they occur.
● Identify reportable signs of respiratory infection.

▪ Prevent infection by using sterile technique while suctioning and by changing ventilator tubing every 24 hours.

▪ Prevent tracheal erosion that can result from an overinflated artificial airway cuff compressing the tracheal wall's vasculature. Use the minimal-leak technique and a cuffed tube with high residual volume (low-pressure cuff), a foam cuff, or a pressure-regulating valve on the cuff. Measure cuff pressure every 8 hours.

▪ Implement measures to prevent tissue necrosis. Position and maintain the nasotracheal tube midline within the nostrils and provide meticulous care. Periodically loosen the tape holding the tube to prevent skin breakdown. Reposition the ET tube from side to side, and retape as needed. Make sure that the ventilator tubing has adequate support.

▪ Monitor for signs of stress ulcers, which are common in the intubated patient, especially in the intensive care unit. Inspect gastric secretions for blood, especially if the patient has a nasogastric tube or reports epigastric tenderness, nausea, or vomiting. Also monitor the patient's hemoglobin level and hematocrit, and check all stools for blood. Give antacids or histamine receptor antagonists, as ordered.

▪ Help the patient communicate without words. Offer him a pen and writing tablet, a word chart, or an alphabet board. (See *Acute respiratory failure teaching topics*.)

ASBESTOSIS

Asbestosis is characterized by diffuse interstitial pulmonary fibrosis resulting from prolonged exposure to airborne asbestos particles. Asbestosis may develop about 15 to 20 years after regular exposure to asbestos ceases. Asbestos exposure also causes pleural plaques and mesotheliomas of the pleura and the peritoneum. A potent cocarcinogen, asbestos heightens a cigarette smoker's risk of lung cancer. In fact, an asbestos worker who smokes is 90 times more likely to develop lung cancer than a smoker who never worked with asbestos.

Asbestosis is a form of pneumoconiosis. It follows prolonged inhalation of respirable asbestos fibers (about 50 microns long and 0.5 micron wide). Sources of exposure include asbestos mining and milling, the construction industry (where asbestos is used in a prefabricated form), and the fireproofing and textile industries. Asbestos is also used in the production of paints, plastics, and brake and clutch linings. Asbestos-related diseases develop in families of asbestos workers as a result of exposure to fibrous dust shaken off workers' clothing at home. Such diseases develop in the general public as a result of exposure to fibrous dust or waste piles from nearby asbestos plants.

Pathophysiology

Asbestosis occurs when lung spaces become filled with asbestos fibers. The inhaled asbestos fibers travel down the airway and penetrate respiratory bronchioles and alveolar walls. Coughing attempts to expel the foreign matter. Mucus production and goblet cells are stimulated to protect the airway from the debris and aid in expectoration. Fibers then become encased in a brown, iron-rich proteinlike sheath in sputum or lung tissue, called *asbestosis bodies.* Chronic irritation by the fibers continues to affect the lower bronchioles and alveoli. The foreign material and inflammation swell airways, and fibrosis develops in response to chronic irritation. Interstitial fibrosis may develop in lower lung zones, affecting lung parenchyma and the pleurae. Raised hyaline plaques may form in the parietal pleura, the diaphragm, and the pleura adjacent to the pericardium. Hypoxia develops as more alveoli and lower airways are affected.

Complications
- Pulmonary fibrosis
- Respiratory failure
- Pulmonary hypertension
- Cor pulmonale

Assessment findings
- The patient typically relates a history of occupational, family, or neighborhood exposure to asbestos fibers.
- The average exposure time is about 10 years.
- The patient may report exertional dyspnea and progressive dyspnea usually over a period of years.
- With extensive fibrosis, the patient may report dyspnea even at rest. In advanced disease, he may complain of a dry cough (which may be productive in smokers), chest pain (usually pleuritic), and recurrent respiratory tract infections.
- Tachypnea and clubbing of the fingers may be seen.
- With auscultation, you may hear characteristic dry crackles in the lung bases.

Diagnostic test results
- Arterial blood gas analysis may reveal decreased partial pressure of arterial oxygen (PaO_2) and decreased partial pressure of arterial carbon dioxide from hyperventilation.
- Chest X-rays may show fine, irregular, and linear diffuse infiltrates. If the patient has extensive fibrosis, X-rays may show lungs with a honeycomb or ground-glass appearance. Films may also show pleural thickening and pleural calcification, bilateral obliteration of costophrenic angles and, in later disease stages, an enlarged heart with a classic "shaggy" border.
- High-resolution computed tomography scan of the thorax may be ordered if chest X-rays are unclear and may reveal fibrotic consolidation.
- Pulmonary function tests may identify decreased vital capacity, forced vital capacity (FVC), and total lung capacity; decreased or normal forced expiratory volume in 1 second

(FEV$_1$); a normal ratio of FEV$_1$ to FVC; and reduced diffusing capacity for carbon monoxide when fibrosis destroys alveolar walls and thickens the alveolocapillary membrane.

Treatment

Chest physiotherapy techniques, such as controlled coughing and postural drainage with chest percussion and vibration, may be implemented to relieve respiratory signs and symptoms and, in advanced disease, manage hypoxia and cor pulmonale.

Aerosol therapy, inhaled mucolytics, and increased fluid intake (at least 3 qt [3 L]/day) may also help relieve respiratory symptoms. Hypoxia requires oxygen administration by cannula or mask (up to 2 L/minute) or by mechanical ventilation if the patient's PaO$_2$ can't be maintained above 40 mm Hg.

Diuretic agents, digoxin preparations, and salt restriction may be necessary for patients with cor pulmonale. Respiratory tract infections require prompt antibiotic therapy. Bronchodilators may be used if reversible obstruction is present.

Nursing interventions

- Provide supportive care, and help the patient adjust to lifestyle changes resulting from chronic illness.
- Be alert for changes in baseline respiratory function. Also watch for changes in sputum quality and quantity, restlessness, increased tachypnea, fever, night sweats, and changes in breath sounds. Report these immediately.
- Perform chest physiotherapy, including postural drainage, chest percussion, and vibration for involved lobes, several times daily.
- Weigh the patient three times per week.
- Provide high-calorie, high-protein foods. Offer small, frequent meals to conserve the patient's energy and prevent fatigue.
- Make sure the patient receives adequate fluids to loosen secretions.
- Schedule respiratory therapy at least 1 hour before or after meals. Provide mouth care after inhalation bronchodilator therapy.

DISCHARGE TEACHING

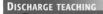

ASBESTOSIS TEACHING TOPICS

● Advise the patient to avoid crowds and people with known infections and to obtain influenza and pneumococcal immunizations.
● If the patient receives home oxygen therapy, explain why he needs it and show him how to operate the equipment.
● If the patient has a transtracheal catheter, teach him how to care for it. Review precautions for catheter use, and urge him to schedule appointments for follow-up care.
● Teach the patient and his family how to perform chest physiotherapy.
● Review the patient's medication regimen with him.
● Encourage the patient to follow a high-calorie, high-protein diet to meet increased energy requirements. Tell him to drink plenty of fluids to prevent dehydration and to help loosen secretions.
● If the patient smokes, encourage him to stop. Provide him with information or counseling, as appropriate.
● Refer the patient for pulmonary rehabilitation, as ordered.
● Encourage the patient to make regular follow-up visits with his physician.
● Teach the patient and his family the signs and symptoms of infection and to call the physician when they occur.

■ Encourage daily activity, and provide diversions as appropriate. Help conserve the patient's energy and prevent fatigue by alternating rest and activity periods.
■ Encourage the patient to stop smoking.
■ Give medication, as ordered, and note the patient's response.
■ Watch for such complications as pulmonary hypertension and cor pulmonale. (See *Asbestosis teaching topics.*)

ASTHMA

Asthma is a chronic lung disease of reversible airway inflammation that may resolve spontaneously or with treatment. It's characterized by obstruction or narrowing of the airways, which are typically inflamed and hyperresponsive to various stimuli. Signs of asthma range from mild wheezing and dyspnea to life-threatening respiratory failure. (See *Determining the severity of asthma,* pages 264 and 265.) Symptoms of bronchial airway inflammation may persist between acute episodes.

Pathophysiology

Asthma that results from sensitivity to specific external allergens is known as *extrinsic*. In cases in which the allergen isn't obvious, asthma is referred to as *intrinsic*. Allergens that cause extrinsic asthma include pollen, animal dander, house dust or mold, kapok or feather pillows, food additives containing sulfites, and any other sensitizing substance. Extrinsic (atopic) asthma usually begins in childhood and is accompanied by other manifestations of atopy (type I, immunoglobulin [Ig] E-mediated allergy), such as eczema and allergic rhinitis. In patients with intrinsic (nonatopic) asthma, no extrinsic allergen can be identified. Most cases are preceded by a severe respiratory tract infection. Irritants, emotional stress, fatigue, exposure to noxious fumes, endocrine changes, and changes in temperature and humidity may aggravate intrinsic asthma. In many patients with asthma, intrinsic and extrinsic asthma coexist. Asthma results in narrowing of the airways, caused by swelling of bronchial mucosa, increased mucus production, and bronchospasm.

Several drugs and chemicals can provoke an asthma attack without using the IgE pathway. They trigger the release of mast cell mediators by way of prostaglandin inhibition. Examples of these substances include aspirin, various nonsteroidal anti-inflammatory drugs (such as indomethacin [Indocin] and aspirin), and tartrazine, a yellow food dye. Exercise may also provoke an asthma attack. In patients with exercise-induced asthma, bronchospasm may follow heat and moisture loss in the upper airways. (See *Asthmatic bronchus,* page 266.)

The allergic response has two phases. When the patient inhales an allergenic substance, sensitized IgE antibodies trigger mast cell degranulation in the lung interstitium, releasing histamine, cytokines, prostaglandins, thromboxanes, leukotrienes, and eosinophil chemotactic factors. Histamine then attaches to receptor sites in the larger bronchi, causing irritation, inflammation, and edema. In the late phase, inflammatory cells flow in. The influx of eosinophils provides additional inflammatory mediators and contributes to local injury. (See *Understanding the progression of an asthma attack,* page 267.)

DETERMINING THE SEVERITY OF ASTHMA

Asthma is classified by severity using these features:
● frequency, severity, and duration of symptoms
● degree of airflow obstruction (spirometry measure) or peak expiratory flow (PEF)
● frequency of nighttime symptoms and the degree that the asthma interferes with daily activities.

Severity can change over time, and even milder cases can become severe in an uncontrolled attack. Long-term therapy depends on whether the patient's asthma is classified as mild intermittent, mild persistent, moderate persistent, or severe persistent. For most patients, quick relief can be obtained by using a short-acting bronchodilator (two to four puffs of a short-acting, inhaled beta$_2$-adrenergic agonist, as needed for symptoms). However, the use of a short-acting bronchodilator more than twice a week in patients with intermittent asthma or daily or increasing use in patients with persistent asthma may indicate the need to initiate or increase long-term control therapy.

Mild intermittent asthma

The signs and symptoms of mild intermittent asthma include:
● daytime symptoms no more than twice a week
● nighttime symptoms no more than twice a month
● lung function testing (either PEF or forced expiratory volume in 1 second) 80% of predicted value or higher
● PEF that varies no more than 20%.

Severe exacerbations, separated by long, symptom-free periods of normal lung function, indicate mild intermittent asthma. A course of systemic corticosteroids is recommended for these exacerbations; otherwise, daily medication isn't required.

Mild persistent asthma

The signs and symptoms of mild persistent asthma include:
● daytime symptoms more than twice a week but less than once a day
● nighttime symptoms more than twice per month
● lung function testing 80% of predicted value or higher
● PEF that varies between 20% and 30%.

The preferred treatment for mild, persistent asthma is a low-dose, inhaled corticosteroid, with alternative treatments including cromolyn (Intal), a leukotriene modifier such as nedocromil (Alocril), or sustained-release theophylline (Slo-Bid).

Moderate persistent asthma

The signs and symptoms of moderate persistent asthma include:
● daily daytime symptoms
● at least weekly nighttime symptoms
● lung function testing 60% to 80% of predicted value
● PEF that varies more than 30%.

DETERMINING THE SEVERITY OF ASTHMA
(continued)

The preferred treatment for moderate persistent asthma is a low- or medium-dose, inhaled corticosteroid combined with a long-acting, inhaled beta$_2$-adrenergic agonist. Alternative treatments include increasing the dosage of the inhaled corticosteroid so that it's within the medium-dose range or replacing the low- or medium-dose inhaled corticosteroid with either a leukotriene modifier or theophylline.

For recurring exacerbations, the preferred treatment is to increase the dosage of the inhaled corticosteroid so that it's within the medium-dose range and to add a long-acting, inhaled beta$_2$-adrenergic agonist. The alternative treatment is to increase the dosage of the inhaled corticosteroid so that it's within the medium-dose range and to add either a leukotriene modifier or theophylline.

Severe persistent asthma
The signs and symptoms of severe persistent asthma include:
- continual daytime symptoms
- frequent nighttime symptoms
- lung function testing is 60% of predicted value or lower
- PEF that varies more than 30%.

The preferred treatment for severe, persistent asthma includes a high-dose, inhaled corticosteroid combined with a long-acting, inhaled beta$_2$-adrenergic agonist. Long-term administration of corticosteroid tablets or syrup (2 mg/kg/day, not to exceed 60 mg/day) may be used to reduce the need for systemic corticosteroid therapy.

Although this common condition can strike at any age, half of all cases first occur in children younger than age 10; in this age-group, asthma affects twice as many boys as girls. Nearly 1 in 13 children has asthma, and this number is increasing worldwide. Emergency department visits, hospitalizations, and deaths resulting from asthma have been increasing for more than 20 years, especially among children and blacks.

Complications
- Status asthmaticus
- Respiratory failure

Assessment findings
- An asthma attack may begin dramatically, with the simultaneous onset of many severe symptoms, or insidiously, with gradually increasing respiratory distress.

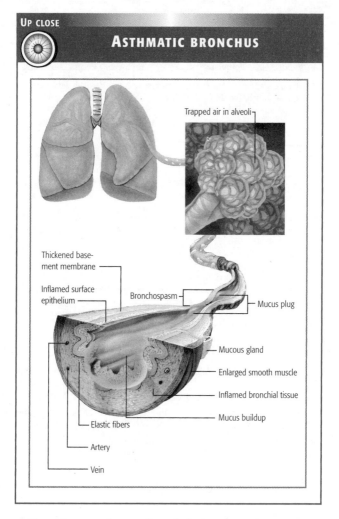

Trapped air in alveoli

Thickened basement membrane

Inflamed surface epithelium

Bronchospasm

Mucus plug

Mucous gland

Enlarged smooth muscle

Inflamed bronchial tissue

Mucus buildup

Elastic fibers

Artery

Vein

■ The asthma attack typically includes progressively worsening shortness of breath, cough, wheezing, and chest tightness or a combination of these signs and symptoms.

UNDERSTANDING THE PROGRESSION OF AN ASTHMA ATTACK

Asthma is an inflammatory disease characterized by bronchospasm and hyperresponsiveness of the airway. These illustrations show the progression of an asthma attack.

1. Histamine (H) attaches to receptor sites in the larger bronchi, where it causes swelling in smooth muscles.

2. Leukotrienes attach to receptor sites in the smaller bronchi and cause swelling of smooth muscle there. Leukotrienes also cause fatty acids called *prostaglandins* to travel through of the bloodstream to the lungs, where they enhance histamine's effects.

3. Histamine stimulates the mucous membranes to secrete excessive mucus, further narrowing the bronchial lumen, as shown.

4. On inhalation (shown at left), the narrowed bronchial lumen can still expand slightly, allowing air to reach the alveoli. On exhalation (shown at right), increased intrathoracic pressure closes the bronchial lumen completely.

5. Mucus fills the lung bases, inhibiting alveolar ventilation, as shown. Blood, shunted to alveoli in other lung parts, still can't compensate for diminished ventilation.

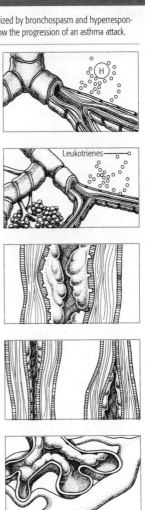

- During an acute attack, the cough sounds tight and dry. As the attack subsides, tenacious mucoid sputum is produced (except in young children, who rarely expectorate).
- Characteristic wheezing may be accompanied by coarse rhonchi, but fine crackles aren't heard unless associated with a related complication.
- Between acute attacks, breath sounds may be normal.
- The intensity of breath sounds in symptomatic patients with asthma is typically reduced. A prolonged phase of forced expiration is typical of airflow obstruction.
- Evidence of lung hyperinflation (use of accessory muscles, for example) is particularly common in children.
- In an acute attack, the patient may experience tachycardia, tachypnea, and diaphoresis.
- In a severe attack, the patient may be unable to speak more than a few words without pausing for breath.
- Cyanosis, confusion, and lethargy indicate impending respiratory failure.

Diagnostic test results

Patients with asthma commonly show these abnormalities in their test results:

- Arterial blood gas (ABG) analysis gives the best indication of the severity of an attack. In patients with acute, severe asthma, the partial pressure of arterial oxygen is less than 60 mm Hg, the partial pressure of arterial carbon dioxide is 40 mm Hg or more, and pH is usually decreased late in the episode.
- Chest X-rays may show hyperinflation with areas of focal atelectasis.
- Complete blood count with differential reveals increased eosinophil count.
- Pulmonary function tests reveal signs of airway obstruction (decreased peak expiratory flow rates and forced expiratory volume in 1 second), low-normal or decreased vital capacity, and increased total lung and residual capacity. However, pulmonary function studies may be normal between attacks.
- Pulse oximetry may reveal decreased arterial oxygen saturation (SaO_2).

Before testing for asthma, rule out other causes of airway obstruction and wheezing. In children, such causes include cystic fibrosis, tumors of the bronchi or mediastinum, and acute viral bronchitis; in adults, other causes include obstructive pulmonary disease, heart failure, and epiglottiditis.

Treatment

The goals of acute asthma treatment are to decrease bronchoconstriction, reduce bronchial airway edema, and increase pulmonary ventilation. After an acute episode, treatment focuses on avoiding or removing precipitating factors, such as environmental allergens or irritants.

If a specific antigen is causing the asthma, the patient may be desensitized through a series of injections of limited amounts of that antigen. The goal is to curb his immune response to the antigen. If an infection is causing the asthma, an antibiotic is prescribed.

For relief of symptoms in adults and children older than age 5, a short-acting, inhaled beta$_2$-adrenergic agonist for bronchodilation may be used, and a short, tapering course of systemic corticosteroids may be needed. The goal of therapy is to control the asthma with minimal or no adverse reactions to the medication.

Acute attacks that don't respond to treatment may require hospital care, an inhaled beta$_2$-adrenergic agonist, inhaled corticosteroids and, possibly, oxygen for hypoxemia. If the patient responds poorly, a systemic corticosteroid and, possibly, subcutaneous epinephrine may help. Beta$_2$-adrenergic agonist inhalation continues hourly. I.V. aminophylline may be added to the regimen, and I.V. fluid therapy is started. A patient who doesn't respond to this treatment, whose airways remain obstructed, and who has increasing respiratory difficulty is at risk for status asthmaticus and may require mechanical ventilation.

Treatment of status asthmaticus consists of aggressive drug therapy: a beta$_2$-adrenergic agonist by nebulizer every 30 to 60 minutes, possibly supplemented with subcutaneous epinephrine, an I.V. corticosteroid, I.V. aminophylline, oxygen administration, I.V. fluid therapy, and intubation and mechanical ventilation for hypercapnic respiratory failure. (See *How status asthmaticus progresses,* page 270.) Although the focus of asthma treatment in the past was alleviating the acute attack, the goal now is to prevent attacks and minimize limitations in activity.

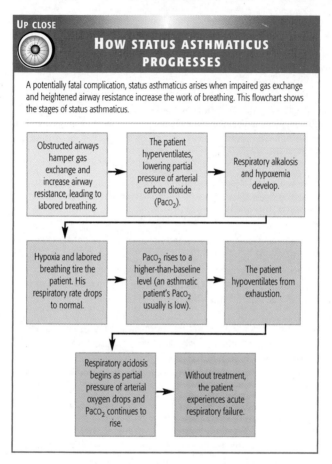

UP CLOSE

HOW STATUS ASTHMATICUS PROGRESSES

A potentially fatal complication, status asthmaticus arises when impaired gas exchange and heightened airway resistance increase the work of breathing. This flowchart shows the stages of status asthmaticus.

Obstructed airways hamper gas exchange and increase airway resistance, leading to labored breathing.

→

The patient hyperventilates, lowering partial pressure of arterial carbon dioxide ($Paco_2$).

→

Respiratory alkalosis and hypoxemia develop.

↓

Hypoxia and labored breathing tire the patient. His respiratory rate drops to normal.

→

$Paco_2$ rises to a higher-than-baseline level (an asthmatic patient's $Paco_2$ usually is low).

→

The patient hypoventilates from exhaustion.

↓

Respiratory acidosis begins as partial pressure of arterial oxygen drops and $Paco_2$ continues to rise.

→

Without treatment, the patient experiences acute respiratory failure.

Medications currently used to prevent exacerbations include a combination of inhaled corticosteroids, inhaled long-acting beta$_2$-adrenergic agonists, leukotriene inhibitors, inhaled anti-inflammatories, and methylxanthines. Treatment of acute attacks still includes inhaled short-acting beta$_2$-adrenergic agonists. The National Institutes of Health now endorse the stepwise approach for managing asthma. Treatment is determined by the severity of the patient's condition:

- Step 1: Mild intermittent
- Step 2: Mild persistent
- Step 3: Moderate persistent
- Step 4: Severe persistent

Nursing interventions

DURING AN ACUTE ATTACK

- Assess the severity of asthma.
- Give the prescribed treatments and assess the patient's response.
- Place the patient in high Fowler's position. Encourage pursed-lip and diaphragmatic breathing. Help the patient to relax.

RED FLAG Monitor the patient's vital signs. Keep in mind that developing or increasing tachypnea may indicate worsening asthma or drug toxicity. Blood pressure readings may reveal a paradoxical pulse, indicating severe asthma. Hypertension may indicate asthma-related hypoxemia.

- Give prescribed humidified oxygen by nasal cannula at 2 L/minute to ease breathing and increase SaO_2. Later, adjust oxygen according to the patient's vital signs and ABG levels.
- Anticipate intubation and mechanical ventilation if the patient fails to maintain adequate oxygenation with increasing $PaCO_2$ levels.
- Monitor serum theophylline levels to make sure they remain in the therapeutic range. Observe your patient for signs and symptoms of theophylline toxicity (vomiting, diarrhea, irritability, and headache) as well as for signs of subtherapeutic dosage (respiratory distress and increased wheezing).
- Observe the frequency and severity of your patient's cough, and note whether it's productive. Then auscultate his lungs, noting adventitious or absent breath sounds. If his cough is unproductive and rhonchi are present, teach him effective coughing techniques. If the patient can tolerate postural drainage and chest percussion, perform these procedures to clear secretions. Suction an intubated patient, as needed.
- Treat dehydration with I.V. fluids until the patient can tolerate oral fluids, which will help make secretions less tenacious.

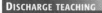

DISCHARGE TEACHING

ASTHMA TEACHING TOPICS

● Teach the patient to avoid known allergens and irritants.
● Describe prescribed drugs, including their names, dosages, actions, adverse effects, and special instructions.
● Teach the patient how to use a metered-dose inhaler.
● If the patient has moderate to severe asthma, explain how to use a peak flowmeter to measure the degree of airway obstruction. Urge him to keep a record of peak flow readings and to bring the record to medical appointments.
● Explain the importance of seeking immediate medical attention if the peak flow drops suddenly (which may forecast severe respiratory problems).
● Tell the patient to seek immediate medical attention if he develops a fever above 100° F (37.8° C), chest pain, shortness of breath without coughing or exercising, or uncontrollable coughing.
● Teach diaphragmatic and pursed-lip breathing and effective coughing techniques.
● Urge the patient to drink at least 3 qt (3 L) of fluids daily to help loosen secretions and maintain hydration.

■ If conservative treatment fails to improve the airway obstruction, anticipate bronchoscopy or bronchial lavage when a lobe or larger area collapses.

DURING LONG-TERM CARE
■ Monitor the patient's respiratory status to detect baseline changes, assess response to treatment, and prevent or detect complications.
■ Auscultate the lungs frequently, noting the degree of wheezing and quality of air movement.
■ Review ABG levels, pulmonary function test results, and SaO_2 readings.
■ If the patient is taking a systemic corticosteroid, observe him for complications, such as an elevated blood glucose level and friable skin and bruising.
■ Cushingoid effects resulting from long-term use of a corticosteroid may be minimized by alternate-day dosing or use of a prescribed inhaled corticosteroid.
■ If the patient is taking an inhaled corticosteroid, watch for signs of candidal infection in the mouth and pharynx. Using

an extender device and rinsing the mouth after each dose may prevent this.

- Observe the patient's anxiety level. Keep in mind that measures to reduce hypoxemia and breathlessness should help relieve anxiety.
- Keep the room temperature comfortable, and use an air conditioner or a fan in hot, humid weather.
- Control exercise-induced asthma by instructing the patient to use a bronchodilator or cromolyn 30 minutes before exercise. Also instruct him to use pursed-lip breathing while exercising. (See *Asthma teaching topics*.)

ATELECTASIS

In atelectasis, alveolar clusters (lobules) or lung segments that expand incompletely may produce a partial or complete lung collapse. This phenomenon effectively removes certain regions of the lung from gas exchange. This allows unoxygenated blood to pass unchanged through these regions and produces hypoxia.

Atelectasis may be chronic or acute. The disorder occurs to some degree in many patients undergoing upper abdominal or thoracic surgery. The prognosis depends on prompt removal of airway obstruction, relief of hypoxia, and reexpansion of the collapsed lung.

Pathophysiology

Atelectasis can result from bronchial occlusion by mucus plugs (a special problem in patients with chronic obstructive pulmonary disease, bronchiectasis, or cystic fibrosis). Mucus plugs may also affect lung expansion in patients who smoke. (Smoking increases mucus production and damages cilia.) The disorder may also result from occlusion caused by foreign bodies, bronchogenic carcinoma, and inflammatory lung disease.

Other causes include respiratory distress syndrome of the neonate, oxygen toxicity, and pulmonary edema, in which changes in alveolar surfactant cause increased surface tension and permit complete alveolar deflation.

External compression, which inhibits full lung expansion, or any condition that makes deep breathing painful may also

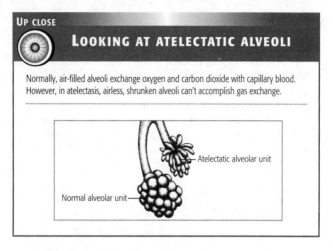

UP CLOSE

LOOKING AT ATELECTATIC ALVEOLI

Normally, air-filled alveoli exchange oxygen and carbon dioxide with capillary blood. However, in atelectasis, airless, shrunken alveoli can't accomplish gas exchange.

Atelectatic alveolar unit

Normal alveolar unit

cause atelectasis. Such compression or pain may result from upper abdominal surgical incisions, rib fractures, pleuritic chest pain, tight chest dressings, and obesity (which elevates the diaphragm and reduces tidal volume).

Lung collapse or reduced expansion may accompany prolonged immobility (which promotes ventilation of one lung area over another) or mechanical ventilation (which supplies constant small tidal volumes without intermittent deep breaths). Central nervous system depression (resulting from drug overdose, for example) eliminates periodic sighing and predisposes the patient to progressive atelectasis. (See *Looking at atelectatic alveoli.*)

Complications
- Hypoxemia
- Acute respiratory failure
- Pneumonia

Assessment findings
- Clinical effects vary with the causes of lung collapse, the degree of hypoxia, and the underlying disease. If atelectasis affects a small lung area, the patient's symptoms may be minimal and transient.

- Inspection may disclose decreased chest wall movement, cyanosis, diaphoresis, substernal or intercostal retractions, and anxiety.
- Palpation may reveal decreased fremitus and mediastinal shift to the affected side.
- Percussion may disclose dullness or flatness over lung fields.
- Auscultation findings may include crackles during the last part of inspiration and decreased (or absent) breath sounds with major lung involvement.
- Auscultation may also reveal tachycardia.
- With massive collapse, the patient may report severe symptoms, such as dyspnea and pleuritic chest pain.

Diagnostic test results

- Arterial blood gas analysis may reveal respiratory acidosis and hypoxemia resulting from atelectasis.
- Bronchoscopy can be used to rule out an obstructing neoplasm or a foreign body if the cause of atelectasis can't be determined.
- Chest X-rays are the primary diagnostic tool, although extensive areas of "microatelectasis" can exist without abnormalities appearing on the films. In widespread atelectasis, X-ray findings define characteristic horizontal lines in the lower lung zones. With segmental or lobar collapse, the films reveal characteristic dense shadows (commonly associated with hyperinflation of neighboring lung zones).
- Pulse oximetry may show deteriorating levels of arterial oxygen saturation.

Treatment

Incentive spirometry every hour, chest percussion, postural drainage, frequent coughing and deep-breathing exercises, and ambulation may improve oxygenation in the patient with atelectasis. If these measures fail, bronchoscopy may help remove secretions. Humidity and bronchodilator medications can improve mucociliary clearance and dilate airways. Mucolytics may also be of some benefit. These drugs may be given by nebulizer or by a mask that establishes continuous positive airway pressure. Alternatively, intermittent positive-pressure breathing therapy may be prescribed.

If the patient has atelectasis secondary to an obstructing neoplasm, he may need surgery or radiation therapy. To minimize the risk of atelectasis after thoracic and abdominal surgery, the patient requires analgesics to facilitate deep breathing.

Nursing interventions

■ Encourage the patient recovering from surgery (or other patients at high risk for atelectasis) to perform coughing and deep-breathing exercises every 1 to 2 hours. To minimize pain during these exercises, hold a pillow tightly over the patient's incisional area. Teach the patient how to do this for himself. Gently reposition the patient often, and help him walk as soon as possible. Provide adequate analgesics to control pain.

■ Monitor mechanical ventilation. Maintain tidal volume at 10 to 15 ml/kg of the patient's body weight to ensure adequate lung expansion. Use the sigh mechanism on the ventilator, if appropriate, to intermittently increase tidal volume at the rate of 3 to 4 sighs/hour.

■ Monitor pulse oximetry for decreases in oxygenation.

■ Help the patient use an incentive spirometer to encourage deep breathing.

■ Humidify inspired air, and encourage adequate fluid intake to mobilize secretions. Use postural drainage and chest percussion to remove secretions.

■ For the intubated or uncooperative patient, provide suctioning, as needed. Give sedatives with care because they depress respirations and the cough reflex. They also suppress sighs. Keep in mind that the patient can cooperate minimally (or not at all) with treatment if he has pain. Administer pain medications appropriately to help the patient's ability to perform coughing and deep-breathing exercises and ambulation.

■ Assess breath sounds and respiratory status frequently. Report changes immediately.

■ Offer ample reassurance and emotional support because the patient's limited breathing capacity may frighten him. (See *Atelectasis teaching topics*.)

DISCHARGE TEACHING

ATELECTASIS TEACHING TOPICS

● Teach the patient how to use the spirometer. Urge him to use it every hour.
● Show the patient and his family how to perform postural drainage and percussion. Instruct the patient to maintain each position for 10 minutes and then perform chest percussion. Let him know when to cough. Teach coughing and deep-breathing exercises to promote ventilation and mobilize secretions.
● Encourage the patient to stop smoking and lose weight, if needed. Refer him to appropriate support groups for help.
● Demonstrate comfort measures to promote relaxation and conserve energy. Advise the patient and his family to alternate periods of rest and activity to promote energy and prevent fatigue.

IDIOPATHIC PULMONARY FIBROSIS

Idiopathic pulmonary fibrosis (IPF) is a chronic and usually fatal interstitial pulmonary disease. About 50% of patients with IPF die within 3 years of diagnosis. Once thought to be a rare condition, it's now diagnosed with much greater frequency. IPF has been known by several other names over the years, including *cryptogenic fibrosing alveolitis, diffuse interstitial fibrosis, idiopathic interstitial pneumonitis,* and *Hamman-Rich syndrome.*

IPF is the result of a series of events that involve inflammatory, immune, and fibrotic processes in the lung. However, despite many studies and hypotheses, the stimulus that begins the progression remains unknown. Viral and genetic causes are suspected but no good evidence has been found to support either theory, although it's clear that chronic inflammation plays an important role. Inflammation develops as a result of the injury and fibrosis that ultimately distorts and impairs the structure and function of the alveolocapillary gas exchange surface.

IPF is slightly more common in men than in women and more likely in smokers than in nonsmokers. Incidence significantly increases with age.

Pathophysiology

Interstitial inflammation consists of alveolar septal infiltrates of lymphocytes, plasma cells, and histocytes. Fibrotic areas are

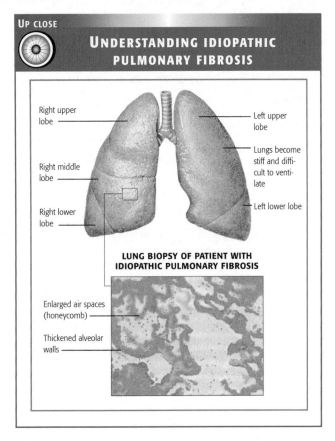

UP CLOSE

UNDERSTANDING IDIOPATHIC PULMONARY FIBROSIS

Right upper lobe

Left upper lobe

Lungs become stiff and difficult to ventilate

Right middle lobe

Right lower lobe

Left lower lobe

LUNG BIOPSY OF PATIENT WITH IDIOPATHIC PULMONARY FIBROSIS

Enlarged air spaces (honeycomb)

Thickened alveolar walls

composed of dense acellular collagen. Areas of honeycombing that form are composed of cystic fibrotic air spaces, frequently lined with bronchiolar epithelium and filled with mucus. Smooth-muscle hyperplasia may occur in areas of fibrosis and honeycombing. (See *Understanding idiopathic pulmonary fibrosis*.)

Complications
- Respiratory failure
- Chronic hypoxemia
- Pulmonary hypertension

- Cor pulmonale
- Polycythemia

Assessment findings

- The usual presenting symptoms of IPF are dyspnea on exertion and a dry, hacking, usually paroxysmal cough.
- Most patients have had these symptoms for several months to 2 years before seeking medical help.
- End-expiratory crackles (sometimes called *Velcro crackles*), especially in the bases of the lungs, are usually heard early in the disease.
- Bronchial breath sounds appear later, when airway consolidation develops.
- Rapid, shallow breathing occurs with exertion or rest, and clubbing has been noted in more than 70% of patients.
- Late in the disease, cyanosis and evidence of pulmonary hypertension (augmented S_2 and S_3 gallop) commonly occur.
- As the disease progresses, profound hypoxemia and severe, debilitating dyspnea are the hallmark signs.

Diagnostic test results

Diagnosis begins with a thorough patient history to exclude more common causes of interstitial lung disease.

- Arterial blood gas (ABG) analysis and pulse oximetry reveal hypoxemia, which may be mild when the patient is at rest early in the disease but may become severe later in the disease. Oxygenation will always deteriorate, usually to a severe level, with exertion.
- Chest X-rays may show one of four distinct patterns: interstitial, reticulonodular, ground-glass, or honeycomb. Although chest X-rays are helpful in identifying the presence of an abnormality, they don't correlate well with histologic findings or pulmonary function tests in determining the severity of the disease. They also don't help distinguish inflammation from fibrosis. However, serial X-rays may help track the progression of the disease.
- High-resolution computed tomography scans provide superior views of the four patterns seen on routine X-ray film and are used routinely to help establish the diagnosis of IPF. They show bibasilar, reticular abnormalities with ground-glass

opacities. Research is currently under way to determine whether the four patterns of abnormality seen on these scans correlate with responsiveness to treatment.

■ Lung biopsy is helpful in the diagnosis of IPF. In the past, an open lung biopsy was the only acceptable procedure and is still the preferred test for complete diagnosis, but now biopsies can be done through a thoracoscope or bronchoscope. Histologic features of the biopsy tissue vary, depending on the stage of the disease and other factors that aren't yet completely understood. The alveolar walls are swollen with chronic inflammatory cellular infiltrate composed of mononuclear cells and polymorphonuclear leukocytes. Intra-alveolar inflammatory cells may be found in early stages. As the disease progresses, excessive collagen and fibroblasts fill the interstitium. In advanced stages, alveolar walls are destroyed and are replaced by honeycombing cysts.

■ Pulmonary function tests show reduced vital capacity and total lung capacity and impaired diffusing capacity for carbon monoxide. Serial pulmonary function tests (especially carbon monoxide diffusing capacity) and ABG values may help track the course of the disease and the patient's response to treatment.

Treatment

Although it can't change the pathology of the disease, oxygen therapy can prevent the problems related to dyspnea and tissue hypoxia in the early stages of the disease process. The patient may require little or no supplemental oxygen while at rest initially, but he'll need more as the disease progresses and during exertion.

No known cure exists. High-dose corticosteroids and cytotoxic drugs may be given to suppress inflammation, but are usually unsuccessful. Recently, interferon-gamma-1B has shown some promise in treating the disease.

Lung transplantation may be successful for younger, otherwise healthy individuals.

IDIOPATHIC PULMONARY FIBROSIS TEACHING TOPICS

● Advise the patient to avoid crowds and people with known infections and to obtain influenza and pneumococcal immunizations.

● If the patient receives home oxygen therapy, explain why he needs it and show him how to operate the equipment.

● If the patient has a transtracheal catheter, teach him how to care for it. Review precautions for catheter use, and urge him to schedule appointments for follow-up care.

● Teach the patient and his family how to perform chest physiotherapy.

● Review the patient's medication regimen with him.

● Encourage the patient to follow a high-calorie, high-protein diet to meet increased energy requirements. Tell him to drink plenty of fluids to prevent dehydration and to help loosen secretions.

● If the patient smokes, encourage him to stop. Provide him with information or counseling, as appropriate.

● Educate the patient and his family about the signs and symptoms of infection and when to call the physician when these occur.

Nursing interventions

■ Explain all diagnostic tests to the patient, who may experience anxiety and frustration about the many tests required to establish the diagnosis.

■ Monitor oxygenation at rest and with exertion. The physician may prescribe one oxygen flow rate for use when the patient is at rest and a higher one for use during exertion to maintain adequate oxygenation. Instruct the patient to increase his oxygen flow rate to the appropriate level for exercise.

■ As IPF progresses, the patient's oxygen requirements increase. He may need a nonrebreathing mask to supply high oxygen percentages. Eventually, maintaining adequate oxygenation may become impossible despite maximum oxygen flow.

■ Most patients need oxygen at home. Make appropriate referrals to discharge planners, respiratory care practitioners, and home equipment vendors to ensure continuity of care.

■ Teach breathing, relaxation, and energy conservation techniques to help the patient manage severe dyspnea. (See *Idiopathic pulmonary fibrosis teaching topics*.)

- Encourage the patient to be as active as possible. Refer him to a pulmonary rehabilitation program.
- Monitor the patient for adverse reactions to drug therapy.
- Teach the patient about prescribed medications, especially adverse effects.
- Teach the patient and his family infection prevention techniques.
- Encourage good nutritional habits. Small, frequent meals with high nutritional value may be needed if dyspnea interferes with eating.
- Provide emotional support for the patient and his family as they deal with the patient's increasing disability, dyspnea, and probable death.

RESPIRATORY DISTRESS SYNDROME

Respiratory distress syndrome (RDS)—also called *hyaline membrane disease*—is the most common cause of neonatal death. The syndrome occurs almost exclusively in infants born before the 37th gestational week (and in about 60% of those born before the 28th week). It's most common in infants of diabetic mothers, those delivered by cesarean section, and those delivered suddenly after antepartum hemorrhage.

In RDS, the premature infant develops widespread alveolar collapse from a surfactant deficiency. Untreated, the syndrome causes death within 72 hours of birth in up to 14% of infants weighing less than 2,500 g (5.5 lb). Aggressive management assisted by mechanical ventilation can improve the prognosis. A few patients who survive are left with bronchopulmonary dysplasia. Mild cases of the syndrome slowly subside after about 3 days.

The immediate cause of RDS is lack of surfactant, a lipoprotein present in alveoli and respiratory bronchioles. In these structures, surfactant helps to lower surface tension, maintain alveolar patency, and prevent collapse, particularly at end expiration.

Pathophysiology

Although neonatal airways are developed by the 27th gestational week, the intercostal muscles are weak, and the alveoli and the capillary blood supplies are immature. Surfactant deficiency causes a higher surface tension. The alveoli can't maintain patency and begin to collapse.

With alveolar collapse, ventilation is decreased and hypoxia develops. The resulting pulmonary injury and inflammatory reaction lead to edema and swelling of the interstitial space, thus impeding gas exchange between the capillaries and the functional alveoli. The inflammation also stimulates production of hyaline membranes composed of white fibrin accumulation in the alveoli. These deposits further reduce gas exchange in the lung and decrease lung compliance, resulting in increased work of breathing.

Decreased alveolar ventilation results in decreased ventilation-perfusion ratio and pulmonary arteriolar vasoconstriction. The pulmonary vasoconstriction can result in increased right cardiac volume and pressure, causing blood to be shunted from the right atrium through a patent foramen ovale to the left atrium. Increased pulmonary resistance also results in deoxygenated blood passing through the ductus arteriosus, bypassing the lungs, and causing a right-to-left shunt. The shunt further increases hypoxia.

Because of immature lungs and an already increased metabolic rate, the infant must expend more energy to ventilate collapsed alveoli. This further increases oxygen demand and contributes to cyanosis. The infant attempts to compensate with rapid shallow breathing, causing an initial respiratory alkalosis as carbon dioxide is expelled. The increased effort at lung expansion causes respirations to slow and respiratory acidosis to occur, leading to respiratory failure.

Complications

- Respiratory insufficiency
- Shock

Assessment findings
- The history typically indicates preterm birth (before 28 gestational weeks) or cesarean delivery.
- The maternal history may include diabetes or antepartum hemorrhage.
- Although the neonate with RDS may breathe normally at first, within minutes to hours after birth, inspection may reveal rapid, shallow respirations with intercostal, subcostal, or sternal retractions, nasal flaring, and audible expiratory grunting.
- The grunting is a natural compensatory mechanism that produces positive end-expiratory pressure (PEEP) to prevent further alveolar collapse.
- Additional findings may include hypotension, peripheral edema, and oliguria.
- In severe disease, the patient may display apnea, bradycardia, and cyanosis (from hypoxemia, left-to-right shunting through the foramen ovale, or right-to-left shunting through atelectatic lung areas).
- Other clinical features are pallor, frothy sputum, and low body temperature (resulting from an immature nervous system and inadequate subcutaneous fat).
- Auscultation typically discloses diminished air entry and crackles, although crackles are rare early in the syndrome.

Diagnostic test results
- Arterial blood gas (ABG) values show a diminished level of partial pressure of arterial oxygen (PaO_2); normal, decreased, or increased level of partial pressure of arterial carbon dioxide; and reduced pH (a combination of respiratory and metabolic acidosis).
- Chest X-rays may be normal for the first 6 to 12 hours in 50% of patients. However, later films show a fine reticulonodular pattern and dark streaks, indicating air-filled, dilated bronchioles.
- The lecithin-sphingomyelin ratio aids in the assessment of prenatal lung development and RDS risk. The test is usually ordered if a cesarean delivery is performed before the 36th gestational week.

Treatment

For prevention of RDS, natural lung surfactant, such as beractant (Survanta), is given to most premature neonates weighing less than 1,250 g (2 lb, 12 oz) at birth or to those having symptoms consistent with surfactant deficiency. The drug is given intratracheally, preferably within 15 minutes of birth, and may be repeated every 6 hours as necessary, up to four doses in 48 hours.

The neonate with RDS requires vigorous respiratory support. Warm, humidified, oxygen-enriched gases are given by oxygen hood or, if such treatment fails, by mechanical ventilation. The neonate with severe RDS may require mechanical ventilation with PEEP or continuous positive airway pressure (CPAP) given by nasal prongs, a tight-fitting face mask or, when necessary, endotracheal tube.

If the neonate can't maintain adequate gas exchange, high-frequency oscillation ventilation may be initiated to provide satisfactory minute volume (the total volume of air breathed in 1 minute) with lower airway pressures.

Treatment may also include:

- radiant warmer or Isolette for thermoregulation
- I.V. fluids and sodium bicarbonate to control acidosis and maintain fluid and electrolyte balance
- tube feedings or total parenteral nutrition to maintain adequate nutrition if the neonate is too weak or unable to eat
- drug therapy with prophylactic antibiotics and diuretics (to reduce pulmonary edema)
- alternative drug therapy—for example, with vitamin E to prevent complications associated with oxygen therapy, and corticosteroids given to the mother to stimulate surfactant production in a fetus at high risk for preterm birth.

Nursing interventions

- Assess the neonate constantly. Monitor ABG levels and fluid intake and output.
- Check for arterial or venous hypotension, as appropriate, if the neonate has an umbilical catheter. Also watch for abnormal central venous pressure and for complications, such as infection, thrombosis, and decreased circulation to the legs.

- If the neonate has a transcutaneous partial pressure of oxygen monitor (an accurate method for determining PaO_2), change the site of the lead placement every 2 to 4 hours to avoid burning the skin.
- Use pulse oximetry to monitor arterial oxygen saturation.
- Weigh the infant once or twice daily.
- Regularly assess skin color, rate and depth of respirations, severity of retractions, nasal flaring, frequency of expiratory grunting, frothing at the lips, and restlessness.
- Regularly assess the effectiveness of oxygen or ventilator therapy. Evaluate every fraction of expired oxygen and PEEP or CPAP change by drawing arterial blood for analysis 20 minutes after each change. Be sure to adjust PEEP or CPAP as indicated by ABG levels.

RED FLAG When the neonate receives mechanical ventilation, watch carefully for signs of barotrauma (increase in respiratory distress, subcutaneous emphysema) and accidental disconnection from the ventilator. Check ventilator settings frequently. Be alert for signals of complications of PEEP or CPAP therapy, such as decreased cardiac output, pneumothorax, and pneumomediastinum.

- Institute infection prevention measures if the infant receives mechanical ventilation.
- Provide suction as necessary. Observe the oxygenation monitor or pulse oximeter before, during, and after suctioning to evaluate the patient's response to this therapy.
- Inspect the skin frequently for signs of breakdown.
- Provide mouth care every 2 hours. Lubricate the infant's nostrils and lips with water-soluble ointment.
- Observe for signs and symptoms of infection resulting from invasive therapies and a weakened immune system.
- As needed, arrange for follow-up care with a neonatal ophthalmologist to detect possible retinal damage from oxygen therapy.

RED FLAG Watch for additional complications of oxygen therapy, such as lung capillary damage, decreased mucus flow, impaired ciliary functioning, and widespread atelectasis. Other problems to watch for include patent ductus arteriosus, heart failure, retinopathy, pulmonary hypertension, necrotizing enterocolitis, and neurologic abnormalities.

DISCHARGE TEACHING

RESPIRATORY DISTRESS SYNDROME TEACHING TOPICS

● Review the patient's medication regimen with the parents, including their names, routes, dosages, adverse effects, and special instructions.

● Explain the function of respiratory devices and equipment. Discuss alarm sounds and mechanical noise, and solicit parent feedback. Encourage them to ask questions and to express their fears and concerns.

● Advise the parents that full recovery may take up to 12 months. When the prognosis is poor, prepare the parents for the neonate's possible death and offer emotional support. When appropriate, refer the parents and family to professional staff, such as pastoral counselors and social workers.

■ Help reduce mortality by detecting RDS early. Recognize intercostal retractions and grunting, especially in a premature infant, as signs of RDS.

■ Make sure the patient receives immediate treatment. (See *Respiratory distress syndrome teaching topics*.)

SARCOIDOSIS

Sarcoidosis is a multisystemic, granulomatous disorder that characteristically produces lymphadenopathy, pulmonary infiltration, and skeletal, liver, eye, or skin lesions.

Sarcoidosis is most common in young adults ages 20 to 40. In the United States, sarcoidosis occurs predominantly among blacks and affects twice as many women as men. Acute sarcoidosis usually resolves within 2 years. Chronic, progressive sarcoidosis, which is uncommon, is associated with pulmonary fibrosis and progressive pulmonary disability.

The cause of sarcoidosis is unknown, but several possibilities exist. The disease may result from a hypersensitivity response—possibly from a T-cell imbalance—to such agents as atypical mycobacteria, fungi, and pine pollen. The incidence is slightly higher within families, suggesting a genetic predisposition. Chemicals may also trigger the disease. (Zirconium or beryllium lead to illnesses that resemble sarcoidosis.)

Pathophysiology

Although the exact mechanism of the disease is unknown, research suggests a T-cell problem and, more specifically, a lymphokine production problem. In other granulomatous diseases, such as tuberculosis (TB), granuloma formation occurs from inadequate pathogen clearance by macrophages. These macrophages require the help of T cells that secrete lymphokines, which in turn activate less effective macrophages to become aggressive phagocytes. Lack of lymphokine secretion by T cells may help explain granuloma formation in sarcoidosis.

Complications

- Pulmonary fibrosis
- Pulmonary hypertension
- Cor pulmonale

Assessment findings

- The patient may report general fatigue and a feeling of malaise, unexplained weight loss, and pain in the wrists, ankles, and elbows.
- She may also complain of breathlessness and shortness of breath on exertion and have a nonproductive cough and substernal pain.
- On inspection, you may observe erythema nodosum, subcutaneous skin nodules with maculopapular eruptions, and punched out lesions on the fingers and toes.
- You may also note weakness and cranial or peripheral nerve palsies.
- When you inspect the nose, you may see extensive nasal mucosal lesions.
- Inspection of the eyes commonly reveals anterior uveitis. Glaucoma and blindness occasionally occur in advanced disease.
- Palpation may reveal bilateral hilar and right paratracheal lymphadenopathy and splenomegaly.
- Such arrhythmias as premature beats may be heard on auscultation.

Diagnostic test results

- A positive Kveim-Siltzbach skin test result points to sarcoidosis. In this test, the patient receives an intradermal injection of an antigen prepared from human sarcoidal spleen or lymph nodes from patients with sarcoidosis. If she has active sarcoidosis, granuloma develops at the injection site in 2 to 6 weeks. When coupled with a skin biopsy at the injection site that shows discrete epithelioid cell granuloma, the test confirms the disease.
- Arterial blood gas (ABG) studies show a decreased partial pressure of arterial oxygen.
- Chest X-rays show bilateral hilar and right paratracheal adenopathy, with or without diffuse interstitial infiltrates. Occasionally, they show large nodular lesions in lung parenchyma.
- Fiberoptic bronchoscopy and lung biopsy may reveal granulomas and positive cultures for mycobacteria and fungi.
- Lymph node, skin, or lung biopsy discloses noncaseating granulomas with negative cultures for mycobacteria and fungi.
- Pulmonary function tests indicate decreased total lung capacity and compliance and reduced diffusing capacity.
- Tuberculin skin tests, fungal serologies, sputum cultures (for mycobacteria and fungi), and biopsy cultures are negative and help rule out infection.

Treatment

Sarcoidosis that doesn't produce symptoms requires no treatment. However, sarcoidosis that causes hypercalcemia, destructive skin lesions, or ocular, respiratory, central nervous system, cardiac, or systemic symptoms (such as fever and weight loss) requires treatment with systemic or topical corticosteroids. Such therapy usually continues for 1 to 2 years, but some patients may need lifelong therapy. A patient with hypercalcemia also needs a low-calcium diet and protection from direct exposure to sunlight.

If the patient has a significant response to the tuberculin skin test that shows TB reactivation, she needs isoniazid (INH) therapy.

Nursing interventions

▨ Watch for and report complications. Also, note abnormal laboratory results (anemia, for example) that could alter patient care.

▨ If the patient has arthralgia, give analgesics, as ordered. Record signs of progressive muscle weakness.

▨ Provide a nutritious, high-calorie diet and plenty of fluids. If the patient has hypercalcemia, speak to the dietitian about a low-calcium diet. Weigh the patient regularly to detect weight loss.

▨ Monitor the patient's respiratory function. Check chest X-rays for the extent of lung involvement, and note and record an increase in sputum volume or bloody sputum. If the patient has pulmonary hypertension or end-stage cor pulmonale, monitor ABG levels, watch for arrhythmias, and give oxygen, as needed.

RED FLAG Because corticosteroids may induce or worsen diabetes mellitus, test the patient's blood via fingersticks for glucose at least every 12 hours at the beginning of corticosteroid therapy. Also, watch for other adverse effects, such as fluid retention, electrolyte imbalance (especially hypokalemia), moon face, hypertension, and personality changes.

▨ During or after corticosteroid withdrawal (particularly if the patient has an infection or other stressor, such as emotional stress or an underlying condition), watch for and report vomiting, orthostatic hypotension, hypoglycemia, restlessness, anorexia, malaise, and fatigue. Remember that the patient on long-term or high-dose therapy is vulnerable to infection.

▨ Listen to the patient's fears and concerns, and remain with her during periods of extreme stress and anxiety. Encourage her to identify actions and care measures that help make her comfortable and relaxed. Perform these measures, and encourage the patient to do so as well.

▨ Whenever possible, include the patient in care decisions, and include her family in all phases of care. (See *Sarcoidosis teaching topics*.)

DISCHARGE TEACHING

SARCOIDOSIS TEACHING TOPICS

● When preparing the patient for discharge, stress the need for compliance with the prescribed steroid therapy. Emphasize the importance of not skipping doses.

● Instruct the patient to take steroids with food.

● Make sure the patient understands the need for regular, careful follow-up examinations and treatment.

● Teach the patient to wear a medical identification bracelet or necklace indicating her corticosteroid therapy.

● Discuss the patient's increased vulnerability to infection, and review ways to minimize exposure to illness.

● Refer the patient with failing vision to community support and resource groups, including the American Foundation for the Blind, if necessary.

SILICOSIS

Silicosis is the most common form of pneumoconiosis. It's a chronic fibrosing disease of the lung characterized by bilateral nodular lesions. It's classified according to the severity of the pulmonary disease and the rapidity of its onset and progression, although it usually occurs as a simple illness that doesn't produce symptoms. (See *Berylliosis: Another type of pneumoconiosis,* page 292.)

Those who work around silica dust, such as foundry workers, boiler scalers, mine workers, quarry workers, and stone cutters, have the highest incidence of the disease. Silica in its pure form occurs in the manufacture of ceramics (flint) and building materials (sandstone). It occurs in mixed form in the production of construction materials (cement). It's also found in powder form (silica flour) in paints, porcelain, scouring soaps, and wood fillers and in the mining of gold, lead, zinc, and iron.

Sand blasters, tunnel workers, and others exposed to high concentrations of respirable silica may develop acute silicosis after 1 to 3 years. Those exposed to lower concentrations of free silica can develop accelerated silicosis, usually after about 10 years of exposure.

The prognosis is good unless the disease progresses to the accelerated form with progressive massive fibrosis.

BERYLLIOSIS: ANOTHER TYPE OF PNEUMOCONIOSIS

Berylliosis—a type of pneumoconiosis—is a systemic granulomatous disease that mainly affects the lungs. It's an occupational disease that commonly affects workers in beryllium alloy, ceramics, foundry, grinder, cathode ray tube, gas mantle, missile, and nuclear reactor industries.

Berylliosis occurs in two forms: acute nonspecific pneumonitis and chronic noncaseating granulomatous disease with interstitial fibrosis, which can cause death from respiratory failure and cor pulmonale. In about 10% of patients with acute berylliosis, chronic disease develops 10 to 15 years after exposure.

SYMPTOMS	DIAGNOSTIC TESTS	TREATMENT
Symptoms of berylliosis include: ● itchy rash ● beryllium ulcer ● swelling and ulceration of the nasal mucosa ● septal perforation ● tracheitis ● bronchitis (dry cough) ● chest tightness ● substernal pain ● tachycardia ● worsening dyspnea.	These tests may help diagnose berylliosis or the extent of respiratory involvement. ● Chest X-rays detect pulmonary edema. ● Pulmonary function studies demonstrate decreased vital capacity as fibrosis stiffens the lungs. ● Arterial blood gas analysis findings indicate diminished partial pressure of arterial oxygen (PaO_2) and carbon dioxide. ● A positive beryllium patch test establishes a patient's hypersensitivity to beryllium but doesn't confirm the diagnosis. ● Positive tissue biopsy and spectrographic analysis support, but don't confirm, the diagnosis. ● Urinalysis may identify beryllium excreted in urine, indicating exposure to the metal.	● A beryllium ulcer requires excision or curettage. ● If the patient has hypoxia, he may need oxygen delivered by nasal cannula or mask (usually 1 to 2 L/minute). ● If the patient has severe respiratory failure, he may need mechanical ventilation if PaO_2 falls below 40 mm Hg. ● The patient with acute berylliosis usually receives corticosteroid therapy in an attempt to alter the disease's progression; maintenance therapy may be lifelong for chronic cases. ● Respiratory symptoms may respond to bronchodilators, increased fluid intake (at least 3 qt [3 L]/day), and chest physiotherapy. ● Diuretic agents, digoxin preparations, and sodium restriction may help the patient with cor pulmonale.

UNDERSTANDING SILICOSIS

Silicosis results when respirable crystalline silica dust, mostly from quartz, is inhaled and deposited in the pulmonary system. The risk depends on the concentration of dust in the atmosphere, the percentage of respirable free silica particles in the dust, and the duration of exposure. Although particles up to 10 microns in diameter can be inhaled, the disease-causing particles deposited in the alveolar space usually have a diameter of only 1 to 3 microns.

Nodules result when alveolar macrophages ingest the silica particles, which they can't process. As a result, the macrophages die and release proteolytic enzymes into the surrounding tissue. The enzymes inflame the tissue, attracting other macrophages and fibroblasts. These produce fibrous tissue to wall off the reaction, resulting in a nodule that has an onionskin appearance.

These nodules develop next to the terminal and respiratory bronchioles. The nodules are concentrated in the upper lung lobes but are commonly accompanied by bullous changes in upper and lower lobes. If the disease doesn't progress, the patient may experience only minimal physiologic disturbances with no disability. Occasionally, however, the fibrotic response accelerates, engulfing and destroying a large area of the lung.

Pathophysiology

Alveolar macrophages engulf respirable particles of free silica, causing release of cytotoxic enzymes. This attracts other macrophages and produces fibrous tissue in the lung parenchyma. Silicosis is associated with a high incidence of tuberculosis (TB). (See *Understanding silicosis*.)

Complications
- Pulmonary fibrosis
- Cor pulmonale
- Ventricular or respiratory failure
- Pulmonary TB

Assessment findings
- The patient has a history of long-term industrial exposure to silica dust.
- He may complain of dyspnea on exertion, which he's likely to attribute to "being out of shape" or "slowing down."

- If the disease has progressed to the chronic and complicated state, the patient may report a dry cough, especially in the morning.
- When you inspect the patient, you may note decreased chest expansion and tachypnea.
- If the patient has advanced disease, he may also have lethargy, malaise, anorexia, and weight loss and may look confused.
- You may percuss areas of increased and decreased resonance.
- On auscultation, you may hear fine to medium crackles, diminished breath sounds, and an intensified ventricular gallop on inspiration—a hallmark of cor pulmonale.

Diagnostic test results

- Arterial blood gas analysis reveals a normal partial pressure of arterial oxygen in simple silicosis, but it may drop significantly below normal in late stages or complicated disease. The patient has a normal partial pressure of arterial carbon dioxide ($PaCO_2$) in the early stages of the disease, but hyperventilation may cause it to drop below normal. If restrictive lung disease develops—particularly if the patient is hypoxic and has severe alveolar ventilatory impairment—$PaCO_2$ may increase above normal.
- Chest X-rays in simple silicosis show small, discrete, nodular lesions distributed throughout both lung fields, although they typically concentrate in the upper lung zones. The lung nodes may appear enlarged and show eggshell calcification. In complicated silicosis, X-rays show one or more conglomerate masses of dense tissue.
- Pulmonary function tests in simple silicosis may be normal, but the patient may demonstrate reduced forced vital capacity (FVC) in complicated silicosis. If the patient has obstructive disease (emphysematous silicosis areas), the forced expiratory volume in 1 second (FEV_1) is reduced. A patient with complicated silicosis also has a reduced FEV_1, but has a normal or high ratio of FEV_1 to FVC. When fibrosis destroys alveolar walls and obliterates pulmonary capillaries or when it thickens the alveolocapillary membrane, the diffusing capacity for carbon monoxide falls below normal. Both restrictive disease and obstructive disease reduce maximal voluntary ventilation.

Treatment

The goal of treatment is to relieve respiratory symptoms, manage hypoxia and cor pulmonale, and prevent respiratory tract infections and irritations. Treatment also includes careful observation for the development of TB.

Daily bronchodilation aerosols and increased fluid intake (at least 3 qt [3 L]/day) relieve respiratory signs and symptoms. Steam inhalation and chest physiotherapy (such as controlled coughing and segmental bronchial drainage) with chest percussion and vibration help clear secretions.

In severe cases, the patient may need oxygen by cannula, mask, or mechanical ventilation (if he can't maintain arterial oxygenation). Antibiotics are needed to treat respiratory tract infection.

Nursing interventions

- Assess for changes in baseline respiratory functioning, including changes in sputum quality and quantity, restlessness, increased tachypnea, and changes in breath sounds. Report changes to the physician immediately.
- Perform chest physiotherapy, including postural drainage and chest percussion and vibration designed for involved lobes, several times per day.
- Provide the patient with a high-calorie, high-protein diet, preferably in small, frequent meals.
- Schedule respiratory therapy at least 1 hour before or after meals. Provide mouth care after bronchodilator therapy.
- Make sure the patient receives enough fluids to loosen secretions.
- Encourage daily activity, and provide the patient with diversional activities, as appropriate. To conserve his energy, alternate periods of rest and activity.
- Give drugs, as ordered. Monitor the patient for desired response and adverse effects.
- Watch for complications, such as pulmonary fibrosis, right ventricular hypertrophy, and cor pulmonale.
- Help the patient adjust to the lifestyle changes associated with a chronic illness. Answer his questions, and encourage him to express his concerns about his illness.

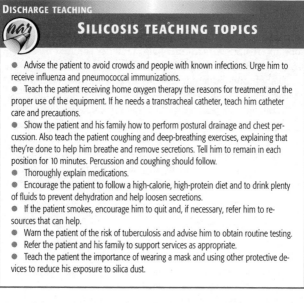

DISCHARGE TEACHING

SILICOSIS TEACHING TOPICS

● Advise the patient to avoid crowds and people with known infections. Urge him to receive influenza and pneumococcal immunizations.

● Teach the patient receiving home oxygen therapy the reasons for treatment and the proper use of the equipment. If he needs a transtracheal catheter, teach him catheter care and precautions.

● Show the patient and his family how to perform postural drainage and chest percussion. Also teach the patient coughing and deep-breathing exercises, explaining that they're done to help him breathe and remove secretions. Tell him to remain in each position for 10 minutes. Percussion and coughing should follow.

● Thoroughly explain medications.

● Encourage the patient to follow a high-calorie, high-protein diet and to drink plenty of fluids to prevent dehydration and help loosen secretions.

● If the patient smokes, encourage him to quit and, if necessary, refer him to resources that can help.

● Warn the patient of the risk of tuberculosis and advise him to obtain routine testing.

● Refer the patient and his family to support services as appropriate.

● Teach the patient the importance of wearing a mask and using other protective devices to reduce his exposure to silica dust.

■ Stay with the patient during periods of extreme stress and anxiety, and include him and his family in care decisions whenever possible.

■ Encourage the patient to stop smoking. (See *Silicosis teaching topics*.)

Vascular lung disorders

Vascular lung disorders affect the vascular structures of the lungs. Normal pulmonary vasculature is a low-pressure, low-resistance system. It includes pulmonary arteries, pulmonary veins, pulmonary capillaries, pulmonary lymphatics, and bronchial circulation.

Conditions that affect any of these vascular components can result in a vascular lung disorder and compromised respiratory function.

COR PULMONALE

The World Health Organization defines chronic cor pulmonale as "hypertrophy of the right ventricle resulting from diseases affecting the function or the structure of the lungs, except when these pulmonary alterations are the result of diseases that primarily affect the left side of the heart or of congenital heart disease." Invariably, cor pulmonale follows some disorder of the lungs, pulmonary vessels, chest wall, or respiratory control center. For example, chronic obstructive pulmonary disease (COPD) produces pulmonary hypertension, which leads to right ventricular hypertrophy and right-sided heart failure. Because cor pulmonale usually occurs late during the course of COPD and other irreversible diseases, the prognosis is generally poor.

About 85% of patients with cor pulmonale have COPD, and 25% of patients with COPD eventually develop cor pulmonale.

Other respiratory disorders that produce cor pulmonale include:

- chronic mountain sickness (living at high altitudes)
- loss of lung tissue after extensive lung surgery
- obesity hypoventilation syndrome (pickwickian syndrome) and upper airway obstruction
- obstructive lung diseases—for example, bronchiectasis and cystic fibrosis
- pulmonary vascular diseases—for example, recurrent thromboembolism, primary pulmonary hypertension, schistosomiasis, and pulmonary vasculitis
- respiratory insufficiency without pulmonary disease—for example, in chest wall disorders such as kyphoscoliosis, neuromuscular incompetence resulting from muscular dystrophy and amyotrophic lateral sclerosis, polymyositis, and spinal cord lesions above the sixth cervical vertebra
- restrictive lung diseases—for example, pneumoconiosis, interstitial pneumonitis, scleroderma, and sarcoidosis.

Cor pulmonale accounts for about 25% of all types of heart failure. It's most common in areas of the world where the incidence of cigarette smoking and COPD is high; cor pulmonale affects middle-age to elderly men more commonly than women, but its incidence in women is increasing. In children, cor pulmonale may be a complication of cystic fibrosis, hemosiderosis, upper airway obstruction, scleroderma, extensive bronchiectasis, neurologic diseases affecting respiratory muscles, or abnormalities of the respiratory control center.

Pathophysiology

Pulmonary capillary destruction and pulmonary vasoconstriction (usually secondary to hypoxia) reduce the area of the pulmonary vascular bed. Thus, pulmonary vascular resistance is increased, causing pulmonary hypertension. To compensate for the extra work needed to force blood through the lungs, the right ventricle dilates and hypertrophies. In response to low oxygen content, the bone marrow produces more red blood cells, causing erythrocytosis. When hematocrit exceeds 55%, blood viscosity increases, further aggravating pulmonary hypertension and increasing the hemodynamic load on the right ven-

WHAT HAPPENS IN COR PULMONALE

Although pulmonary restrictive disorders (such as fibrosis or obesity), obstructive disorders (such as bronchitis), or primary vascular disorders (such as recurrent pulmonary emboli) may cause cor pulmonale, these disorders share this common pathway.

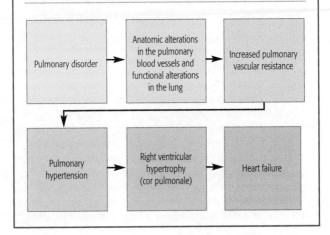

tricle. Right-sided heart failure is the result. (See *What happens in cor pulmonale.*)

Complications
- Right- and left-sided heart failure
- Hepatomegaly
- Edema
- Ascites
- Pleural effusions
- Thromboembolism

Assessment findings
- As long as the heart can compensate for the increased pulmonary vascular resistance, clinical features reflect the underlying disorder and occur mostly in the respiratory system.

They include chronic productive cough, exertional dyspnea, wheezing, fatigue, and weakness.

■ Progression of cor pulmonale is associated with dyspnea (even at rest) that worsens on exertion, tachypnea, orthopnea, edema, weakness, and right upper quadrant discomfort.

■ Signs of cor pulmonale and right-sided heart failure include dependent edema, distended jugular veins, prominent parasternal or epigastric cardiac impulse, hepatojugular reflux, ascites, tachycardia, and an enlarged, tender liver.

■ Decreased cardiac output may cause a weak pulse and hypotension.

■ Chest examination yields various findings, depending on the underlying cause of cor pulmonale.

 – In COPD, auscultation reveals wheezing, rhonchi, and diminished breath sounds.

 – When the disease is secondary to upper airway obstruction or damage to central nervous system respiratory centers, chest findings may be normal, except for a right ventricular lift, gallop rhythm, and loud pulmonic component of S_2.

 – Tricuspid insufficiency produces a pansystolic murmur heard at the lower left sternal border; its intensity increases on inspiration, distinguishing it from a murmur resulting from mitral valve disease.

 – A right ventricular early murmur that increases on inspiration can be heard at the left sternal border or over the epigastrium.

 – A systolic pulmonic ejection click may also be heard.

■ Alterations in level of consciousness may occur.

Diagnostic test results

■ Arterial blood gas (ABG) analysis shows decreased partial pressure of arterial oxygen (PaO_2) (typically less than 70 mm Hg and usually no more than 90 mm Hg on room air).

■ Chest X-ray shows large central pulmonary arteries and suggests right ventricular enlargement by rightward enlargement of the heart's silhouette on an anterior chest X-ray.

■ Echocardiography or angiography demonstrates right ventricular enlargement; echocardiography can estimate pulmonary

artery pressure (PAP) while also ruling out structural and congenital lesions.
- Electrocardiogram frequently shows arrhythmias, such as premature atrial and ventricular contractions and atrial fibrillation during severe hypoxia; it may also show right bundle-branch block, right axis deviation, prominent P waves and inverted T waves in right precordial leads, and right ventricular hypertrophy.
- PAP measurements show increased right ventricular and pulmonary artery pressures, stemming from increased pulmonary vascular resistance. Right ventricular systolic and pulmonary artery systolic pressures will exceed 30 mm Hg. Pulmonary artery diastolic pressure will exceed 15 mm Hg.
- Pulmonary function tests show results consistent with the underlying pulmonary disease. Hematocrit is typically greater than 50%.

Treatment

Treatment of cor pulmonale is designed to reduce hypoxemia, increase the patient's exercise tolerance and, when possible, correct the underlying condition.

In addition to bed rest, treatment may include:
- antibiotics when respiratory infection is present; culture and sensitivity of sputum specimens aid in selection of antibiotics
- anticoagulants, as indicated, to reduce the risk of thromboembolism
- low-sodium diet, restricted fluid intake, and diuretics such as furosemide [Lasix] to reduce edema
- oxygen by mask or cannula in concentrations ranging from 24% to 40%, depending on PaO_2, as necessary; in acute cases, therapy may also include mechanical ventilation; patients with underlying COPD generally shouldn't receive high concentrations of oxygen because of possible subsequent respiratory depression
- phlebotomy to reduce the red blood cell count if polycythemia is present

COR PULMONALE TEACHING TOPICS

● Make sure the patient understands the importance of maintaining a low-sodium diet, weighing himself daily, and watching for increased edema. Teach him to detect edema by pressing the skin over a shin with one finger, holding it for a second or two, then checking for a finger impression. Increased weight, increased edema, or respiratory difficulty should be reported to the practitioner.

● Instruct the patient to plan for frequent rest periods and to perform breathing exercises regularly.

● If the patient needs supplemental oxygen therapy at home, refer him to an agency that can help obtain the required equipment and, as necessary, arrange for follow-up examinations.

● If the patient has been placed on anticoagulant therapy, emphasize the need to watch for bleeding (epistaxis, hematuria, bruising) and to report signs to the physician. Also encourage him to return for periodic laboratory tests to monitor International Normalized Ratio, platelet count, hematocrit, hemoglobin level, and prothrombin time.

● Because pulmonary infection commonly exacerbates chronic obstructive pulmonary disease and cor pulmonale, tell the patient to watch for and immediately report early signs of infection, such as increased sputum production, change in sputum color, increased coughing or wheezing, chest pain, fever, fatigue, and tightness in the chest. Tell the patient to avoid crowds and anyone known to have pulmonary infections, especially during the flu season. Patients should receive Pneumovax and an annual influenza vaccine.

● Warn the patient to avoid substances that may depress the ventilatory drive, such as sedatives and alcohol.

■ potent pulmonary artery vasodilators (such as diazoxide [Proglycem], nitroprusside [Nitropress], hydralazine [Apresoline], angiotensin-converting enzyme inhibitors, calcium channel blockers, or prostaglandins) in primary pulmonary hypertension.

Depending on the underlying cause, some variations in treatment may be indicated. For example, a tracheotomy may be necessary if the patient has an upper airway obstruction. Steroids may be used in patients with a vasculitis autoimmune phenomenon or acute exacerbations of COPD.

Nursing interventions

■ Plan the diet carefully with the patient and the staff dietitian. Because the patient may lack energy and tire easily when eating, plan for small, frequent meals rather than three heavy ones.

■ Prevent fluid retention by limiting the patient's fluid intake to 1 to 2 qt (1 to 2 L)/day and providing a low-sodium diet.

■ Monitor serum potassium levels closely if the patient is receiving diuretics.

■ Reposition bedridden patients often to prevent atelectasis.

■ Provide meticulous respiratory care, including oxygen therapy and, for COPD patients, pursed-lip breathing exercises. Periodically measure ABG levels and watch for signs of impending respiratory failure, such as change in pulse rate, labored respirations, changes in mental status, and fatigue. (See *Cor pulmonale teaching topics*.)

PULMONARY EDEMA

Pulmonary edema is a common complication of cardiac disorders. It's marked by an accumulation of fluid in extravascular spaces of the lung. The disorder may occur as a chronic condition, or it may develop quickly and rapidly become fatal.

Pulmonary edema usually results from left-sided heart failure caused by arteriosclerotic, cardiomyopathic, hypertensive, or valvular heart disease. (See *How pulmonary edema develops,* page 304.)

Other factors that may predispose the patient to pulmonary edema include:

■ barbiturate or opiate poisoning

■ heart failure

■ infusion of excessive volumes of I.V. fluids or an overly rapid infusion

■ impaired pulmonary lymphatic drainage (from Hodgkin's disease or obliterative lymphangitis after radiation)

■ inhalation of irritating gases

■ mitral stenosis and left atrial myxoma (which impair left atrial emptying)

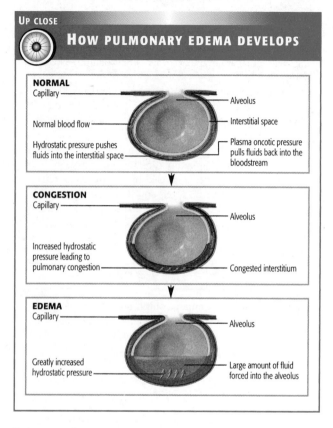

UP CLOSE

HOW PULMONARY EDEMA DEVELOPS

NORMAL
Capillary — — Alveolus
Normal blood flow — — Interstitial space
Hydrostatic pressure pushes fluids into the interstitial space — — Plasma oncotic pressure pulls fluids back into the bloodstream

CONGESTION
Capillary — — Alveolus
Increased hydrostatic pressure leading to pulmonary congestion — — Congested interstitium

EDEMA
Capillary — — Alveolus
Greatly increased hydrostatic pressure — — Large amount of fluid forced into the alveolus

- pneumonia
- pulmonary venoocclusive disease.

Normally, pulmonary capillary hydrostatic pressure, capillary oncotic pressure, capillary permeability, and lymphatic drainage are in balance. When this balance changes or the lymphatic drainage system is obstructed, fluid infiltrates into the lung and pulmonary edema results. If pulmonary capillary hydrostatic pressure increases, the compromised left ventricle requires increased filling pressures to maintain adequate cardiac output. These pressures are transmitted to the left atrium, pulmonary veins, and pulmonary capillary bed, forcing fluids and solutes from the intravascular compartment into the interstitium of the lungs. As the interstitium overloads with fluid, fluid floods the peripheral alveoli and impairs gas exchange.

If colloid osmotic pressure decreases, the hydrostatic force that regulates intravascular fluids (the natural pulling force) is lost because there's no opposition. Fluid flows freely into the interstitium and alveoli, impairing gas exchange and leading to pulmonary edema.

Blockage of the lymph vessels can result from compression by edema or tumor fibrotic tissue and by increased systemic venous pressure. Hydrostatic pressure in the large pulmonary veins increases, the pulmonary lymphatic system can't drain correctly into the pulmonary veins, and excess fluid moves into the interstitial space. Pulmonary edema then results from fluid accumulation.

Capillary injury, such as occurs in acute respiratory distress syndrome (ARDS) or with inhalation of toxic gases, increases capillary permeability. The injury causes plasma proteins and water to leak out of the capillary and move into the interstitium, increasing the interstitial oncotic pressure, which is normally low. As interstitial oncotic pressure begins to equal capillary oncotic pressure, the water begins to move out of the capillary and into the lungs, resulting in pulmonary edema.

Complications
- Respiratory acidosis
- Metabolic acidosis
- Cardiac or respiratory arrest

Assessment findings
- The patient's history may include a predisposing factor for pulmonary edema.
- The patient typically complains of a persistent cough.
- He may report getting a cold and being dyspneic on exertion.
- He may experience paroxysmal nocturnal dyspnea and orthopnea.
- On inspection, you may note restlessness and anxiety.

- With severe pulmonary edema, the patient's breathing may be visibly labored and rapid.
- His cough may sound intense and produce frothy, bloody sputum.
- In advanced stages, his level of consciousness decreases.
- Jugular vein distention is present.
- In acute pulmonary edema, the skin feels sweaty, cold, and clammy.
- Auscultation reveals crepitant crackles and a diastolic (S_3) gallop.
- In severe pulmonary edema, you may hear wheezing as the alveoli and bronchioles fill with fluid.
- Additional findings include worsening tachycardia, more profuse crackles, decreasing blood pressure, thready pulse, and decreased cardiac output. In advanced pulmonary edema, breath sounds diminish.

Diagnostic test results

Clinical features of pulmonary edema permit a working diagnosis. Diagnostic tests provide the following information:

- Arterial blood gas (ABG) analysis usually shows hypoxia with variable partial pressures of arterial carbon dioxide, depending on the patient's degree of fatigue. ABG results may also reveal metabolic acidosis.
- Chest X-rays show diffuse haziness of the lung fields and, usually, cardiomegaly and pleural effusion.
- Echocardiogram may reveal weak heart muscle, leaking or narrow heart valves, or fluid surrounding the heart.
- Electrocardiography may provide evidence of previous or current myocardial infarction.
- Pulmonary artery catheterization is used to identify left-sided heart failure (indicated by elevated pulmonary artery wedge pressures). These findings help to rule out ARDS, in which wedge pressure usually remains normal.
- Pulse oximetry may reveal decreasing levels of arterial oxygen saturation.

Treatment

Treatment goals are to reduce extravascular fluid, improve gas exchange and myocardial function and, if possible, correct underlying disease. High concentrations of oxygen can be given by cannula or mask. (Typically, the patient with pulmonary edema doesn't tolerate a mask.) If the patient's arterial oxygen levels remain too low, positive pressure ventilation can increase oxygen delivery to the tissues and usually improves his acid-base balance. Bronchodilators, such as beta$_2$-agonists inhalants, help decrease bronchospasm. Diuretics, such as furosemide (Lasix) or bumetanide (Bumex), may also be used to promote ventilation and increase urinary production.

Treatment of myocardial dysfunction includes positive inotropic agents to enhance contractility. Pressor agents may also be given to enhance contractility and to promote vasoconstriction in peripheral vessels.

Morphine (Duramorph) may reduce anxiety and dyspnea and dilate the systemic venous bed, promoting blood flow from pulmonary circulation to the periphery.

RED FLAG Using morphine in the patient with respiratory distress can compromise respirations. Have resuscitation equipment available in the event of a cardiac arrest.

Other treatments include phlebotomy and sublingual nitroglycerin, I.V. nitrates or angiotensin-converting enzyme inhibitors.

Nursing interventions

- Help the patient relax to promote oxygenation and control bronchospasm.
- Reassure the patient, who's likely to be frightened by his inability to breathe normally. Provide emotional support to his family as well.
- Place the patient in high Fowler's position to enhance lung expansion.
- Give oxygen as ordered.
- Assess the patient's condition frequently, and document his responses to treatment. Monitor ABG and pulse oximetry values, oral and I.V. fluid intake, urine output and, in the patient

with a pulmonary artery catheter, pulmonary end-diastolic and artery wedge pressures. Check the cardiac monitor often. Report changes immediately.

- Watch for complications of treatment, such as electrolyte depletion. Also watch for complications of oxygen therapy and mechanical ventilation.
- Monitor vital signs every 15 to 30 minutes while giving vaso-active medication in dextrose 5% in water by I.V. drip. During use, protect the solution from light by wrapping the bottle or bag with aluminum foil.
- Carefully record the time and the amount of morphine given. (See *Pulmonary edema teaching topics.*)

PULMONARY EMBOLISM

Pulmonary embolism is an obstruction of the pulmonary arterial bed that occurs when a mass—such as a dislodged thrombus—lodges in a pulmonary artery branch, partially or completely obstructing it. This causes a ventilation-perfusion ($\dot{V}/\dot{Q}$) mismatch, resulting in hypoxemia as well as intrapulmonary shunting.

The prognosis varies. Although the pulmonary infarction that results from embolism may be so mild that it doesn't cause symptoms, massive embolism (more than 50% obstruction of pulmonary arterial circulation) and pulmonary infarction can cause rapid death.

UNDERSTANDING THROMBUS FORMATION

Thrombus formation results from vascular wall damage, venous stasis, or hypercoagulability of the blood. Trauma, clot dissolution, sudden muscle spasm, intravascular pressure changes, or a change in peripheral blood flow can cause the thrombus to loosen or fragmentize. Then the thrombus, now called an embolus, floats to the heart's right side and enters the lung through the pulmonary artery. There, the embolus may dissolve, continue to fragmentize, or grow.

By occluding the pulmonary artery, the embolus prevents alveoli from producing enough surfactant to maintain alveolar integrity. As a result, alveoli collapse and atelectasis develops. If the embolus enlarges, it may clog most or all pulmonary vessels and cause death.

Pathophysiology

In most patients, pulmonary embolism results from a dislodged thrombus (blood clot) that originates in the leg veins. More than one-half of such thrombi arise in the deep veins of the legs; usually multiple thrombi arise. Other, less common sources of thrombi include the pelvic, renal, and hepatic veins, the right side of the heart, and the upper extremities. (See *Understanding thrombus formation.*)

Rarely, pulmonary embolism results from other types of emboli, including bone, air, fat, amniotic fluid, tumor cells, or a foreign object, such as a needle, catheter part, or talc (from drugs intended for oral administration that are injected I.V. by substance abusers).

The risk increases with long-term immobility, chronic pulmonary disease, heart failure or atrial fibrillation, thrombophlebitis, polycythemia vera, thrombocytosis, cardiac arrest, defibrillation, cardioversion, autoimmune hemolytic anemia, sickle cell disease, varicose veins, recent surgery, age older than 40, osteomyelitis, pregnancy, lower extremity fractures or surgery, burns, obesity, vascular injury, cancer, and hormonal contraceptive use. (See *Pulmonary emboli,* page 310. Also see *Who's at risk for pulmonary embolism?* page 311.)

PULMONARY EMBOLI

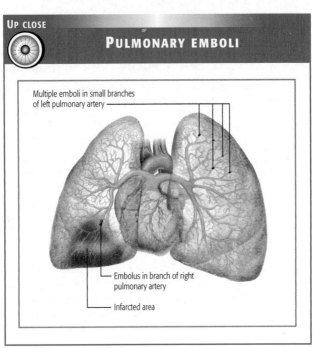

Multiple emboli in small branches of left pulmonary artery

Embolus in branch of right pulmonary artery

Infarcted area

Complications

- Pulmonary infarction (lung tissue death)
- Emboli extension
- Hepatic congestion and necrosis
- Pulmonary abscess
- Shock
- Acute respiratory distress syndrome
- Massive atelectasis
- Venous overload
- $\dot{V}/\dot{Q}$ mismatch
- Death

Assessment findings

- When you begin your assessment, you may find the patient has tachycardia, dyspnea, chest pain, and tachypnea.

WHO'S AT RISK FOR PULMONARY EMBOLISM?

Many disorders and treatments increase the risk for pulmonary embolism. Risk is particularly high for patients who have had surgery. The anesthetic used during surgery can injure lung vessels, and surgery or prolonged bed rest can promote venous stasis, further compounding the risk.

Predisposing disorders
- Autoimmune hemolytic anemia
- Cardiac disorders
- Diabetes mellitus
- History of thromboembolism, thrombophlebitis, or vascular insufficiency
- Infection
- Long-bone fracture
- Lung disorders, especially chronic types
- Manipulation or disconnection of central lines
- Osteomyelitis
- Polycythemia
- Sickle cell disease

Venous stasis
- Age older than 40

- Burns
- Obesity
- Orthopedic casts
- Prolonged bed rest or immobilization
- Recent childbirth

Venous injury
- I.V. drug abuse
- I.V. therapy
- Leg or pelvic fractures or injuries
- Surgery, particularly of the legs, pelvis, abdomen, or thorax

Increased blood coagulability
- Cancer
- Use of high-estrogen hormonal contraceptives

- If circulatory collapse has occurred, the patient has a weak, rapid pulse rate and hypotension.
- The patient's history may reveal a predisposing condition.
- The patient may complain that he gets acutely short of breath which may be associated with pleuritic or anginal type pain.
- The severity of these symptoms depends on the extent of damage. The signs and symptoms produced by small or fragmented emboli depend on their size, number, and location. If the embolus totally occludes the main pulmonary artery, cardiac arrest may occur.
- The patient may have a low-grade fever.
- On inspection, you may note a productive cough, possibly producing blood-tinged sputum.

- Less commonly, you may observe chest splinting, massive hemoptysis, leg edema and, with a large embolus, cyanosis, syncope, and distended jugular veins.
- If you observe restlessness—a sign of hypoxia—the patient may have circulatory collapse.
- Palpation may reveal a warm, tender area in the extremities, a possible area of thrombosis.
- On auscultation, you may hear a transient pleural friction rub and crackles at the embolus site.
- You may also note an S_3 and S_4 gallop, with increased intensity of the pulmonic component of S_2.
- In pleural infarction, the patient's history may include heart disease and left-sided heart failure.
- He may complain of sudden, sharp pleuritic chest pain accompanied by progressive dyspnea.

Diagnostic test results

- Arterial blood gas (ABG) analysis sometimes reveals respiratory alkalosis, hypoxemia, and a widened arterial-alveolar oxygen difference.
- Chest X-ray helps to rule out other pulmonary diseases, although it's inconclusive in the 1 to 2 hours after embolism. It may also show areas of atelectasis, an elevated diaphragm, pleural effusion, a prominent pulmonary artery and, occasionally, the characteristic wedge-shaped infiltrate that suggests pulmonary infarction. Sinus tachycardia and nonspecific ST changes may be seen. Electrocardiography is abnormal in 70% of patients with pulmonary embolism.
- Electrocardiography helps to distinguish pulmonary embolism from myocardial infarction.
- D-dimer by enzyme-linked immunosorbent assay rules out deep vein thrombosis.
- Lung perfusion scan (lung scintiscan) can show a pulmonary embolus, and ventilation scan (usually performed with a lung perfusion scan) confirms the diagnosis.
- Pulmonary angiography may show a pulmonary vessel filling defect or an abrupt vessel ending, both of which indicate pulmonary embolism. This is the most definitive test, but it's only used if the diagnosis can't be confirmed any other way

and anticoagulant therapy would put the patient at significant risk.

▓ Thoracentesis may rule out empyema, a sign of pneumonia, if the patient has pleural effusion.

Treatment

The goal of treatment is to maintain adequate cardiovascular and pulmonary function until the obstruction resolves and to prevent any recurrence. (Most emboli resolve within 10 to 14 days.)

Treatment for an embolism caused by a thrombus generally consists of oxygen therapy as needed and anticoagulation with heparin to inhibit new thrombus formation. The patient on heparin therapy needs daily or frequent coagulation studies (partial thromboplastin time [PTT]). Low-molecular-weight heparin has been used successfully for I.M. injections. The patient may also receive warfarin for 6 to 12 months or longer depending on his risk factors and etiology. His International Normalized Ratio should be monitored daily and then biweekly.

If the patient has a massive pulmonary embolism and shock, he may need fibrinolytic therapy with urokinase, streptokinase, or a tissue plasminogen activator. Initially, these thrombolytic agents dissolve clots within 12 to 24 hours. Seven days later, these drugs lyse clots to the same degree as heparin therapy alone.

If the embolus causes hypotension, the patient may need a vasopressor. A septic embolus requires antibiotic therapy, not anticoagulants, and evaluation for the infection's source, most likely endocarditis.

If the patient can't take anticoagulants or develops recurrent emboli during anticoagulant therapy, surgery in the form of a vena cava filter may be performed.

To prevent postoperative venous thromboembolism, the patient may require a vascular compression device applied to his legs.

If the patient has a fat embolus, oxygen therapy is needed. He may also need mechanical ventilation, corticosteroids and, if pulmonary edema arises, diuretics.

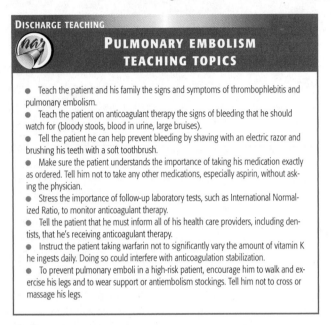

DISCHARGE TEACHING

PULMONARY EMBOLISM TEACHING TOPICS

- Teach the patient and his family the signs and symptoms of thrombophlebitis and pulmonary embolism.
- Teach the patient on anticoagulant therapy the signs of bleeding that he should watch for (bloody stools, blood in urine, large bruises).
- Tell the patient he can help prevent bleeding by shaving with an electric razor and brushing his teeth with a soft toothbrush.
- Make sure the patient understands the importance of taking his medication exactly as ordered. Tell him not to take any other medications, especially aspirin, without asking the physician.
- Stress the importance of follow-up laboratory tests, such as International Normalized Ratio, to monitor anticoagulant therapy.
- Tell the patient that he must inform all of his health care providers, including dentists, that he's receiving anticoagulant therapy.
- Instruct the patient taking warfarin not to significantly vary the amount of vitamin K he ingests daily. Doing so could interfere with anticoagulation stabilization.
- To prevent pulmonary emboli in a high-risk patient, encourage him to walk and exercise his legs and to wear support or antiembolism stockings. Tell him not to cross or massage his legs.

Nursing interventions

- As ordered, give oxygen by nasal cannula or mask. If the patient has worsening dyspnea, check his ABG levels. If breathing is severely compromised, provide endotracheal intubation with assisted ventilation as ordered.
- Give heparin, as ordered, by I.V. push or continuous drip. Monitor coagulation studies frequently. Effective heparin therapy raises PTT to about 2 to 2½ times normal.
- During heparin therapy, watch closely for epistaxis, petechiae, and other signs of abnormal bleeding. Check the patient's stools for occult blood. Don't give I.M. injections.
- After the patient stabilizes, encourage him to move about, and assist with isometric and range-of-motion exercises. Check his temperature and the color of his feet to detect venous stasis. Never vigorously massage his legs; this could cause thrombi to dislodge.

- Apply antiembolism stockings to promote venous return.
- Watch for possible anticoagulant treatment complications, including gastric bleeding, stroke, and hemorrhage.
- If the patient has pleuritic chest pain, give the ordered analgesic.
- Provide the patient with diversional activities to promote rest and relieve restlessness. (See *Pulmonary embolism teaching topics.*)

PULMONARY HYPERTENSION

In both the rare primary form and the more common secondary form, a resting systolic pulmonary artery pressure (PAP) greater than 30 mm Hg and a mean PAP greater than 18 mm Hg indicates pulmonary hypertension.

Primary or idiopathic pulmonary hypertension is characterized by increased PAP and increased pulmonary vascular resistance, both without an obvious cause. This form is most common in women between ages 20 and 40 and is usually fatal within 3 to 4 years; mortality is highest in pregnant women.

Secondary pulmonary hypertension results from existing cardiac or pulmonary disease. The prognosis in secondary pulmonary hypertension depends on the severity of the underlying disorder.

The cause of primary pulmonary hypertension is unknown, but the tendency for the disease to occur in families points to a hereditary defect. It also occurs more commonly in those with collagen disease and is thought to result from altered immune mechanisms. (See *Changes in pulmonary hypertension*, page 316.)

Pathophysiology

In primary pulmonary hypertension, the smooth muscle in the pulmonary artery wall hypertrophies, narrowing the small pulmonary arteries (arterioles) or obliterating them completely. Fibrous lesions also form around the vessels, impairing distensibility and increasing vascular resistance. Pressures in the left ventricle, which receives blood from the lungs, remain normal.

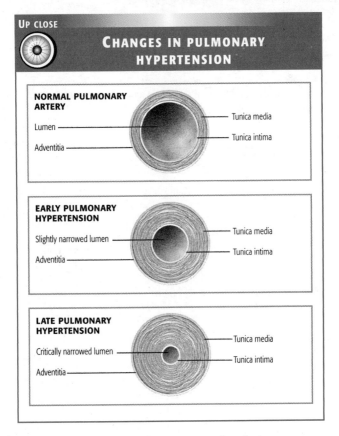

UP CLOSE

CHANGES IN PULMONARY HYPERTENSION

NORMAL PULMONARY ARTERY

Lumen

Adventitia

Tunica media

Tunica intima

EARLY PULMONARY HYPERTENSION

Slightly narrowed lumen

Adventitia

Tunica media

Tunica intima

LATE PULMONARY HYPERTENSION

Critically narrowed lumen

Adventitia

Tunica media

Tunica intima

However, the increased pressures generated in the lungs are transmitted to the right ventricle, which supplies the pulmonary artery. Eventually, the right ventricle fails (cor pulmonale). Although oxygenation isn't severely affected initially, hypoxia and cyanosis eventually occur. Death results from cor pulmonale.

Alveolar hypoventilation can result from diseases caused by alveolar destruction or from disorders that prevent the chest wall from expanding sufficiently to allow air into the alveoli. The resulting decreased ventilation increases pulmonary vascular resistance. Hypoxemia resulting from this ventilation-perfusion mismatch also causes vasoconstriction, further increasing vascular resistance and resulting in pulmonary hypertension.

Coronary artery disease or mitral valvular disease causing increased left ventricular filling pressures may cause secondary pulmonary hypertension. Ventricular septal defect and patent ductus arteriosus cause secondary pulmonary hypertension by increasing blood flow through the pulmonary circulation through left-to-right shunting. Pulmonary emboli and chronic destruction of alveolar walls, as in emphysema, cause secondary pulmonary hypertension by obliterating or obstructing the pulmonary vascular bed. Secondary pulmonary hypertension can also occur by vasoconstriction of the vascular bed, such as through hypoxemia and acidosis. Conditions resulting in vascular obstruction can cause pulmonary hypertension because blood isn't allowed to flow appropriately through the vessels.

Secondary pulmonary hypertension can be reversed if the disorder is resolved. If hypertension persists, hypertrophy occurs in the medial smooth muscle layer of the arterioles. The larger arteries stiffen, and hypertension progresses. Pulmonary pressures begin to equal systemic blood pressure, causing right ventricular hypertrophy and eventually cor pulmonale.

Primary cardiac diseases may be congenital or acquired. Congenital defects cause a left-to-right shunt, rerouting blood through the lungs twice and causing pulmonary hypertension. Acquired cardiac diseases, such as mitral insufficiency or aortic stenosis, result in left-sided heart failure that diminishes the flow of oxygenated blood from the lungs. This increases pulmonary vascular resistance and right ventricular pressure.

Complications
- Cor pulmonale
- Cardiac failure
- Cardiac arrest

Assessment findings
The patient with primary pulmonary hypertension may have no signs or symptoms until pulmonary vascular damage be-

comes severe. (In fact, the disorder may not be diagnosed until autopsy.)

- Usually, a patient with pulmonary hypertension complains of increasing dyspnea on exertion, weakness, syncope, and fatigue.
- He may also have difficulty breathing, feel short of breath, and report that breathing causes pain. Such signs may result from left-sided heart failure.
- Inspection may show signs of right-sided heart failure, including ascites and jugular vein distention.
- The patient may appear restless and agitated and have a decreased level of consciousness (LOC).
- He may be confused and have memory loss.
- You may observe decreased diaphragmatic excursion and respiration, and the point of maximal impulse may be displaced beyond the midclavicular line.
- On palpation, you may note signs of right-sided heart failure such as peripheral edema.
- The patient typically has an easily palpable right ventricular lift and a reduced carotid pulse.
- He may also have a palpable and tender liver and tachycardia.
- Auscultation findings are specific to the underlying disorder but may include narrow splitting of S_2, accentuated P_2 and, possibly, a systolic click.
- You may also hear decreased breath sounds and loud tubular sounds.
- The patient may have decreased blood pressure.

Diagnostic test results

- Arterial blood gas (ABG) studies reveal hypoxemia (decreased partial pressure of arterial oxygen).
- Cardiac catheterization discloses increased PAP, with a systolic pressure greater than 30 mm Hg.
- Echocardiography allows the assessment of ventricular wall motion and possible valvular dysfunction. It can also demonstrate right ventricular enlargement, abnormal septal configuration consistent with right ventricular pressure overload, and a reduction in left ventricular cavity size.

- Electrocardiography in right-sided heart failure shows right axis deviation and tall or peaked P waves in inferior leads.
- Perfusion lung scan may produce normal or abnormal results, with multiple patchy and diffuse filling defects that don't suggest pulmonary thromboembolism.
- Pulmonary angiography reveals filling defects in pulmonary vasculature such as those that develop with pulmonary emboli.
- Pulmonary function tests may show decreased flow rates and increased residual volume in underlying obstructive disease; in underlying restrictive disease, they may show reduced total lung capacity.
- Radionuclide imaging allows assessment of right and left ventricular functioning, and open lung biopsy may be used to determine the type of disorder.
- Pulmonary tissue biopsy may be done to confirm venoocclusive disease.
- Chest X-ray may show pulmonary artery enlargement and right atrial and ventricular enlargement.

Treatment

Oxygen therapy decreases hypoxemia and resulting pulmonary vascular resistance. For patients with right-sided heart failure, treatment also includes fluid restriction, cardiac glycosides to increase cardiac output, and diuretics to decrease intravascular volume and extravascular fluid accumulation. Vasodilators and calcium channel blockers can reduce myocardial work load and oxygen consumption. Bronchodilators and beta-adrenergic agents may also be prescribed. A patient with primary pulmonary hypertension usually responds to epoprostenol (PGI_2) as a continuous home infusion.

For a patient with secondary pulmonary hypertension, treatment must also aim to correct the underlying cause. If that isn't possible and the disease progresses, the patient may need a heart-lung transplant.

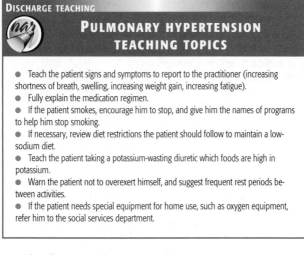

Nursing interventions

■ Give oxygen therapy, as ordered, and observe the patient's response. Report signs of increasing dyspnea so the physician can adjust treatment accordingly.

■ Monitor ABG levels for acidosis and hypoxemia. Report any change in the patient's LOC immediately.

■ When caring for a patient with right-sided heart failure, especially one receiving diuretics, record weight daily, carefully measure intake and output, and explain all medications and diet restrictions. Check for increasing jugular vein distention, which may signal fluid overload.

■ Monitor the patient's vital signs, especially blood pressure and heart rate. If hypotension or tachycardia develops, notify the physician. If the patient has a pulmonary artery catheter, monitor PAP and pulmonary artery wedge pressure, as ordered, and report changes.

■ Make sure the patient alternates periods of rest and activity to reduce the body's oxygen demand and prevent fatigue.

■ Before discharge, help the patient adjust to the limitations imposed by this disorder.

- Listen to the patient's fears and concerns, and remain with him during periods of extreme stress and anxiety.
- Answer the patient's questions as best you can. Encourage him to identify care measures and activities that make him comfortable and relaxed. Perform these measures, and encourage the patient to do so as well.
- Include the patient in care decisions, and include his family members in all phases of his care. (See *Pulmonary hypertension teaching topics*.)

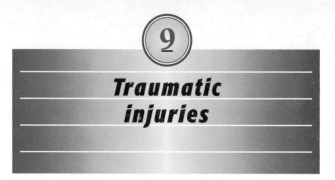

9

Traumatic injuries

Traumatic respiratory injuries are commonly life-threatening and have been a factor contributing to more than 25% of trauma-related deaths. They include asphyxia, chest trauma (blunt and penetrating), inhalation injury, near drowning, and pneumothorax.

ASPHYXIA

Asphyxia is a condition of insufficient oxygen and accumulating carbon dioxide in the blood and tissues. It results from interference with respiration. Asphyxia leads to cardiopulmonary arrest and is fatal without prompt treatment.

Pathophysiology

Asphyxia results from any internal or external condition or substance that inhibits respiration, including:

- hypoventilation that stems from opioid abuse, medullary disease or hemorrhage, respiratory muscle paralysis, or cardiopulmonary arrest
- intrapulmonary obstruction associated with airway obstruction, pulmonary edema, pneumonia, and near drowning
- extrapulmonary obstruction, as in tracheal compression from a tumor, pneumothorax, strangulation, trauma, or suffocation
- inhalation of toxic agents, resulting from carbon monoxide poisoning, smoke inhalation, and excessive oxygen inhalation.

Complications
- Neurologic damage
- Death

Assessment findings
The patient's history (obtained from a family member, friend, or emergency personnel) reveals the cause of asphyxia. Signs and symptoms depend on the duration and degree of asphyxia.
- On general observation, the patient typically appears anxious, agitated or confused, and dyspneic, with prominent neck muscles.
- Other common signs and symptoms include wheezing, stridor, altered respiratory rate (apnea, bradypnea, occasional tachypnea, and decreasing pulse oximetry), and a fast, slow, or absent pulse.
- Inspection may reveal little or no air moving in or out of the nose and mouth. You may note intercostal rib retractions as the intercostal muscles pull against resistance.
- You may note pale skin and, depending on the severity of the asphyxia, cyanosis in mucous membranes, lips, and nail beds.
- Trauma-induced asphyxia may cause erythema and petechiae on the upper chest, up to the neck and face.
- In late-stage carbon monoxide poisoning, mucous membranes appear cherry red.
- Auscultation reveals decreased or absent breath sounds.

Diagnostic test results
- Arterial blood gas (ABG) analysis, the most important test, indicates decreased partial pressure of arterial oxygen (less than 60 mm Hg) and increased partial pressure of arterial carbon dioxide (more than 50 mm Hg).
- Chest X-rays may detect a foreign body, pulmonary edema, atelectasis, or pneumothorax.
- Pulmonary function tests may indicate respiratory muscle weakness.
- Toxicology tests may show drugs, chemicals, or abnormal hemoglobin levels.

Treatment

Asphyxia requires immediate respiratory support with cardiopulmonary resuscitation (CPR), endotracheal (ET) intubation,
supplemental oxygen, mechanical ventilation, and pulse oximetry as needed. It also calls for prompt treatment of the underlying cause, such as bronchoscopy for extraction of a foreign
body; an opioid antagonist, such as naloxone (Narcan), for
opioid overdose; or gastric lavage for poisoning.

Nursing interventions

- If a foreign body is blocking the patient's airway, perform abdominal thrust.
- In an unconscious patient, the tongue may obstruct the airway. You may be able to open the airway by simply repositioning the patient.
- If the patient has no spontaneous respirations and no pulse,
  begin CPR.
- If needed, assist with ET intubation to provide an airway, and
  give supplemental oxygen or provide mechanical ventilation
  as ordered. Monitor ABG levels, the best indicator of oxygenation and acid-base status.
- Ensure I.V. access, monitor I.V. fluids, and obtain laboratory
  specimens as ordered.
- If the patient ingested poison, insert a nasogastric tube or an
  Ewald tube for lavage.
- Give medications for opioid overdose such as naloxone as ordered.
- Monitor the patient's cardiac status, vital signs, and neurologic status throughout treatment.

- Continually reassure the patient throughout treatment because respiratory distress is terrifying.
- If asphyxia was intentionally induced, such as carbon monoxide poisoning, refer the patient to a psychiatrist. (See *Asphyxia teaching topics.*)

CHEST TRAUMA

Chest trauma accounts for almost one-half of all trauma occurrences and almost one-fourth of all trauma-related deaths. Chest trauma is commonly classified as penetrating or blunt, depending on the type of injury. Penetrating chest trauma involves an injury by a foreign object, such as a knife (most common stabbing injury), bullet (most common missile injury), or other pointed object that penetrates the thorax. These are considered open injuries because the thoracic cavity is exposed to pressure from the outside atmosphere. Blunt chest trauma, which is considered a closed chest injury, results from sudden compression or positive pressure inflicted by a direct blow to the organ and surrounding tissue. Blunt chest trauma commonly occurs in motor vehicle accidents (when the chest strikes the steering wheel), falls, or crushing injury.

Typically, penetrating chest trauma is fairly limited, usually involving isolated organs and lacerated tissues. In some cases, however, extensive tissue damage can occur if a bullet implodes in the chest cavity. Blunt chest trauma can cause extensive injury to the chest wall, lung, pleural space, and great vessels. Injuries resulting from blunt chest trauma include pulmonary contusion, rib fractures, pneumothorax, hemothorax, and rupture of the diaphragm or great vessels. (See *Injuries associated with chest trauma,* pages 326 to 331.) Blunt injuries are associated with multisystem organ injuries and carry a higher mortality than penetrating injuries.

Pathophysiology
Injuries to the chest usually involve one or more of the following:
- hypovolemia resulting from massive blood loss

(Text continues on page 330.)

INJURIES ASSOCIATED WITH CHEST TRAUMA

INJURY	PATHOPHYSIOLOGIC MECHANISM OF INJURY
Pneumothorax	Blunt or penetrating injury allowing air to accumulate in the pleural space
Tension pneumothorax	Blunt or penetrating injury allowing air to accumulate in the pleural space without a way to escape, leading to complete lung collapse
Hemothorax	Blunt or penetrating trauma allowing blood to accumulate in the pleural space
Chylothorax	Blunt or penetrating trauma usually to the thoracic duct or lymphatics allowing lymphatic fluid to drain and accumulate in the pleural space
Pneumomediastinum	Blunt or penetrating trauma allowing air to accumulate in the mediastinum
Flail chest	Blunt trauma resulting in rib or sternal fractures leading to instability of the chest

ASSESSMENT FINDINGS	TREATMENT CONSIDERATIONS
• Dyspnea • Chest pain • Decreased or absent breath sounds • Chest X-ray positive for air between visceral and parietal pleura	• Chest tube insertion
• Severe dyspnea • Restlessness • Cyanosis • Tracheal shift to unaffected side • Distended jugular veins • Absence of breath sounds on affected side • Tachycardia • Hypotension • Distant heart sounds • Hypoxemia	• Emergency lung reexpansion; possible thoracotomy for penetrating injury • Chest tube insertion
• Dyspnea • Tachycardia • Tachypnea • Cool clammy skin • Hypotension • Diminished capillary refill • Absent breath sounds on affected side • Chest X-ray positive for blood accumulation	• Chest tube insertion with possible autotransfusion
• Chest X-ray positive for pleural effusion (although may not be evident for 2 to 4 weeks) after injury	• Chest tube insertion • Possible thoracotomy to ligate thoracic duct
• Dyspnea • Chest pain	• Chest tube placement with repair of underlying injury
• Dyspnea • Labored shallow respirations • Chest wall pain • Crepitus from body fragments (subcutaneous emphysema)	• Symptomatic and supportive care • Prevention of hemothorax and pneumothorax

(continued)

INJURIES ASSOCIATED WITH CHEST TRAUMA
(continued)

INJURY	PATHOPHYSIOLOGIC MECHANISM OF INJURY
Flail chest *(continued)*	
Pulmonary contusion	Blunt trauma injuring lung tissue with the potential to cause respiratory failure
Tracheobronchial tear	Blunt trauma causing injury to the tracheobronchial tree, possibly leading to airway obstruction and tension pneumothorax
Diaphragmatic rupture	Blunt trauma causing a tear in the diaphragm, possibly allowing abdominal contents to herniate into the thorax
Cardiac contusion	Blunt trauma resulting in bruising of the cardiac muscle

ASSESSMENT FINDINGS	TREATMENT CONSIDERATIONS
● Asymmetrical (paradoxical) chest movements ● Chest X-ray positive for fractures	
● Dyspnea ● Restlessness ● Hemoptysis ● Tachycardia ● Crackles ● Decreased lung compliance ● Atelectasis ● Arterial blood gas analysis revealing hypoxemia and hypercarbia ● Chest X-ray revealing local or diffuse patchy, poorly outlined densities or irregular linear infiltrates	● Intubation and mechanical ventilation ● Hemodynamic monitoring ● Possible thoracotomy if massive hemorrhage suspected
● Dyspnea ● Palpable fracture, hoarseness, and subcutaneous edema (laryngeal fracture) ● Noisy breathing, labored respirations, and altered level of consciousness (tracheal injury) ● Hemoptysis, subcutaneous emphysema, and possible tension pneumothorax (bronchial injury)	● Emergency surgical repair of injury
● Chest pain referred to the shoulder ● Dyspnea ● Diminished breath sounds ● Bowels sounds audible in chest ● Tachypnea ● Chest X-ray positive for tear	● Surgical repair
● Chest discomfort ● Electrocardiogram abnormalities (unexplained sinus tachycardia, atrial fibrillation, bundle branch block, ST segment changes) ● Serial creatine kinase levels revealing possible cardiac muscle damage	● Supportive and symptomatic care

(continued)

INJURIES ASSOCIATED WITH CHEST TRAUMA
(continued)

INJURY	PATHOPHYSIOLOGIC MECHANISM OF INJURY
Cardiac tamponade	Blunt or penetrating trauma allowing blood to accumulate in the pericardial sac, ultimately impairing venous return and cardiac output
Great vessel rupture	Blunt trauma resulting in injury to major blood vessels such as the aorta

- hypoxemia resulting from airway alteration; damage to the chest muscles, lung parenchyma or ribs; severe hemorrhage; collapse of the lungs; or pneumothorax
- cardiac failure resulting from an increase in intrathoracic pressure or subsequent cardiac injury, such as cardiac tamponade or contusion.

Tissue damage caused by penetrating trauma, such as an impaled object or foreign body, is related to the object size as well as the depth and velocity of penetration. For example, penetrating chest trauma by a bullet has many variables. The extent of injury depends on the distance at which the weapon was fired, the type of ammunition, the velocity of the ammunition, and the entrance and (if present) exit wounds. Other factors to consider when assessing a penetrating chest injury include the type of weapon—for example, the caliber, barrel, and length of a gun, and the powder composition. An intact bullet causes less damage than a bullet that explodes on impact. A bullet that explodes within the chest may break up and scatter fragments,

ASSESSMENT FINDINGS	TREATMENT CONSIDERATIONS
● Dyspnea ● Midthoracic pain ● Tachycardia ● Tachypnea ● Hypotension, distended jugular veins, and muffled heart sounds (Beck's triad) ● Paradoxical pulse	● Pericardiocentesis
● Dyspnea ● Hoarseness ● Stridor ● Absent femoral pulses ● Retrosternal or interscapular pain ● Widening mediastinum	● Transfusion ● Surgical repair

burn tissue, fracture bone, disrupt vascular structures, or cause a bullet embolism.

Injury resulting from blunt chest trauma is related to the amount of force, compression, and cavitation. Blunt force that strikes the chest wall at high velocity fractures the ribs and transfers that force to underlying organ and lung tissue. The direct impact of force is transmitted internally, and the energy is dissipated to internal structures. The flexibility or elasticity of the chest wall directly affects the degree of injury. The first and second ribs take an enormous amount of blunt force to fracture and therefore are associated with significant intrathoracic injuries.

AGE AWARE Because the chest in the frail older person is inflexible and fragile, injury and death, even from minor chest trauma, are more likely.

Complications
■ Acute respiratory distress syndrome
■ Bronchopleural fistula

- Ventilator-induced lung injury such as barrel trauma
- Infection
- Pneumonia
- Pulmonary emboli

Assessment findings

The patient's history reveals a recent injury to the chest, and the patient may complain of dyspnea and chest pain. Other clinical features vary with the complications caused by the chest injury.

FRACTURES

- A patient with a sternal fracture—usually a transverse fracture located in the middle or upper sternum—may complain of persistent chest pain, even at rest.
- A patient with a rib fracture may complain of tenderness over the fracture site and pain that worsens with deep breathing and movement.
- Inspection reveals shallow, splinted respirations (a result of the painful breathing).
- Palpation reveals slight edema and crepitus over the fracture site.
- You may note hypoventilation on auscultation.

HEMOTHORAX

- If the patient develops hemothorax, he'll report chest pain after the injury, along with some form of respiratory distress.
- Depending on the seriousness of hemothorax, inspection may show no obvious respiratory distress, mild respiratory distress, or severe dyspnea with restlessness and pallor or cyanosis.
- The patient may have asymmetrical chest movements and flat jugular veins.
- In massive hemothorax, you may observe bloody sputum or hemoptysis.
- Palpation of hemothorax may reveal unilateral decreased fremitus and decreased chest expansion on inspiration.
- If hemothorax is small, percussion won't detect changes.
- If hemothorax is moderate or massive, percussion reveals dullness over the area of fluid collection.

- Auscultation may reveal unilateral diminished breath sounds or, in more severe hemothorax, unilateral absent breath sounds.
- The patient with moderate or massive hemothorax also has hypotension and tachycardia.

PNEUMOTHORAX
- If the patient develops pneumothorax, he'll usually complain of acute, sharp chest pain and shortness of breath.
- Inspection of the patient may show an obviously increased respiratory rate, cyanosis, agitation and, possibly, asymmetrical chest expansion.
- Percussion reveals unilateral hyperresonance. On auscultation, breath sounds are diminished or absent on the affected side.
- You'll also note a crunching sound that occurs with each heartbeat—Hamman's sign, which indicates mediastinal air accumulation.

TENSION PNEUMOTHORAX
- If tension pneumothorax develops, the patient may complain of acute chest pain.
- On inspection, you may observe cyanosis, increasing dyspnea, tracheal deviation, distended jugular veins, and asymmetrical or paradoxical neck movement.
- Palpation confirms the tracheal deviation and may disclose subcutaneous crepitus in the neck and upper chest area.
- Percussion usually reveals unilateral hyperresonance.
- On auscultation, you'll note unilateral absent breath sounds, muffled heart sounds, and hypotension.

FLAIL CHEST
- A patient who develops flail chest may report severe pain (from the rib fractures) and extreme shortness of breath.
- On inspection, you may note that he appears restless.
- You may also see bruising and disfigurement in the chest area; rapid, shallow respirations; cyanosis; and paradoxical chest movements. (See *Paradoxical breathing in flail chest,* page 334.)
- Palpation may reveal tachycardia, bony crepitus at the fracture site, and subcutaneous crepitus.

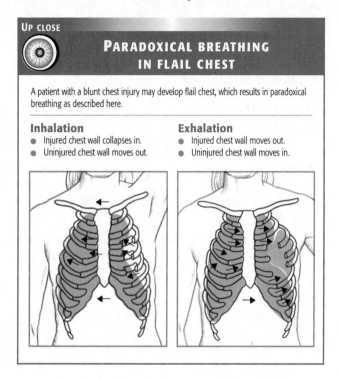

UP CLOSE

PARADOXICAL BREATHING IN FLAIL CHEST

A patient with a blunt chest injury may develop flail chest, which results in paradoxical breathing as described here.

Inhalation
- Injured chest wall collapses in.
- Uninjured chest wall moves out.

Exhalation
- Injured chest wall moves out.
- Uninjured chest wall moves in.

■ Auscultation may show hypotension and diminished breath sounds.

PULMONARY CONTUSIONS
■ In a patient with pulmonary contusions, assessment findings include hemoptysis, pallor or cyanosis, dyspnea and, possibly, signs of airway obstruction.

MYOCARDIAL CONTUSIONS
■ Myocardial contusions may produce tachycardia, ecchymosis, chest pain, and electrocardiogram (ECG) abnormalities.

DIAPHRAGMATIC RUPTURE
■ Diaphragmatic rupture causes severe respiratory distress and death.

■ If the patient doesn't receive immediate treatment, assessment reveals a decrease in the vital capacity and serious circulatory changes—the result of herniation of the abdominal contents into the thorax.

Diagnostic test results

■ Angiography reveals aortic laceration or rupture.
■ Blood studies show that serum levels of aspartate aminotransferase, alanine aminotransferase, lactate dehydrogenase, creatine kinase (CK), and the isoenzyme CK-MB are elevated.
■ Chest X-rays may confirm rib and sternal fractures, pneumothorax, flail chest, pulmonary contusions, lacerated or ruptured aorta, tension pneumothorax (mediastinal shift), diaphragmatic rupture, lung compression, or atelectasis with hemothorax.
■ Contrast studies and liver and spleen scans detect diaphragmatic rupture.
■ Echocardiography, computed tomography scans, and nuclear heart and lung scans show the extent of injury.
■ With cardiac damage, such as a pericardial contusion or tamponade, the ECG may show right bundle-branch block. Arrhythmias, conduction abnormalities, and ST-wave changes may occur in myocardial contusions.

Treatment

Blunt chest injuries call for controlling bleeding and maintaining a patent airway, adequate ventilation, and fluid and electrolyte balance. Further treatment depends on the specific injury and complications:

FRACTURES

Single fractured ribs are managed conservatively with mild analgesics and follow-up examinations to check for indications of a pneumothorax or hemothorax. To prevent atelectasis, the patient should perform incentive spirometry, deep breathing, and coughing for lung expansion. Intercostal nerve blocks may help with more severe fractures.

PNEUMOTHORAX

Treatment for pneumothorax involves inserting a spinal, 14G, or 16G needle into the second intercostal space at the midclavicular line to release pressure. Then the physician inserts a chest tube in the affected side to normalize pressure and reexpand the lung. The patient also receives oxygen and I.V. fluids. He may require intubation and mechanical ventilation.

SHOCK

Shock related to hemothorax calls for I.V. infusion of lactated Ringer's or normal saline solution. If the patient loses more than 1,500 ml of blood or more than 30% of circulating blood volume, he'll also need a transfusion of packed red blood cells or an autotransfusion. He may also require intubation, mechanical ventilation and, possibly, a thoracotomy. Chest tubes are inserted into the fifth or sixth intercostal space at the midaxillary line to remove blood.

FLAIL CHEST

Treatment of flail chest may include endotracheal (ET) intubation and mechanical ventilation with positive pressure. The patient may also receive I.V. muscle relaxants. If he requires controlled ventilation, he'll receive a neuromuscular blocking agent. If an air leak occurs, he may need surgery for flail chest.

PULMONARY CONTUSIONS

Pulmonary contusions are managed with colloids to replace volume and maintain oncotic pressure. (Steroid use is controversial.) The patient may also need ET intubation and mechanical ventilation as well as antibiotics, diuretics, and analgesics.

MYOCARDIAL CONTUSIONS

Myocardial contusions call for cardiac and hemodynamic monitoring to detect arrhythmias and prevent cardiogenic shock. Drug therapy depends on the type of arrhythmia. Treatment is similar to that for myocardial infarction (MI).

MYOCARDIAL RUPTURE, SEPTAL PERFORATION, AND OTHER CARDIAC LACERATIONS

Myocardial rupture, septal perforation, and other types of cardiac lacerations require immediate surgical repair. Less severe ventricular wounds require use of a digital or balloon catheter. Atrial wounds require a clamp or balloon catheter.

The patient with an aortic rupture or laceration who reaches the hospital alive needs immediate surgery with synthetic grafts or anastomosis used to repair the damage. He requires a large amount of I.V. fluids (lactated Ringer's solution) and whole blood along with oxygen at a very high rate. A pneumatic anti-shock garment is applied, and he's promptly taken to the operating room.

For a patient with a diaphragmatic rupture, a nasogastric tube is inserted to temporarily decompress the stomach, and he's prepared for surgical repair.

Nursing interventions

- Closely monitor any patient with a blunt chest injury.
- Frequently check pulses (including peripheral pulses) and level of consciousness. Also evaluate the color and temperature of skin, depth of respiration, use of accessory muscles, and length of inhalation compared with exhalation.
- Look for a tracheal shift—a sign of tension pneumothorax. Also look for distended jugular veins and paradoxical chest motion. Listen to the patient's heart and breath sounds carefully, and palpate for subcutaneous emphysema and fractured ribs.
- For simple rib fractures, give mild analgesics, encourage bed rest, and apply heat. Don't strap or tape the chest.
- Anticipate the need to insert chest tubes, especially if bleeding is prolonged. To prevent atelectasis, frequently turn the patient, and encourage him to perform coughing and deep breathing.
- For more severe fractures, assist with administration of intercostal nerve blocks. (Obtain X-rays before and after this treatment to rule out pneumothorax.)
- For pneumothorax, assist during placement of the chest tube. Give oxygen and I.V. fluids as ordered.

DISCHARGE TEACHING

CHEST TRAUMA TEACHING TOPICS

- Reinforce the physician's explanation of the patient's condition and treatment plan. Make sure the patient and his family understand the care that's required.
- Teach the patient incentive spirometry and postural drainage techniques.
- Teach the patient breathing exercises to maintain effective pulmonary function. Explain the need for turning, coughing, and deep breathing.
- Discuss the medications prescribed for pain, including their adverse effects.
- Teach splinting techniques for turning, deep breathing, and ambulation.
- Encourage the patient not to smoke. Explain that smoking increases tracheobronchial secretions and decreases blood oxygen saturation.
- Teach the patient with rib or sternal fractures that pain will persist for several weeks. Instruct him to take analgesics as prescribed.
- Advise the patient to notify the practitioner if pain worsens or is accompanied by fever, a productive cough, and shortness of breath. These may indicate infection.
- Tell the patient to avoid contact sports until the pain is resolved and the practitioner permits him to resume such activities.

- For flail chest, place the patient in semi-Fowler's position. Oxygenate the patient, and anticipate intubation and controlled mechanical ventilation after emergency chest tube insertion. Observe for signs of tension pneumothorax. Suction the patient as needed. Start I.V. therapy, and observe closely for signs of excessive or insufficient fluid resuscitation and of acid-base imbalance. If paralytic agents are needed while the patient is mechanically ventilated, make sure to give analgesics and sedation to control pain and anxiety.

- For hemothorax, assist with chest tube insertion, observe the volume and consistency of chest drainage, and give oxygen. Begin autotransfusion if indicated. Monitor and document vital signs and blood loss. Immediately report falling blood pressure, rising pulse rate, and uncontrolled hemorrhage, all of which require a thoracotomy to stop the bleeding.

- For pulmonary contusions, monitor blood gas levels to ensure adequate ventilation. Provide oxygen therapy, mechanical ventilation, chest tube care, and I.V. therapy as needed. Give ordered colloids, analgesics, and corticosteroids.

- For suspected cardiac contusion, care is essentially the same as for a patient with an MI. Cardiac monitoring or telemetry

detects arrhythmias, and the patient should be carefully monitored for signs of cardiogenic shock. Impose bed rest in
semi-Fowler's position (unless contraindicated). Give oxygen,
analgesics, and supportive drugs such as digoxin (Lanoxin),
as ordered, to control heart failure or supraventricular arrhythmia. Watch for cardiac tamponade, which calls for peri-
cardiocentesis.

■ If the patient has decreased mobility, reposition him at least
every 2 hours to maintain skin integrity. Inspect his skin and
keep it clean and dry. (See *Chest trauma teaching topics*.)

INHALATION INJURY

Inhalation injuries result from trauma to the pulmonary system
after inhalation of toxic substances or of gases that are nontoxic
but interfere with cellular respiration. Inhaled exposure forms
include fog, mist, fumes, dust, gas, vapor, or smoke. Inhalation
injuries commonly accompany burns.

Inhalation injuries have a variety of causes.

THERMAL INHALATION
Pulmonary complications remain the leading cause of death following thermal trauma. This type of trauma is commonly caused
by the inhalation of hot air or steam. Mortality exceeds 50%
when inhalation injury accompanies burns of the skin. Suspect
this type of injury with reports of flames in a confined area, even
if burns on the surface aren't visible.

CHEMICAL INHALATION
A variety of gases may be generated during the burning of materials. The acids and alkalis released from the burning can produce chemical burns when inhaled. The inhaled substances can
reach the respiratory tract as insoluble gases and lead to permanent damage.

Synthetic materials also produce gases that can be toxic.
Plastic material has the ability to produce toxic vapors when
heated or burned. The inhalation of chemicals in a powder or
liquid form without burning is also capable of causing pulmonary damage. Substances such as ammonia, chlorine, sulfur

dioxide, and hydrogen chloride are considered pulmonary irritants.

CARBON MONOXIDE POISONING

Carbon monoxide is a colorless, odorless, tasteless gas produced as a result of combustion and oxidation. Poisoning from carbon monoxide can occur from inhalation of small amounts of this gas over a long period or the inhalation of large amounts in a short period. Carbon monoxide is considered a chemical asphyxiant. Accidental poisoning can occur from exposure to heaters, smoke from a fire, or use of a gas lamp, gas stove, or charcoal grill in a small, poorly ventilated area.

Pathophysiology

The pathophysiology of each type of inhalation injury varies.

THERMAL INHALATION

The entire respiratory tract is at risk for damage from thermal inhalation injury; however, injury rarely progresses to the lungs. The area of greatest damage is the upper airway, where inhaled hot air or steam is rapidly cooled. Reflective closure of the vocal cords and laryngeal spasm usually prevent full inhalation of the hot air or steam, limiting injury to the lower respiratory tract. Steam inhalation is more harmful than hot air inhalation because water holds heat longer than dry air.

CHEMICAL INHALATION

Irritating gases (chlorine, hydrogen chloride, nitrogen dioxide, phosgene, and sulfur dioxide) combine with water in the lungs to form corrosive acids. These acids cause denaturation of proteins, cellular damage, and edema of the pulmonary tissues. Smoke inhalation injuries generally fall into this category. Chemical burns to the airway are similar to burns on the skin, except that they're painless because the tracheobronchial tree is insensitive to pain. The inhalation of small amounts of noxious chemicals can damage the alveoli and bronchi.

CARBON MONOXIDE POISONING

Several gases, such as carbon monoxide and hydrogen cyanide, aren't directly toxic to the respiratory system. However, these gases interfere with cellular respiration. Carbon monoxide has a greater attraction to hemoglobin than oxygen. When carbon monoxide enters the blood, it binds with the hemoglobin to form carboxyhemoglobin. Carboxyhemoglobin reduces the oxygen-carrying capacity of the hemoglobin. This results in decreased oxygenation to the cells and tissues.

Assessment findings

Physical findings with an inhalation injury vary depending on the gas or substance inhaled and the length of exposure.

THERMAL INHALATION

- The entire respiratory tract has the potential to be damaged by this type of inhalation injury, but injury rarely progresses to the lungs.
- Ulcerations, erythema, and edema of the mouth and epiglottis are the initial symptoms noted with this type of injury.
- Edema may rapidly progress to upper airway obstruction.
- Stridor, wheezing, crackles, increased secretions, hoarseness, and shortness of breath may also be noted.
- If there was direct thermal injury to the upper airway, burns of the face and lips, burned nasal hairs, and laryngeal edema will be present.

CHEMICAL INHALATION

- The most common effects of smoke or chemical inhalation include atelectasis, pulmonary edema, and tissue anoxia.
- Respiratory distress usually occurs early in the course of smoke inhalation secondary to hypoxia.
- Patients who at first show no respiratory difficulties may suddenly develop respiratory distress.
- Keep intubation and mechanical ventilation equipment available for immediate use.

CARBON MONOXIDE POISONING

- Carboxyhemoglobin reduces the oxygen-carrying capacity of hemoglobin. This typically causes a bright red flush of the face and cherry red lips.

OXYGEN SATURATION IN CARBON MONOXIDE POISONING

When assessing for carbon monoxide poisoning, be aware that pulse oximetry devices measure oxygenated and deoxygenated hemoglobin but don't measure dysfunctional hemoglobin, such as carboxyhemoglobin. Therefore, the oxygen saturation levels in the presence of carbon monoxide poisoning will be within normal ranges as the carboxyhemoglobin levels aren't measured.

- The symptoms of carbon monoxide poisoning vary with the concentration of carboxyhemoglobin. (See *Oxygen saturation in carbon monoxide poisoning.*)
- Mild poisoning generally indicates a carbon monoxide level between 11% and 20%. Symptoms at this level typically include headache, decreased cerebral function, decreased visual acuity, and slight shortness of breath.
- Moderate poisoning indicates a carbon monoxide level between 21% and 40%. Symptoms at this concentration include headache, tinnitus, nausea, drowsiness, dizziness, altered mental status, confusion, stupor, irritability, hypotension, tachycardia, electrocardiogram (ECG) changes, and changes in skin color.
- Severe poisoning is defined as a carbon monoxide level between 41% and 60%. Symptoms include coma, convulsions, and generalized instability.
- In the final stage (fatal poisoning), the carbon monoxide level reaches 61% to 80%, and death results.

Diagnostic test results
- Arterial blood gas analysis provides valuable information on the acid-base status, ventilation, and oxygenation status of the patient.
- Initial blood studies include a complete blood count, liver function studies, and electrolyte, blood urea nitrogen and creatinine levels. Obtaining these studies will provide baseline data for analysis.

- Cardiac monitoring will monitor ischemic changes. A depressed ST segment on ECG is a common finding in the moderate stage of carbon monoxide poisoning.
- A chest X-ray will also be performed and evaluated.
- In patients with suspected carbon monoxide poisoning, a carboxyhemoglobin level will be obtained.

Treatment

Obtain a history of the exposure, and attempt to identify the toxic agent. Immediately provide oxygen to the patient. Intubation and mechanical ventilation may be required if the patient demonstrates severe respiratory distress or an altered state of mentation. Upper airway edema requires emergency endotracheal intubation. Bronchodilators, antibiotics, and I.V. fluids may be prescribed.

The preferred treatment for carbon monoxide poisoning is administration of 100% humidified oxygen, continued until carboxyhemoglobin levels fall to the nontoxic range of 10%. Chest physiotherapy may assist in expectoration of necrotic tissue from the lungs.

The use of hyperbaric oxygen for carbon monoxide poisoning remains controversial, although it's known that it lowers carboxyhemoglobin levels more rapidly than humidified oxygen. Fluid resuscitation is an important component of managing inhalation injury, but careful monitoring of fluid status is essential due to the risk of pulmonary edema development.

Nursing interventions

- Remove the patient's clothing. Prevent self-contamination from the toxic substance if there's a possibility that any is on the patient's clothing.
- Establish an I.V. access for medication, blood products, and fluid administration.
- Obtain laboratory specimens to evaluate ventilation, oxygenation, and baseline values.
- Obtain chest X-ray, ECG, and pulmonary function studies.
- Implement cardiac monitoring to assess for ischemic changes or arrhythmias.
- Monitor for signs of pulmonary edema that may accompany fluid resuscitation.

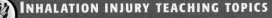

■ In the event of bronchospasm, provide oxygen, bronchodilators via a nebulizer and, possibly, aminophylline (Truphylline).
■ Monitor fluid balance and intake and output closely.
■ Give antibiotics as prescribed.
■ Assess lung sounds frequently, and notify the physician immediately of changes in lung sounds or oxygenation.
■ Provide a supportive and educational environment for the patient, his family, and significant others.
■ Monitor laboratory studies for changes that may indicate multisystem complications. (See *Inhalation injury teaching topics*.)

NEAR DROWNING

In near drowning, the victim survives (at least temporarily) the physiologic effects of submersion in fluid. Hypoxemia and acidosis are the primary problems in victims of near drowning.

The three forms of near drowning are dry near drowning, in which the victim doesn't aspirate fluid but suffers respiratory obstruction or asphyxia (10% to 15% of patients); wet near drowning, in which the victim aspirates fluid and suffers from asphyxia or secondary changes from fluid aspiration (about 85% of patients); and secondary near drowning, in which the victim suffers recurrence of respiratory distress (usually aspiration pneumonia or pulmonary edema) from minutes to 2 days after a near-drowning incident.

Pathophysiology
Regardless of the tonicity of the fluid aspirated, hypoxemia is the most serious consequence of near drowning, followed by meta-

bolic acidosis. Other consequences depend on the kind of water aspirated. After freshwater aspiration, changes in the character of lung surfactant result in exudation of protein-rich plasma into the alveoli. This, plus increased capillary permeability, leads to pulmonary edema and hypoxemia

After saltwater aspiration, the hypertonicity of sea water exerts an osmotic force, which pulls fluid from pulmonary capillaries into the alveoli. The resulting intrapulmonary shunt causes hypoxemia. The pulmonary capillary membrane may be injured and may induce pulmonary edema. In wet and secondary near drowning, pulmonary edema and hypoxemia occur as a result of aspiration.

Regardless of the type of near drowning (freshwater or saltwater), aspiration of contaminants can occur. The victim may aspirate chlorine, mud, algae, weeds, and other foreign material. Saltwater aspiration is considered more dangerous because salt water contains more types of disease-causing bacteria. These contaminants may lead to obstruction, aspiration pneumonia, and pulmonary fibrosis.

A protective effect may be seen in cold water submersion (exposure to temperatures 69.8° F [21° C]). Rapid body cooling results in cardiac arrest and decreased tissue oxygen demand. The protective effect is most pronounced in children and may be due to the large ratio of body surface area to mass. Because water rapidly conducts heat away from the body, even persons who drown in warm water may suffer from hypothermia. (See *Physiologic changes in near drowning,* page 346.)

Complications
- Neurologic impairment
- Seizure disorders
- Pulmonary edema
- Renal damage
- Bacterial aspiration
- Cardiac complications (arrhythmias and decreased blood pressure)

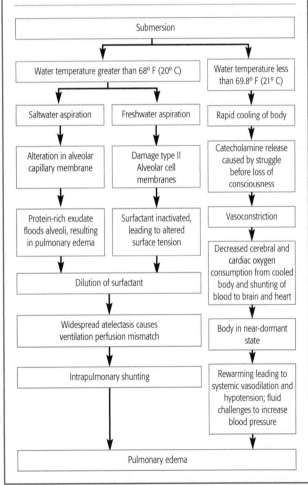

PHYSIOLOGIC CHANGES IN NEAR DROWNING

The flowchart below shows the primary cellular alterations that occur during near drowning. Separate pathways are shown for saltwater and freshwater incidents. Hypothermia presents a separate pathway that may preserve neurologic function by decreasing the metabolic rate. All pathways lead to diffuse pulmonary edema.

Submersion

Water temperature greater than 68° F (20° C)

Water temperature less than 69.8° F (21° C)

Saltwater aspiration → Freshwater aspiration → Rapid cooling of body

Alteration in alveolar capillary membrane

Damage type II Alveolar cell membranes

Catecholamine release caused by struggle before loss of consciousness

Protein-rich exudate floods alveoli, resulting in pulmonary edema

Surfactant inactivated, leading to altered surface tension

Vasoconstriction

Dilution of surfactant

Decreased cerebral and cardiac oxygen consumption from cooled body and shunting of blood to brain and heart

Widespread atelectasis causes ventilation perfusion mismatch

Body in near-dormant state

Intrapulmonary shunting

Rewarming leading to systemic vasodilation and hypotension; fluid challenges to increase blood pressure

Pulmonary edema

Assessment findings

■ The patient's history (obtained from a family member, friend, or emergency personnel) reveals the cause of the near drowning.
■ The patient may display an array of signs and symptoms.
■ If he's conscious, he may complain of a headache or substernal chest pain.
■ Your initial assessment of the patient's vital signs may detect fever; rapid, slow, or absent pulse; shallow, gasping, or absent respirations; confusion; and seizures.
■ If the patient was exposed to cold temperatures, he may experience hypothermia.
■ On initial observation, the patient may be unconscious, semiconscious, or awake.
■ If he's awake, he usually appears apprehensive, irritable, restless, or lethargic, and he may vomit. Inspection may reveal cyanosis or pink, frothy sputum (indicating pulmonary edema).
■ Palpation of the abdomen may disclose abdominal distention.
■ Auscultation of the lungs may reveal crackles, rhonchi, wheezing, or apnea.
■ You may note tachycardia, an irregular heartbeat (arrhythmias), or cardiac arrest when you auscultate the heart.
■ The patient may also experience hypotension.

Diagnostic test results

Supportive tests include:
■ arterial blood gas (ABG) analysis to determine the degree of hypoxia, intrapulmonary shunt, and acid-base balance
■ blood urea nitrogen and creatinine levels and urinalysis to evaluate renal function
■ cervical spine X-ray to rule out fracture
■ complete blood count to determine hemolysis
■ electrocardiogram (ECG) to detect myocardial ischemia
■ serial chest X-rays to evaluate pulmonary changes
■ serum electrolyte levels to monitor electrolyte balance.

Treatment

Prehospital care includes stabilizing the patient's neck and spine to prevent further injury, cardiopulmonary resuscitation (CPR) as needed, and administration of supplemental oxygen.

After the patient reaches the hospital, resuscitation continues. His oxygenation and circulation are maintained. X-rays confirm cervical spine integrity, and the patient's blood pH and electrolyte imbalances are corrected. If he's hypothermic, steps are taken to rewarm him.

ABG results help guide pulmonary therapy and determine the need for sodium bicarbonate to treat metabolic acidosis.

If the patient can't maintain an open airway, has abnormal ABG levels and pH, or doesn't have spontaneous respirations, he may need endotracheal (ET) intubation and mechanical ventilation. If he develops bronchospasm, he may need bronchodilators. Central venous pressure or pulmonary artery wedge pressure (PAWP) indicates the need for fluid replacement and cardiac drug therapy. The patient may also require standard treatment for pulmonary edema. Nasogastric (NG) tube drainage prevents vomiting, and an indwelling urinary catheter allows monitoring of urine output.

Nursing interventions

- Continue CPR as indicated. Assist with ET intubation, if needed, and give supplemental oxygen.
- If the patient has been submerged in cold water, use a bladder probe or a pulmonary artery line thermistor to determine his core body temperature.
- If the patient is hypothermic, start rewarming procedures during resuscitation. Don't stop resuscitation until the patient's body temperature ranges between 86° and 90.3° F (30° to 32.4° C).
- Protect the cervical spine until fracture is ruled out.
- Ensure peripheral I.V. access, and give I.V. fluids as needed.
- If ordered, insert an NG tube to remove swallowed water and reduce the risk of vomiting and aspiration.
- Insert an indwelling urinary catheter to monitor urine output. Metabolic acidosis may develop to compensate for impaired renal function.

- Assess ABG levels and obtain an ECG. The patient probably needs continuous cardiac monitoring.
- Continually monitor the patient's vital signs and neurologic status. He may have central nervous system damage despite treatment for hypoxia and shock.
- Obtain baseline serum electrolyte levels; continue monitoring these levels.
- If the patient has a central line in place, closely monitor all hemodynamic parameters, including cardiac output, central venous pressure, PAWP, heart rate, and arterial blood pressure.
- Give bronchodilator and antibiotic agents as ordered. (See *Near drowning teaching topics.*)

PNEUMOTHORAX

Pneumothorax is characterized by an accumulation of air or gas between the parietal and visceral pleurae. The amount of air or gas trapped in the intrapleural space determines the degree of lung collapse. In tension pneumothorax, the air in the pleural space is under higher pressure than air in adjacent lung and vascular structures. Without prompt treatment, tension or large pneumothorax results in fatal pulmonary and circulatory impairment.

Pathophysiology

Spontaneous pneumothorax usually occurs in otherwise healthy adults ages 20 to 40. It may be caused by air leakage from ruptured congenital blebs adjacent to the visceral pleural surface, near the apex of the lung. Secondary spontaneous pneumothorax is a complication of underlying lung disease, such as chronic obstructive pulmonary disease, asthma, cystic fibrosis, tuberculosis, and whooping cough. Spontaneous pneumothorax may also occur in interstitial lung disease, such as eosinophilic granuloma or lymphangiomyomatosis.

Traumatic pneumothorax may result from insertion of a central venous line, thoracic surgery, or a penetrating chest injury, such as a gunshot or knife wound. It may follow a transbronchial biopsy, or may occur during thoracentesis or a closed pleural biopsy. When traumatic pneumothorax follows a penetrating chest injury, it commonly coexists with hemothorax (blood in the pleural space).

In tension pneumothorax, positive pleural pressure develops as a result of traumatic pneumothorax. When air enters the pleural space through a tear in lung tissue and is unable to leave by the same vent, each inspiration traps air in the pleural space, resulting in positive pleural pressure. This causes collapse of the ipsilateral lung and marked impairment of venous return, which can severely compromise cardiac output, and may cause a mediastinal shift. Decreased filling of the great veins of the chest results in diminished cardiac output and lowered blood pressure. (See *Effects of pneumothorax*.)

Pneumothorax can also be classified as open or closed. In open pneumothorax (usually the result of trauma), air flows between the pleural space and the outside of the body. In closed pneumothorax, air reaches the pleural space directly from the lung.

Complications
- Fatal pulmonary and circulatory impairment

Assessment findings
- The patient's history reveals sudden, sharp, pleuritic pain.
- The patient may report that chest movement, breathing, and coughing exacerbate the pain. He may also report shortness of breath.
- Inspection typically reveals asymmetrical chest wall movement with overexpansion and rigidity on the affected side.

EFFECTS OF PNEUMOTHORAX

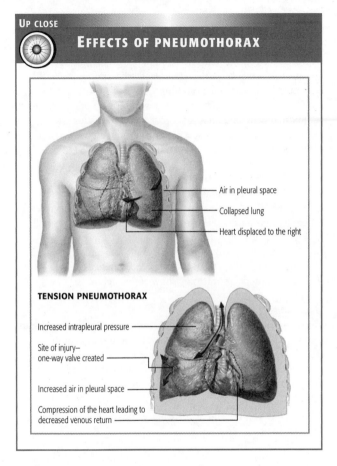

Air in pleural space

Collapsed lung

Heart displaced to the right

TENSION PNEUMOTHORAX

Increased intrapleural pressure

Site of injury–
one-way valve created

Increased air in pleural space

Compression of the heart leading to
decreased venous return

- The patient may appear cyanotic with circumoral cyanosis as a first sign.
- In tension pneumothorax, he may have distended jugular veins and pallor, and he may exhibit anxiety. (Test results may confirm increased central venous pressure.)
- Palpation may reveal crackling beneath the skin, indicating subcutaneous emphysema (air in tissues) and decreased vocal fremitus.

- In tension pneumothorax, palpation may disclose tracheal deviation away from the affected side and a weak and rapid pulse.
- Percussion may reveal hyperresonance on the affected side, and auscultation may disclose decreased or absent breath sounds over the collapsed lung.
- The patient may be hypotensive with tension pneumothorax.
- Spontaneous pneumothorax that releases only a small amount of air into the pleural space may not cause signs or symptoms.

Diagnostic test results
- Arterial blood gas analysis may show hypoxemia, possibly accompanied by respiratory acidosis and hypercapnia. Arterial oxygen saturation levels may decrease initially but typically return to normal within 24 hours.
- Chest X-rays reveal air in the pleural space and, possibly, a mediastinal shift, which confirms the diagnosis.
- Pulse oximetry results may show early decline.

Treatment
Typically, treatment is conservative for spontaneous pneumothorax with no signs of increased pleural pressure (indicating tension pneumothorax), with lung collapse less than 30%, and with no dyspnea or other indications of physiologic compromise. Such treatment consists of bed rest, careful monitoring (blood pressure and pulse and respiratory rates), oxygen administration and, possibly, aspiration of air with a large-bore needle attached to a syringe.

If more than 30% of the lung collapses, treatment to reexpand the lung includes placing a thoracostomy tube in the second or third intercostal space in the midclavicular line. The thoracostomy tube then connects to an underwater seal or to low-pressure suction.

Recurring spontaneous pneumothorax requires thoracotomy and pleurectomy. These procedures prevent recurrence by causing the lung to adhere to the parietal pleura. Traumatic and tension pneumothorax require chest tube drainage; traumatic pneumothorax may also require surgical repair. Analgesics may be prescribed.

Nursing interventions

■ Listen to the patient's fears and concerns. Offer reassurance as appropriate. Remain with the patient during periods of extreme stress and anxiety. Encourage him to identify actions and care measures that promote comfort and relaxation. Be sure to perform these measures, and encourage the patient and his family to do so as well. Include the patient and his family in care-related decisions whenever possible.

■ Keep the patient as comfortable as possible, and give analgesics as needed. The patient with pneumothorax usually feels most comfortable sitting upright.

■ Watch for complications signaled by pallor, gasping respirations, and sudden chest pain. Carefully monitor vital signs at least every hour for indications of shock, increasing respiratory distress, or mediastinal shift. Listen for breath sounds over both lungs.

■ Make sure the suction set-up is functioning appropriately when the patient has a chest tube inserted. Watch for signs of tension pneumothorax. These include decreasing blood pressure and increasing pulse and respiratory rates, which could be fatal without prompt treatment. If the patient doesn't have a chest tube connected to suction (also called *water seal drainage*), monitor for recurrence of pneumothorax and recollapse of the lung. If this occurs, obtain a portable chest X-ray immediately.

FOR CHEST TUBE INSERTION

■ To facilitate chest tube insertion, place the patient in high Fowler's position, semi-Fowler's position, supine, or have him lie on his unaffected side with his arms overhead. During chest tube insertion, urge him to control the urge to cough and gasp. However, after the chest tube is placed, encourage him to cough and breathe deeply (at least once per hour) to facilitate lung expansion.

■ Change the dressings around the chest tube insertion site at least every 24 hours. Keep the insertion site clean, and watch for signs of infection. Be careful not to reposition or dislodge the tube. If the tube dislodges, immediately place a petroleum gauze dressing over the opening to prevent rapid lung col-

PNEUMOTHORAX TEACHING TOPICS

● Reassure the patient. Explain what pneumothorax is, what causes it, and all diagnostic tests and procedures.

● Discuss the potential for recurrent spontaneous pneumothorax, and review its signs and symptoms. Emphasize the need for immediate medical intervention if these should occur.

● If the patient has an underlying chronic respiratory disease, teach him the signs and symptoms of pneumothorax.

● The patient with a chronic lung disorder should also be encouraged to stop smoking, avoid high altitudes, scuba diving, or flying in unpressurized aircraft to prevent the recurrence of pneumothorax.

lapse; however, use extreme caution. If the lung has a hole or tear (evidenced by bubbling in the water-seal chamber), tension pneumothorax may be created by a tight dressing placement.

■ Watch for continuing air leakage (bubbling). This indicates the lung defect's failure to heal, which may necessitate surgery. Also, watch for increasing subcutaneous emphysema by checking around the neck and at the tube's insertion site for crackling beneath the skin. For the patient receiving mechanical ventilation, watch for difficulty in breathing in time with the ventilator. Also watch for pressure changes on the ventilator gauges.

FOR THORACOTOMY

■ Urge the patient to control coughing and gasping during the procedure.

■ Monitor vital signs frequently after thoracotomy. Also, for the first 24 hours, assess respiratory status by checking breath sounds hourly. Observe the chest tube site for leakage, and note the amount and color of drainage. Walk the patient, as ordered (usually on the first postoperative day), to promote deep inspiration and lung expansion. (See *Pneumothorax teaching topics.*)

Neoplastic disorders

Neoplastic growths may be benign or malignant, depending on their ability to invade and metastasize to other areas of the body. Neoplastic thoracic disorders include laryngeal and lung cancer, and mesotheliomas.

LARYNGEAL CANCER

Squamous cell carcinoma constitutes about 95% of laryngeal cancers. Rare laryngeal cancer forms—adenocarcinoma and sarcoma—account for the rest. The disease affects males about nine times more commonly than females, and most patients are between ages 50 and 65.

Patterns of metastasis in laryngeal cancer reflect the organ anatomy. Tumors of the glottis (true vocal cords) tend to remain localized because the underlying tissues lack lymph nodes. Supraglottic tumors, however, typically spread through the lymphatics to adjacent areas. Although these tumors can metastasize to distant sites, such as the lungs, localized disease may threaten survival because of airway problems. (See *A look at laryngeal cancer*, page 356.)

The cause of laryngeal cancer is unknown. Major risk factors include smoking and heavy alcohol consumption. Minor risk factors include chronic inhalation of noxious fumes and familial disposition.

Laryngeal cancer is classified by its location:
- supraglottis (false vocal cords)
- glottis (true vocal cords)

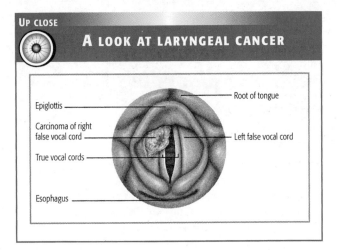

A LOOK AT LARYNGEAL CANCER

Epiglottis

Carcinoma of right false vocal cord

True vocal cords

Esophagus

Root of tongue

Left false vocal cord

■ subglottis (rare downward extension from vocal cords).

Pathophysiology

Initially, the mucosa is exposed to an irritating substance and develops into a tougher mucosa by increasing its thickness or by the development of a keratin layer. Cellular changes also lead to the growth of abnormal epithelial cells that eventually become malignant. These areas of epithelial cells are commonly white and patchy or red and patchy. Metastasis of cancer of the head and neck depends on the primary site of the tumor and usually spreads to the mucosa, muscle, and bone. Systemic metastasis through the blood and lymphatic system is also possible. When this occurs, it's typically to the lung or liver.

Complications

■ Increasing dysphagia
■ Pain
■ Airway obstruction

Assessment findings

Varied assessment findings in laryngeal cancer depend on the tumor's location and its stage.

STAGE I

■ With stage I disease, the patient may complain of local throat irritation or hoarseness that lasts about 2 weeks.

STAGES II AND III

■ In stages II and III, he usually reports hoarseness.
■ He may also have a sore throat, and his voice volume may be reduced to a whisper.

STAGE IV

■ In stage IV, he typically reports pain radiating to his ear, dysphagia, and dyspnea.
■ In advanced stage IV disease, palpation may detect a neck mass or enlarged cervical lymph nodes.

Diagnostic test results

■ Biopsy identifies malignant cells.
■ Chest X-ray identifies metastasis.
■ Laryngoscopy allows definitive staging by obtaining multiple biopsy specimens to establish primary diagnosis, to determine the extent of the disease, and to identify additional premalignant lesions or second primary lesions.
■ Xeroradiography, laryngeal tomography, computed tomography scan, and laryngography confirm the presence of a mass.

Treatment

Early lesions may respond to laser surgery or radiation therapy; advanced lesions to laser surgery, radiation therapy, and chemotherapy. Treatment aims to eliminate cancer and preserve speech. If speech preservation isn't possible, speech rehabilitation may include esophageal speech or prosthetic devices. Surgical techniques to construct a new voice box are experimental. (See *Reviewing alternative speech methods*, page 358.)

In early disease, laser surgery destroys precancerous lesions; in advanced disease, it can help clear obstructions. Other surgical procedures vary with tumor size and include cordectomy, partial or total laryngectomy, supraglottic laryngectomy, and total laryngectomy with laryngoplasty.

REVIEWING ALTERNATIVE SPEECH METHODS

During convalescence, your patient may work with a speech pathologist who can teach him new ways to speak using various communication techniques such as those below.

Esophageal speech

By drawing air in through the mouth, trapping it in the upper esophagus, and releasing it slowly while forming words, the patient can again communicate by voice. With training and practice, a highly motivated patient can master esophageal speech in about a month. Recognize that speech will sound choppy at first, but with increasing skill, words will flow more smoothly and understandably.

Because esophageal speech requires strength, an elderly patient or one with asthma or emphysema may find it too physically demanding. Because it also requires frequent sessions with a speech pathologist, a chronically ill patient may find esophageal speech overwhelming.

Artificial larynges

The throat vibrator and the Cooper-Rand device are basic artificial larynges. Both types vibrate to produce speech that's easy to understand, although it sounds monotonous and mechanical.

Tell the patient to operate a throat vibrator by holding it against his neck. A pulsating disk in the device vibrates the throat tissue as the patient forms words with his mouth. The throat vibrator may be difficult to use immediately after surgery, when the patient's neck wounds are still sore.

The Cooper-Rand device vibrates sounds piped into the patient's mouth through a thin tube, which the patient positions in the corner of his mouth. Easy to use, this device may be preferred soon after surgery.

Surgically implanted prostheses

Most surgical implants generate speech by vibrating when the patient manually closes the tracheostomy, forcing air upward. One such device is the Blom-Singer voice prosthesis. Only hours after it's inserted through an incision in the stoma, the patient can speak in a normal voice. The surgeon may implant the device when radiation therapy ends or within a few days (or even years) after laryngectomy.

To speak, the patient covers his stoma while exhaling. Exhaled air travels through the trachea, passes through an airflow port on the bottom of the prosthesis, and exits through a slit at the esophageal end of the prosthesis. This creates the vibrations needed to produce sound.

Not all patients are eligible for tracheoesophageal puncture, the procedure in which the prosthesis is inserted. Considerations include the extent of the laryngectomy, pharyngoesophageal muscle status, stomal size and location, and the patient's mental and emotional status, visual and auditory acuity, hand-eye coordination, bimanual dexterity, and self-care skills.

Radiation therapy alone or combined with surgery is effective but can result in complications, including airway obstruction, pain, taste changes, and chronic dry mouth (xerostomia).

Chemotherapeutic agents may include methotrexate (Rheumatrex), cisplatin (Platinol-AQ), bleomycin (Blenoxane), fluorouracil (Adrucil), and paclitaxel (Taxol).

Nursing interventions

■ Provide supportive psychological, preoperative, and postoperative care to reduce complications and speed recovery.

■ Encourage the patient to discuss his concerns before surgery. Help him choose a temporary, alternative way to communicate, such as writing or using sign language or an alphabet board. If appropriate, arrange for a laryngectomee to visit him.

AFTER PARTIAL LARYNGECTOMY

■ Give I.V. fluids and, usually, tube feedings for the first 2 days after surgery; then resume oral fluids. Keep the tracheostomy tube (inserted during surgery) in place until tissue edema subsides.

■ Make sure the patient doesn't use his voice until the physician gives permission (usually 2 to 3 days postoperatively). Then caution the patient to whisper until he heals completely.

AFTER TOTAL LARYNGECTOMY

■ As soon as the patient returns to his room from surgery, position him on his side, and elevate his head 30 to 45 degrees. If he has tissue flaps to close the wound, position him so that the side with the flaps isn't dependent. When you move him, remember to support the back of his neck to prevent tension on sutures and possible wound dehiscence.

■ If the patient has a laryngectomy tube in place, care for it as you would a tracheostomy tube. Shorter and thicker than a tracheostomy tube, the laryngectomy tube stays in place until the stoma heals (about 7 to 10 days).

■ Watch the stoma for crusting and secretions, which can cause skin breakdown. To prevent crusting, provide adequate room

RECOGNIZING AND MANAGING COMPLICATIONS OF LARYNGEAL SURGERY

When your patient returns from surgery, you'll need to monitor his recovery, watching carefully for such complications as fistula formation, a ruptured carotid artery, and stenosis of the tracheostomy site.

Fistula formation

Warning signs of fistula formation include redness, swelling, and secretions on the suture line. The fistula may form between the reconstructed hypopharynx and the skin. This eventually heals spontaneously, although the process may take weeks or months.

Feed the patient who has a fistula through a nasogastric tube. Otherwise, food will leak through the fistula and delay healing.

Ruptured carotid artery

Bleeding, an important sign of a ruptured carotid artery, may occur in a patient who received preoperative radiation therapy or one with a fistula that constantly bathes the carotid artery with oral secretions.

If rupture occurs, apply pressure to the site. Call for help immediately, and take the patient to the operating room for carotid ligation.

Tracheostomy stenosis

Constant shortness of breath alerts you to tracheostomy stenosis, which may occur weeks to months after laryngectomy.

Management includes fitting the patient with successively larger tracheostomy tubes until he can tolerate insertion of a full-sized one.

humidification. Remove crusts with petroleum jelly, antimicrobial ointment, and moist gauze.

■ Monitor vital signs. Be especially alert for fever, which indicates infection. Record fluid intake and output, and watch for dehydration. Also, be alert for and report postoperative complications. (See *Recognizing and managing complications of laryngeal surgery.*)

■ Provide frequent mouth care. Clean the patient's tongue and the sides of his mouth with a soft toothbrush or a terry washcloth, and rinse his mouth with a deodorizing mouthwash. If a patient is receiving radiotherapy or chemotherapy, avoid al-

LARYNGEAL CANCER TEACHING TOPICS

● Advise the patient to eat small, frequent meals at first until he can swallow better.

● Tell him to avoid straining during bowel movements to reduce stress and pressure on his stoma and sutures.

● If the patient smoked before surgery, advise him to quit.

● Also, prepare the patient for other functional losses. Forewarn him that he won't be able to smell aromas, blow his nose, whistle, gargle, sip, or suck on a straw.

● Reassure the patient that speech rehabilitation measures (including laryngeal speech, esophageal speech, an artificial larynx, and various mechanical devices) may help him communicate again.

● Encourage the patient to take advantage of services and information offered by the American Speech-Language-Hearing Association, the International Association of Laryngectomees, the American Cancer Society, and the local chapter of the Lost Chord Club.

cohol mouthwashes. Normal saline mouth rinses cleanse and maintain moisture.

■ Suction gently. Unless ordered otherwise, don't attempt deep suctioning, which could penetrate the suture line. Suction through both the tube and the patient's nose because the patient can no longer blow air through his nose. Suction his mouth gently.

■ After inserting a drainage catheter (usually connected to a blood drainage system or a GI drainage system), don't stop suction without the physician's consent. After removing the catheter, check the dressings for drainage.

■ Give analgesics as ordered. Keep in mind that opioid analgesics depress respiration and inhibit coughing.

■ If the physician orders nasogastric (NG) tube feedings, check tube placement, and elevate the patient's head to prevent aspiration. Be ready to perform suction after NG tube removal or oral fluid intake because the patient may have difficulty swallowing.

■ Support the patient through inevitable grieving. If his depression becomes severe, consider referring him for appropriate counseling. (See *Laryngeal cancer teaching topics.*)

LUNG CANCER

Two broad categories of lung cancer are small-cell lung cancer (also called *oat cell lung cancer*) and non-small-cell lung cancer. These categories reflect different behavior patterns and determine treatment approach. Squamous cell, large-cell, and adenocarcinoma compose the majority of non-small-cell lung cancer.

As with many solid tumors, prognosis for lung cancer depends on the stage at diagnosis. Unfortunately, most patients have advanced disease at diagnosis, reflecting the 14% 5-year survival rate. Lung cancer is the most common cause of cancer death in men and women.

Most experts agree that lung cancer is attributable to inhalation of carcinogenic pollutants by a susceptible host. Most susceptible are those persons who smoke or who work with or near asbestos.

Pollutants in tobacco smoke cause progressive lung cell degeneration. Lung cancer is 10 times more common in smokers than in nonsmokers; 90% of lung cancer patients are current or former smokers.

Cancer risk is determined by the number of cigarettes smoked daily, the depth of inhalation, how early in life smoking began, and the nicotine content of the cigarettes. Two other factors also increase susceptibility: exposure to carcinogenic industrial and air pollutants (asbestos, uranium, arsenic, nickel, iron oxides, chromium, radioactive dust, and coal dust), and familial susceptibility.

Pathophysiology

Lung cancer usually begins with the transformation of one epithelial cell of the airway. The bronchi in general, and certain specific portions of the bronchi, such as the segmental bifurcation and sites of mucus production, are thought to be more vulnerable to injury from carcinogens. As a lung tumor grows, it can partially or completely obstruct the airway, resulting in lobar collapse distal to the tumor. A lung tumor can also cause hemorrhage, causing hemoptysis. Early metastasis may occur to other thoracic structures, such as hilar lymph nodes or the medi-

DETERMINING PACK-YEARS

Patients who smoke cigarettes are at a higher risk for such respiratory diseases as lung cancer, emphysema, and bronchitis. Use this formula to calculate pack-years and assess a patient's risk for lung disease:

number of years smoked × number of packs smoked daily = pack-years.

For example, a patient who smokes 2 packs of cigarettes daily for 42 years has accumulated 84 pack-years.

Normally, the more pack-years, the greater the risk for lung disease.

astinum. Distant metastasis can occur to the brain, liver, bone, and adrenal glands.

Complications

- Tracheal obstruction
- Esophageal compression with dysphagia
- Phrenic nerve paralysis with hemidiaphragm elevation and dyspnea
- Sympathetic nerve paralysis with Horner syndrome
- Eighth cervical and first thoracic nerve compression with ulnar and Pancoast's syndrome (shoulder pain radiating to the ulnar nerve pathways); lymphatic obstruction with pleural effusion
- Hypoxemia
- Anorexia and weight loss
- Cachexia
- Hypertrophic osteoarthropathy
- Superior vena cava syndrome
- Spinal cord compression

Assessment findings

Because early lung cancer may cause no symptoms, the disease is usually advanced when it's diagnosed. While taking the patient's history, be sure to assess his exposure to carcinogens. If he's a smoker, determine pack-years. (See *Determining pack-years.*)

Chief complaints may include:
- hoarseness

- coughing
- dyspnea
- hemoptysis.

Other things you may notice at examination:

- The patient becomes short of breath when he walks or exerts himself.
- You may also observe finger clubbing; edema of the face, neck, and upper torso; dilated chest and abdominal veins (superior vena cava syndrome); weight loss; and fatigue.
- Palpation may reveal enlarged lymph nodes, especially in the neck, and an enlarged liver.
- Percussion findings may include dullness over the lung fields in a patient with pleural effusion.
- Auscultation may disclose decreased breath sounds, wheezing, and pleural friction rub (with pleural effusion). (See *Additional findings in lung cancer.*)

Diagnostic test results

- Bronchoscopy can identify the tumor site. Bronchoscopic washings provide material for cytologic and histologic study. The flexible fiber-optic bronchoscope increases test effectiveness.
- Chest X-rays usually show an advanced lesion and can detect a lesion up to 2 years before signs and symptoms appear. Findings may indicate tumor size and location.
- Computed tomography scan of the chest may help to delineate the tumor's size and its relationship to surrounding structures.
- Cytologic sputum analysis, which is 75% reliable, requires a sputum specimen expectorated from the lungs and tracheobronchial tree, not from postnasal secretions or saliva.
- Needle biopsy of the lungs relies on biplanar fluoroscopic visual control to locate peripheral tumors before withdrawing a tissue specimen for analysis. This procedure confirms the diagnosis in 80% of patients.
- Tissue biopsy of metastatic sites (including supraclavicular and mediastinal nodes and pleura) helps to assess disease extent. Based on histologic findings, staging determines the disease's extent and prognosis and helps direct treatment.

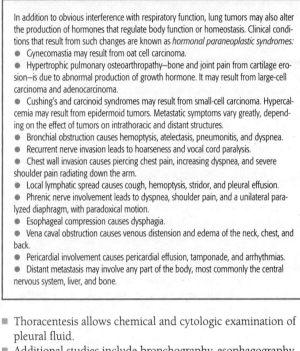

ADDITIONAL FINDINGS IN LUNG CANCER

In addition to obvious interference with respiratory function, lung tumors may also alter the production of hormones that regulate body function or homeostasis. Clinical conditions that result from such changes are known as *hormonal paraneoplastic syndromes:*

● Gynecomastia may result from oat cell carcinoma.

● Hypertrophic pulmonary osteoarthropathy—bone and joint pain from cartilage erosion—is due to abnormal production of growth hormone. It may result from large-cell carcinoma and adenocarcinoma.

● Cushing's and carcinoid syndromes may result from small-cell carcinoma. Hypercalcemia may result from epidermoid tumors. Metastatic symptoms vary greatly, depending on the effect of tumors on intrathoracic and distant structures.

● Bronchial obstruction causes hemoptysis, atelectasis, pneumonitis, and dyspnea.

● Recurrent nerve invasion leads to hoarseness and vocal cord paralysis.

● Chest wall invasion causes piercing chest pain, increasing dyspnea, and severe shoulder pain radiating down the arm.

● Local lymphatic spread causes cough, hemoptysis, stridor, and pleural effusion.

● Phrenic nerve involvement leads to dyspnea, shoulder pain, and a unilateral paralyzed diaphragm, with paradoxical motion.

● Esophageal compression causes dysphagia.

● Vena caval obstruction causes venous distension and edema of the neck, chest, and back.

● Pericardial involvement causes pericardial effusion, tamponade, and arrhythmias.

● Distant metastasis may involve any part of the body, most commonly the central nervous system, liver, and bone.

▪ Thoracentesis allows chemical and cytologic examination of pleural fluid.

▪ Additional studies include bronchography, esophagography, and angiocardiography (contrast studies of the bronchial tree, esophagus, and cardiovascular tissues).

▪ Tests to detect metastasis include bone scan (abnormal findings may lead to a bone marrow biopsy, which is typically recommended in patients with small-cell carcinoma), positron emission tomography (PET) scan, computed tomography scan of the brain, liver function studies, and gallium scans of the liver and spleen. PET scan should be performed to exclude metastatic disease before subjecting the patient to a thoracotomy.

Treatment

Various combinations of surgery, radiation therapy, and chemotherapy improve both the prognosis and patient survival. Because lung cancer is usually advanced at diagnosis, most treatment is palliative.

Surgery is the primary treatment for stage I, stage II, or selected stage III non-small-cell lung cancer, unless the tumor is inoperable or other conditions (such as cardiac disease or poor lung function) rule out surgery. Surgery may involve partial lung removal (wedge resection, segmental resection, lobectomy, radical lobectomy) or total removal (pneumonectomy, radical pneumonectomy).

Preoperative radiation therapy and chemotherapy may reduce tumor bulk to allow for surgical resection and may also improve response rates. Radiation therapy is ordinarily recommended for stage I and stage II lesions if surgery is contraindicated, and for stage III disease confined to the involved hemithorax and the ipsilateral supraclavicular lymph nodes. The standard treatment for stage III disease in good performance status patients is concurrent chemotherapy and radiation therapy.

Multiple chemotherapy combinations have been used in non-small-cell lung cancer. If the patient is in reasonably good shape, a platinum-based drug combination is preferred. Cisplatin (Platinol-AQ) and carboplatin (Paraplatin) have similar activity, but cisplatin is more toxic to the kidneys. A variety of drugs can be combined with platinum-based drugs with comparable efficacy, including etoposide (Toposar), paclitaxel (Taxol), docetaxel (Taxotere), gemcitabine (Gemzar), and vinorelbine (Navelbine).

A new classification of anticancer drugs called "target agents" act on specific molecular targets influencing cancer growth.

Small-cell lung cancer is generally not treated by surgery because it's considered a systemic disease. When the cancer is limited to the chest area, concurrent chemotherapy and radiation therapy are given. However, if distant metastasis has occurred, chemotherapy alone is offered. Drugs used in small cell lung cancer include cisplatin, carboplatin, etoposide, irinotecan (Camptosar), and topotecan (Hycamtin).

Immunotherapy is still being studied. Nonspecific treatment programs using bacille Calmette-Guérin vaccine or, possibly, *Corynebacterium parvum* offer the most promise.

In laser therapy, a laser beam is directed through a bronchoscope to destroy local tumors.

Nursing interventions

- Give comprehensive supportive care and provide patient teaching to minimize complications and speed the patient's recovery from surgery, radiation therapy, and chemotherapy.
- Urge the patient to voice his concerns and schedule time to answer his questions. Be sure to explain procedures before performing them. This will help reduce the patient's anxiety.
- Before and after surgery, give ordered analgesics as necessary.

AFTER THORACIC SURGERY

- Maintain a patent airway and monitor chest tubes to reestablish normal intrathoracic pressure and prevent postoperative and pulmonary complications.
- Monitor vital signs and watch for and report abnormal respirations and other changes.
- Suction the patient often and encourage him to begin deep breathing and coughing as soon as possible. Check secretions often. Initially, sputum will appear thick and dark with blood, but it should become thinner and grayish yellow within 1 day.
- Monitor and document amount and color of closed chest drainage. Keep chest tubes patent and draining effectively. Watch for fluctuation in the water seal chamber on inspiration and expiration, indicating that the chest tube remains patent. Watch for air leaks and report them immediately. Position the patient on the surgical side to promote drainage and lung reexpansion.
- Watch for and report foul-smelling discharge or excessive drainage on surgical dressings. Usually, you'll remove the dressing after 24 hours, unless the wound appears infected.
- Monitor intake and output. Maintain adequate hydration.

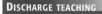

LUNG CANCER TEACHING TOPICS

- Warn an outpatient to avoid tight clothing, sunburn, and harsh ointments on his chest. Teach him exercises to prevent shoulder stiffness.
- If the patient is receiving chemotherapy or radiation therapy, explain possible adverse effects of these treatments. Teach him ways to avoid complications such as infection. Also review reportable adverse effects.
- Educate high-risk patients about ways to reduce their chances of developing lung cancer or recurrent cancer.
- Refer smokers to local branches of the American Cancer Society or Smokenders. Provide information about group therapy, individual counseling, and hypnosis.
- Urge all heavy smokers older than age 40 to have a chest X-ray annually and cytologic sputum analysis every 6 months. Also encourage patients who have recurring or chronic respiratory tract infections, chronic lung disease, or a nagging or changing cough to seek prompt medical evaluation.

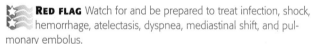

RED FLAG Watch for and be prepared to treat infection, shock, hemorrhage, atelectasis, dyspnea, mediastinal shift, and pulmonary embolus.

- To help prevent pulmonary embolus, apply antiembolism stockings, and encourage the patient to perform range-of-motion exercises.

FOR CHEMOTHERAPY

- Ask the dietary department to provide soft, nonirritating, protein-rich foods. Encourage the patient to eat high-calorie, between-meal snacks.
- Give antiemetics and antidiarrheals as needed.
- Schedule patient care to help the patient conserve his energy.
- Monitor red blood cell count for bone marrow suppression, and institute precautions as necessary such as using an electric razor for shaving if the patient's platelet count is low.

FOR RADIATION THERAPY

- Provide meticulous skin care to minimize skin breakdown. (See *Lung cancer teaching topics*.)

MESOTHELIOMAS

Mesotheliomas, which originate in the serosal lining of the pleural cavity, account for less than 10% of all cancer-related deaths. Incidence is high, however, in asbestos workers and their immediate families and among people who live along major routes used for transporting large quantities of asbestos.

Mesotheliomas have a latency period ranging from 20 to 45 years from exposure to tumor discovery, usually occur in people older than age 50, and are invariably fatal. Typically, less than 2 years pass between the onset of symptoms and death.

Pathophysiology

The link between this tumor and asbestos exposure is well established. Predisposition, chronic inflammation, radiation, recurrent lung infection seldom account for a mesothelioma. Smoking alone doesn't increase the risk for developing a mesothelioma; coupled with asbestos exposure, it increases the risk by about 50%.

It's unknown whether a mesothelioma begins in the visceral or parietal pleura; in animals, tumor-causing asbestos fibers migrate to mesothelial cells, penetrating the pleura. From there, the pleural lymphatics carry them to the pleural surface. Signs and symptoms result from pleural effusion, restricted lung function, tumor mass, infection, and advanced disease.

Complications

- Severe dyspnea
- Infection
- Complications of immobility (skin breakdown)

Assessment findings

- The patient's history will probably reveal asbestos exposure at some time in his life.
- His chief complaints may be chest pain and dyspnea.
- Other complaints include cough, hoarseness, anorexia, weight loss, weakness, and fatigue.

- Vital signs may reflect an elevated temperature. Inspection reveals shortness of breath and, in some cases, finger clubbing.
- You may discover dullness over lung fields on chest percussion and diminished chest sounds on auscultation.

Diagnostic tests

- Chest X-rays exhibit nodular, irregular, unilateral pleural thickening and varying degrees of unilateral pleural effusion.
- Computed tomography scan of the chest defines the tumor's extent.
- Open pleural biopsy is necessary to obtain a specimen. Then histologic study can confirm the diagnosis.

Treatment

No standard treatment exists for a mesothelioma. Surgery, radiation therapy, chemotherapy, and a combination of treatments are usually tried, but they seldom control the disease.

If surgery is performed, a pleurectomy is the usual procedure. Postoperative radiation has also been useful. Cisplatin (Platinol-AQ) and mitomycin (Mutamycin) were the most successful chemotherapy drug combinations but were quite toxic. Pemetrexate (Alimta) was recently approved in combination with cisplatin (for mesothelioma) and is usually tolerated well.

Nursing interventions

- Listen to the patient's fears and concerns. Give clear, concise explanations of all procedures and actions, and remain with him during periods of severe anxiety. Encourage him to identify actions that promote comfort. Then be sure to perform them and to encourage the patient and his family to help. Include the patient in decisions related to his care whenever possible.
- Give ordered pain medication as required. Monitor and document the medication's effectiveness.
- Perform comfort measures, such as repositioning and relaxation techniques.
- Monitor respiratory status. Provide oxygen, as ordered, and assist the patient to a comfortable position (Fowler's position,

MESOTHELIOMA TEACHING TOPICS

● Show the patient how to perform relaxation techniques. Also demonstrate breathing and positioning variations to ease the dyspnea associated with progressive disease.
● Teach the patient measures (such as increasing fluid intake) to minimize adverse effects of treatment.
● When appropriate, teach the patient and his family procedures to maximize breathing and prevent the complications of immobility.
● Explain how to practice meticulous hand washing and sterile techniques to avoid infection.
● Refer the patient to the social services department, support groups, and community or professional mental health resources to help him and his family cope with terminal illness.

for example) that allows for maximal chest expansion to relieve respiratory distress.

■ If mobility decreases, turn the patient frequently. Provide skin care, particularly over bony prominences. Encourage him to be as active as possible.

■ Prevent infection. Adhere to strict sterile technique when suctioning the patient, changing dressings or I.V. tubing, and performing any type of invasive procedure. Monitor body temperature and white blood cell count closely.

■ Monitor I.V. fluid intake to avoid circulatory overload and pulmonary congestion.

■ Watch for treatment complications by observing and listening to the patient. Also monitor laboratory studies and vital signs. Perform appropriate nursing measures to prevent or alleviate complications. Report complications. (See *Mesothelioma teaching topics*.)

Emergencies and complications

Respiratory compromise, resulting from respiratory emergencies, is a leading cause of morbidity and mortality. Such *emergencies* include airway obstruction, anaphylaxis, bronchospasm, respiratory arrest, and respiratory depression; such *complications* include respiratory acidosis and alkalosis.

EMERGENCIES
AIRWAY OBSTRUCTION

Maintaining a patent airway is vital to life, and the body uses coughing as its main mechanism to clear the airway. However, coughing may be ineffective in clearing the airway in some disease states, or even under normal healthy conditions, if an obstruction is present.

A patient's airway can become obstructed or compromised by vomitus, food, his teeth, blood, or saliva; however, the most common cause of airway obstruction is the tongue. That's because muscle tone decreases when a person is unconscious or unresponsive, which increases the potential for the tongue and epiglottis to obstruct the airway.

Upper airway obstruction may also be caused by edema in associated anatomical structures. For example, edema of the tongue (caused by surgery or trauma), laryngeal edema, and smoke inhalation edema can all lead to an obstruction. Other potential causes of upper airway obstruction include:
- peritonsillar, retropharyngeal, or pharyngeal abscesses
- tumors of the head or neck, space-occupying lesions
- tenacious secretions in the airway, bacterial or viral infections

- cerebral disorders (stroke)
- trauma to the face, trachea, larynx, or mediastinum, resulting in blood into nasopharynx
- aspiration of a foreign object, including blood (if ruptured esophageal varices) or bits of food
- fire or inhalation burns on the head, face, or neck area
- croup
- epiglottiditis
- laryngospasms, laryngeal edema related to endotracheal intubation (after extubation)
- anaphylaxis.

Pathophysiology
Upper airway obstruction is an interruption in the flow of air through the nose, mouth, pharynx, or larynx. Prompt detection and intervention can prevent a partial airway obstruction from progressing to a complete airway obstruction. However, if not recognized early, it may progress to respiratory and cardiac arrest—a life-threatening situation—and cardiopulmonary resuscitation will be required.

Complications
- Cardiac and respiratory arrest
- Coma
- Death

Assessment findings
Signs of a partial airway obstruction can include diaphoresis, tachycardia, coughing, increased work of breathing with increased use of accessory muscles, and elevated blood pressure; however, the patient may also be asymptomatic. With a complete airway obstruction, the following symptoms may be observed:
- restlessness
- choking
- gasping for air
- wheezing, whistling, or another unusual breath sound that indicates difficulty breathing
- cyanosis or pallor
- cessation of coughing; the individual can't make any sounds

- change in level of consciousness (LOC) or progression to unconsciousness
- agitation, panic, or increasing anxiety
- hypoxia and hypercapnia
- cardiac arrest.

Diagnostic test results

Physical examination may indicate decreased breath sounds. Tests, although not usually necessary to diagnose an upper airway obstruction, may include the following:

- X-rays (such as chest and neck X-rays), bronchoscopy, and laryngoscopy reveal the type and site of the obstruction.
- Computed tomography scanning may be ordered to rule out a tumor, a foreign body, or an infection or trauma.

Treatment

Treatment focuses on relieving the obstruction and generating oxygenation. (See *Opening an obstructed airway.*)

Prompt assessment should focus on determining the cause of the obstruction. When an obstruction is related to the tongue or an accumulation of tenacious secretions, place the head in a slightly extended position and insert an oral airway. If the patient has a complete airway obstruction, can't cough or speak, and a foreign body obstruction is suspected, a series of abdominal thrusts are performed in an attempt to remove the foreign object. (See *Obstructed airway management,* pages 376 to 378.)

If an upper airway obstruction is deemed an emergency, the following procedures are warranted.

CRICOTHYROTOMY

Cricothyrotomy involves the excision of the cricothyroid membrane below the thyroid cartilage and the cricoid ring. A tracheostomy tube is placed through this opening to keep the newly created airway open until a tracheotomy can be performed. The tube is typically uncuffed and has an inner diameter large enough for a small catheter. This procedure is used when no other option is available to establish an airway; for example, if the setting is outside of the hospital. It should be converted to a tracheostomy if the patient still needs airway support after 24 hours. (See *Performing an emergency cricothyrotomy,* pages 379 and 380.)

OPENING AN OBSTRUCTED AIRWAY

To open an obstructed airway, use the head-tilt, chin-lift maneuver or the jaw-thrust maneuver, as described here.

Head-tilt, chin-lift maneuver

In many cases of airway obstruction, the muscles controlling the patient's tongue have relaxed, causing the tongue to obstruct the airway. If the patient doesn't appear to have a neck injury, use the head-tilt, chin-lift maneuver to open his airway. Use these four steps to carry out this maneuver:

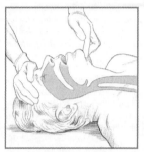

● Place your hand closest to the patient's head on his forehead.
● Apply firm pressure—firm enough to tilt the patient's head back.
● Place the fingertips of your other hand under the bony portion of the patient's lower jaw, near the chin.
● Lift the patient's chin. Be sure to keep his mouth partially open (as shown at right). Avoid placing your fingertips on the soft tissue under the patient's chin because this may inadvertently obstruct the airway you're trying to open.

Jaw-thrust maneuver

If you suspect a neck injury, use the jaw-thrust maneuver to open the patient's airway. Use these four steps to carry out this maneuver:

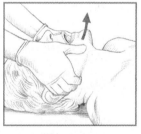

● Kneel at the patient's head with your elbows on the ground.
● Rest your thumbs on the patient's lower jaw near the corners of his mouth, pointing your thumbs toward his feet.
● Place your fingertips around the lower jaw.
● To open the airway, lift the lower jaw with your fingertips (as shown at right).

ENDOTRACHEAL INTUBATION

Endotracheal (ET) intubation involves the insertion of a tube into the trachea through the nose (nasotracheal intubation) or the mouth (orotracheal intubation). Many facilities have guidelines limiting the use of nasotracheal intubation for specific pa-

(Text continues on page 378.)

OBSTRUCTED AIRWAY MANAGEMENT

An obstructed airway causes anoxia, which in turn leads to brain damage and death in 4 to 6 minutes. The Heimlich maneuver uses an upper-abdominal thrust to create sufficient diaphragmatic pressure in the static lung below the foreign body to expel the obstruction. The Heimlich maneuver is used in conscious adult patients and in children older than age 1. However, the abdominal thrust is contraindicated in pregnant women, markedly obese patients, and infants younger than age 1. For such patients, use a chest thrust, which forces air out of the lungs to create an artificial cough.

These maneuvers are contraindicated in a patient with mild airway obstruction, when the patient can maintain adequate ventilation to dislodge the foreign body by effective coughing, and in an infant. However, if the patient has poor air exchange and increased breathing difficulty, a silent cough, cyanosis, or the inability to speak or breathe, take immediate action to dislodge the obstruction.

Conscious adult with mild airway obstruction

● Ask the person who's coughing or using the universal distress sign (clutching the neck between the thumb and fingers) if she's choking. If she indicates that she is but can speak and cough forcefully, she has good air exchange and should be encouraged to continue to cough. Remain with the person and monitor her.

Conscious adult with severe airway obstruction

● Ask the person, "Are you choking?" If the patient nods yes and has signs of se-

vere airway obstruction, tell her that you'll help dislodge the foreign body.

● Stand behind the patient and wrap your arms around her waist. Make a fist with one hand, and place the thumb side against her abdomen in the midline, slightly above the umbilicus and well below the xiphoid process. Grasp your fist with the other hand (as shown below).

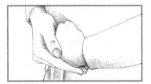

● Squeeze the patient's abdomen with quick inward and upward thrusts. Make each thrust a separate and distinct movement, forceful enough to create an artificial cough that will dislodge an obstruction (as shown below).

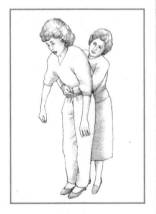

OBSTRUCTED AIRWAY MANAGEMENT *(continued)*

● Make sure that you have a firm grasp on the patient because she may lose consciousness and need to be lowered to the floor. Support her head and neck to prevent injury, and continue as described.

● Repeat the thrusts until the foreign body is expelled.

● If the patient becomes unconscious, contact the emergency medical service (EMS) and follow the interventions for relieving an obstructed airway in an unconscious person. If the victim of an airway obstruction becomes unconscious, the lay rescuer should lower the patient to the ground and immediately contact the EMS and begin cardiopulmonary resuscitation (CPR). Studies demonstrate that chest thrusts generated higher sustained airway pressure than pressure generated by abdominal thrusts. For this reason, it's believed that chest compressions alone may relieve the obstruction in the unconscious victim.

Unresponsive adult

● Lower the patient to the ground and immediately contact the EMS.

● Begin CPR.

● Each time the airway is opened using a head-tilt, chin-lift maneuver, look for an object in the patient's mouth.

● Remove the object, if present.

● Attempt to ventilate the patient and follow with 30 chest compressions.

● The blind finger sweep is no longer recommended by the American Heart Association; it should be used only when a foreign body can be seen in the mouth. Studies have shown that blind finger sweeps may result in injury to the patient's mouth and throat or to the rescuer's fingers, and there's no evidence as to its effectiveness. In addition, the tongue-jaw lift is no longer used. Open the patient's mouth using a head-tilt, chin-lift maneuver.

Obese or pregnant adult

● If the patient is conscious, stand behind her and place your arms under her armpits and around her chest.

● Place the thumb side of your clenched fist against the middle of the sternum, avoiding the margins of the ribs and the xiphoid process. Grasp your fist with your other hand and perform a chest thrust with enough force to expel the foreign body. Continue until the patient expels the obstruction or loses consciousness (as shown below).

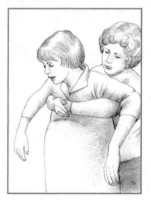

● If the patient loses consciousness, carefully lower her to the floor.

● Then, follow the same steps you would use for the unresponsive adult.

(continued)

OBSTRUCTED AIRWAY MANAGEMENT *(continued)*

Conscious child with severe airway obstruction

- If the child is conscious and can stand but can't cough or make a sound, perform abdominal thrusts using the same technique you would with an adult.

Unresponsive child

- Use the same techniques you would for the unresponsive adult.

Conscious infant

- Place the conscious infant face down so that he's straddling your arm with his head lower than his trunk. Rest your forearm on your thigh and deliver five forceful back blows with the heel of your hand between the infant's shoulder blades (as shown below).

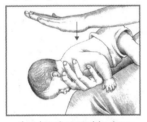

- If you haven't removed the obstruction, place your free hand on the infant's back. Supporting his neck, jaw, and chest with your other hand, turn him over onto your thigh. Keep his head lower than his trunk.

- Position your fingers. To do so, imagine a line between the infant's nipples and place the index finger of your free hand on his sternum, just below this imaginary line. Then place your middle and ring fingers next to your index finger and lift the index finger off his chest. Deliver five quick chest thrusts as you would for chest compression at a rate of approximately one per second.

- Never perform a blind finger sweep on a child or an infant because you risk pushing the foreign body farther back into the airway. Also, abdominal thrusts aren't recommended for infants because they may damage the liver.

- If the airway obstruction persists, repeat the five back blows and five chest thrusts until the obstruction is relieved or the infant becomes unresponsive.

Unresponsive infant

- Use the same techniques you would for the unresponsive adult.
- Continue until the obstruction is relieved or help arrives.

tient populations, including certain types of trauma, head and neck surgery, and difficult intubations. Nasotracheal intubation not only increases patient discomfort but increases the risk of sinus infection.

TRACHEOTOMY

Tracheotomy involves incising the skin over the trachea, thus creating a surgical wound for placement of a tube to establish an

PERFORMING AN EMERGENCY CRICOTHYROTOMY

To perform an emergency cricothyrotomy, first put on sterile gloves and clean the patient's neck with a sterile gauze pad soaked in chlorhexidine solution. To reduce the risk of contamination, use a circular motion, working outward from the incision site.

● Locate the precise insertion site by sliding your thumb and fingers down to the thyroid gland. You'll know you've located its outer borders when the space between your fingers and thumb widens.

● Move your finger across the center of the gland, over the anterior edge of the cricoid ring.

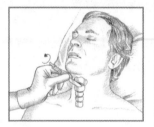

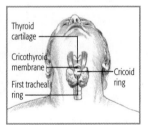

Thyroid cartilage
Cricothyroid membrane
First tracheal ring
Cricoid ring

Using a scalpel

● Make a horizontal incision, less than ½" (1.3 cm) long, in the cricothyroid membrane just above the cricoid ring.

● Insert a dilator to prevent tissue from closing around the incision. If a dilator isn't available, insert the handle of the scalpel and rotate it 90 degrees (as shown at top of next column).

● If a small tracheostomy tube (#6 or smaller) is available, insert it into the opening and secure it to help maintain a patent airway. If a tracheostomy tube isn't available, tape the dilator or scalpel han-

dle in place until a tracheostomy tube is available.

● If the patient can breathe spontaneously, attach a humidified oxygen source to the tracheostomy tube with a T tube; if he can't, attach a handheld resuscitation bag. You'll need to inflate the cuff of the tracheostomy tube with a syringe to provide positive-pressure ventilation.

● Auscultate bilaterally for breath sounds, and take the patient's vital signs.

● Dispose of the gloves properly and wash your hands.

Using a needle

● Attach a 10-ml syringe to a 14G (or larger) through-the-needle or over-the-needle catheter. Then insert the catheter into the cricothyroid membrane just above the cricoid ring.

● Direct the catheter downward at a 45-degree angle, as shown at top of next page, to the trachea to avoid damaging the vocal cords. Maintain negative pressure by pulling back the syringe plunger as you advance the catheter. You'll know the catheter has entered the trachea when air enters the syringe.

(continued)

PERFORMING AN EMERGENCY CRICOTHYROTOMY *(continued)*

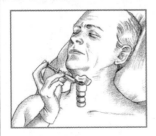

● When the catheter reaches the trachea, advance it and remove the needle and syringe. Tape the catheter in place.
● Attach the catheter hub to one end of the I.V. extension tubing. At the other end, attach a hand-operated release valve or a pressure-regulating adjustment valve. Connect the entire assembly to an oxygen source.
● Press the release valve to introduce oxygen into the trachea and inflate the lungs. When you can see that they're inflated, release the valve to allow passive exhalation. Adjust the pressure-regulating valve to the minimum pressure needed for adequate lung inflation.
● Auscultate bilaterally for breath sounds, and take the patient's vital signs.
● Dispose of the gloves properly and wash your hands.

COMBATING TRACHEOTOMY COMPLICATIONS

This chart lists possible tracheotomy complications along with measures to prevent, detect, and treat them.

COMPLICATION	PREVENTION
Aspiration	● Evaluate the patient's ability to swallow. ● Elevate his head and inflate the cuff during feeding and for 30 minutes afterward. ● Keep head of bed elevated ≥ 30 degrees
Bleeding at tracheotomy site	● Don't pull on the tracheostomy tube; don't allow ventilator tubing to do so. ● If the dressing adheres to the wound, wet it with hydrogen peroxide and remove it gently.

airway (tracheostomy). (See *Combating tracheotomy complications*.) However, this procedure may also be performed electively to prevent damage to the larynx such as when mechanical ventilation is necessary for more than 1 week.

Nursing interventions

The following serve as guidelines when caring for a patient with an upper airway obstruction.

- Recognize that an upper airway obstruction is a medical emergency.
- Assess for the cause of the obstruction.
- Assess breath sounds.
- Monitor chest X-rays and arterial blood gas results after the obstruction is relieved.
- Observe for "seesaw" respirations, use of accessory muscles, or retractions.
- Apply pulse oximetry to assess the patient's oxygenation status, and administer oxygen, as needed.

DETECTION	TREATMENT
● Assess for dyspnea, tachypnea, rhonchi, crackles, excessive secretions, and fever.	● Obtain a chest X-ray, if ordered. ● Suction excessive secretions. ● Give antibiotics, if necessary.
● Check dressings regularly; slight bleeding is normal, especially if the patient has a bleeding disorder.	● Keep the cuff inflated to prevent edema and blood aspiration. Give humidified oxygen. ● Document the character of bleeding. Check for prolonged clotting time. ● As ordered, assist with Gelfoam application or ligation of a small bleeder.

(continued)

COMBATING TRACHEOTOMY COMPLICATIONS *(continued)*

COMPLICATION	PREVENTION
Infection at tracheotomy site	● Always use strict sterile technique. ● Thoroughly clean all tubing. ● Change the nebulizer or humidifier jar and all tubing according to hospital policy. ● Collect sputum and wound drainage specimens for culture.
Pneumothorax	● Assess for subcutaneous emphysema, which may indicate pneumothorax. Notify the practitioner if this occurs.
Subcutaneous emphysema	● Make sure the cuffed tube is patent and properly inflated. ● Avoid displacement by securing ties and using lightweight ventilator tubing and swivel valves.
Tracheal malacia	● Avoid excessive cuff pressures. ● Avoid suctioning beyond the end of the tube.

■ Continually assess for stridor, cyanosis, and changes in LOC, and notify the practitioner immediately.

■ Perform abdominal thrusts if a foreign object obstruction is suspected.

■ Prepare for a cricothyrotomy if the setting is outside of the health care environment.

■ Prepare for ET intubation or a tracheotomy if an airway can't be established.

■ Anticipate cardiac arrest if the obstruction isn't cleared promptly.

DETECTION	TREATMENT
● Check for purulent, foul-smelling drainage from the stoma. ● Be alert for other signs and symptoms of infection, including fever, malaise, increased white blood cell count, and local pain.	● As ordered, obtain culture specimens and give antibiotics. ● Inflate the tracheostomy cuff to prevent aspiration. ● Suction the patient frequently; avoid cross-contamination. ● Change dressings when soiled.
● Auscultate for decreased or absent breath sounds. ● Check for tachypnea, pain, and subcutaneous emphysema.	● If ordered, prepare for chest tube insertion. ● Obtain a chest X-ray, as ordered, to evaluate pneumothorax or to check placement of the chest tube.
● Be aware that subcutaneous emphysema is most common in mechanically ventilated patients. ● Palpate the neck for crepitus, listen for air leakage around the cuff, and check the site for unusual swelling.	● Be sure to inflate the cuff properly or use a larger tube. ● Suction the patient, and clean the tube to remove blockage. ● Document the extent of crepitus.
● Note a dry, hacking cough and blood-streaked sputum when the tube is being manipulated.	● Minimize trauma from tube movement. ● Keep tracheostomy cuff pressure below 18 mm Hg.

ANAPHYLAXIS

Anaphylaxis is a dramatic, acute atopic reaction marked by the sudden onset of rapidly progressive urticaria and respiratory distress. A severe reaction may initiate vascular collapse, leading to systemic shock and, possibly, death.

Anaphylactic reactions result from systemic exposure to sensitizing drugs or other specific antigens. Such substances may be serums (usually horse serum), vaccines, allergen extracts (such as pollen), enzymes (L-asparaginase), hormones, penicillin and other antibiotics, sulfonamides, local anesthetics, salicylates, polysaccharides (such as iron dextran), diagnostic chemicals (sodium dehydrocholate, radiographic contrast media), foods (chocolate, legumes, nuts, berries, seafood, egg albumin) and sulfite-containing food additives, insect venom (honeybees, wasps, hornets, yellow jackets, fire ants, and certain spiders) and, rarely, a ruptured hydatid cyst.

The most common anaphylaxis-causing antigen is penicillin. This drug induces a reaction in 1 to 4 of every 10,000 patients treated with it. Penicillin is also most likely to induce anaphylaxis after parenteral administration or prolonged therapy.

Pathophysiology

An anaphylactic reaction requires previous sensitization or exposure to the specific antigen. After initial exposure to an antigen, the immune system responds by producing specific immunoglobulin (Ig) antibodies in the lymph nodes. Helper T cells enhance this process. These IgE antibodies then bind to membrane receptors located on mast cells (found throughout connective tissue, typically near small blood vessels) and basophils.

When the body encounters the antigen again, the IgE antibodies, or cross-linked IgE receptors, recognize the antigen as foreign. This activates a series of cellular reactions that trigger degranulation—the release of chemical mediators (such as histamine, prostaglandins, and platelet-activating factor) from mast cell stores. IgG or IgM enters the reaction and activates the release of complement factors. (See *What happens in anaphylaxis.*)

Complications

- Death minutes to hours after the first symptoms (although a delayed or persistent reaction may occur for up to 24 hours)
- Respiratory obstruction
- Systemic vascular collapse

Assessment findings

Signs and symptoms of anaphylaxis may include:

- exposure to an antigen
- feeling of impending doom or fright
- apprehension
- restlessness
- cyanosis

WHAT HAPPENS IN ANAPHYLAXIS

An anaphylactic reaction requires previous sensitization or exposure to the specific antigen. The following illustrates the anaphylactic process.

1. Response to the antigen

Immunoglobulin (Ig) M and IgG recognize the antigen as a foreign substance and attach themselves to it.

The process to destroy the antigen (the *complement cascade*) begins but can't finish, either because of insufficient amounts of the protein catalyst A or because the antigen inhibits certain complement enzymes. The patient exhibits no signs or symptoms at this stage.

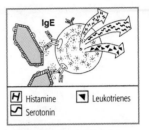

H Histamine　　◢ Leukotrienes
◿ Serotonin

3. Intensified response

The activated IgE stimulates mast cells located in connective tissue along the venule walls. These mast cells release more histamine (H) and eosinophil chemotactic factor of anaphylaxis (ECF-A). These substances produce disruptive lesions, which weaken the venules.

Itchy, red skin; wheals; and swelling appear. Signs and symptoms worsen.

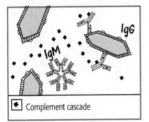

◆ Complement cascade

2. Released chemical mediators

The antigen's continued presence or reintroduction activates IgE, which promotes the release of mediators, including histamine, serotonin, and leukotrienes.

The sudden release of histamine causes vasodilation and increases capillary permeability, resulting in a loss of circulating plasma, thus decreasing blood pressure. The patient begins to exhibit sudden nasal congestion; itchy, watery eyes; flushing; sweating; weakness; and anxiety.

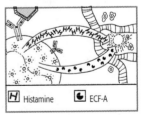

H Histamine　　● ECF-A

4. Distress

In the lungs, the histamine causes endothelial cells to burst and endothelial tissue to tear away from surrounding tissue. Fluids leak into the alveoli, and leukotrienes prevent alveoli from expanding, thereby reducing pulmonary compliance.

(continued)

WHAT HAPPENS IN ANAPHYLAXIS *(continued)*

Tachypnea, crowing, use of accessory muscles for breathing, and cyanosis signal respiratory distress. Resulting neurologic signs and symptoms include severe anxiety, change in level of consciousness and, possibly, seizures.

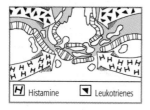

| H Histamine | ◤ Leukotrienes |

5. Deterioration

Meanwhile, basophils and mast cells begin to release prostaglandins and bradykinin, with histamine and serotonin,

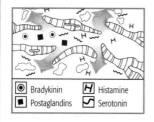

| ◉ Bradykinin | H Histamine |
| ■ Postaglandins | ∿ Serotonin |

increasing vascular permeability and causing fluids to leak from the vessels. Circulatory shock can result in minutes.

Shock; confusion; cool, pale skin; generalized edema; tachycardia; and hypotension signal rapid vascular collapse.

6. Failed compensatory mechanism

Damage to endothelial cells causes basophils and mast cells to release heparin. Eosinophils release arylsulfatase B (to neutralize the leukotrienes), phospholipase D (to neutralize heparin), and cyclic adenosine monophosphate and the prostaglandins E_1 and E_2 (to increase the metabolic rate). However, this response can't reverse anaphylaxis.

Hemorrhage, disseminated intravascular coagulation, and cardiopulmonary arrest result.

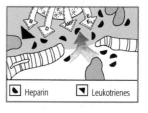

| ◤ Heparin | ◤ Leukotrienes |

- cool, clammy skin
- erythema
- edema
- tachypnea
- weakness
- sweating
- sneezing
- dyspnea
- nasal pruritus

- urticaria
- well-circumscribed, discrete cutaneous wheals with erythematous, raised, serpiginous borders and blanched centers
- giant hives
- complaints of a lump in the throat
- hoarseness or stridor
- wheezing, dyspnea, and complaints of chest tightness, suggestive of bronchial obstruction
- severe abdominal cramps, nausea, and diarrhea
- urinary urgency and incontinence
- dizziness, drowsiness, headache, restlessness, and seizures
- hypotension, shock and, sometimes, angina and cardiac arrhythmias.

Diagnostic test results

No tests are required to identify anaphylaxis. The patient's history and presenting signs and symptoms establish the diagnosis. If signs and symptoms occur without a known allergic stimulus, other possible causes of shock, such as acute myocardial infarction, status asthmaticus, and heart failure, must be ruled out.

Skin testing may help to identify a specific allergen. However, because skin tests can cause serious reactions, a scratch test should be performed first in high-risk situations.

Treatment

Always an emergency, anaphylaxis requires an *immediate* injection of aqueous epinephrine given every 5 to 15 minutes, as needed, to control symptoms and maintain blood pressure.

In the early stages of anaphylaxis, when the patient remains conscious and normotensive, epinephrine may be administered I.M. If the patient has severe hypotension or cardiac arrest, I.V. epinephrine is indicated.

A patent airway must be established and endotracheal intubation or tracheotomy may be needed if laryngeal edema occurs. Oxygen administration is vital to maintain oxygenation to the tissues. If the patient's systolic blood pressure can't be maintained above 90 mm Hg, vasopressors can be used.

If cardiac arrest occurs, cardiopulmonary resuscitation must be initiated at once.

Nursing interventions

- Provide supplemental oxygen and observe the patient's response. If hypoxia continues, prepare to help insert an artificial airway.
- Insert a peripheral I.V. line for administering emergency drugs and large volumes of crystalloids.
- After the initial emergency, give other medications, as ordered, such as subQ epinephrine, longer-acting epinephrine, a corticosteroid, and I.V. diphenhydramine for urticaria.
- In severe reactions when the patient is unconscious and hypotensive, give the drug I.V., as ordered.

> **RED FLAG** Rapid infusion of aminophylline can cause or aggravate severe hypotension.

- Watch for early signs of laryngeal edema, such as stridor, hoarseness, and dyspnea.
- Assist with ventilation, closed-chest cardiac massage, and sodium bicarbonate administration, as ordered.
- Watch for hypotension and shock. As ordered, maintain circulatory volume with volume expanders (plasma, plasma expanders, normal saline solution, and albumin). As prescribed, give an I.V. vasopressor, norepinephrine, and dopamine to stabilize blood pressure. Monitor blood pressure, central venous pressure, and urine output.
- Continually reassure the patient, and explain all tests and treatments to reduce his fear and anxiety. If necessary, reorient the patient to the situation and his surroundings.
- If the patient undergoes skin or scratch testing, monitor him for signs of a serious allergic response. Keep emergency resuscitation equipment nearby during and after the test.
- Advise the patient to carry an anaphylaxis kit whenever he's outdoors. Urge him to familiarize himself with the kit and to know how to use it before the need arises. (See *Using an anaphylaxis kit.*)
- If the patient must receive a drug to which he's allergic, prevent a severe reaction by making sure he receives careful desensitization, with gradually increasing doses of the antigen or with advance administration of a corticosteroid. A patient with a history of allergies should receive a drug with high anaphylactic potential only after cautious pretesting for sensi-

USING AN ANAPHYLAXIS KIT

If the practitioner prescribes an anaphylaxis kit for the patient to use in an emergency, explain to the patient that the kit contains everything he needs to treat an allergic reaction: two epinephrine autoinjectors, alcohol swabs, a tourniquet, and antihistamine tablets.

Instruct the patient to notify the practitioner at once if anaphylaxis occurs (or to ask someone else to call him) and to use the anaphylaxis kit as follows:

Getting ready
● Take the epinephrine autoinjector from the kit. Don't remove the cap, however, until ready to use.
● Next, clean about 4″ (10 cm) of the skin on your arm or thigh with an alcohol swab. (If you're right-handed, clean your left arm or thigh. If you're left-handed, clean your right arm or thigh.)

Injecting the epinephrine
● Position the black tip of the epinephrine autoinjector over the injection site.
● Firmly push the device into the injection site. A loud clicking sound indicates that the device is injecting the medication, so hold the injector in place for 10 seconds.
● Remove the autoinjector, and dispose of it properly.
    Note: The practitioner can determine the correct dosage and administration for infants and children younger than age 12.

Removing the insect's stinger
● Quickly remove the insect's stinger if it's visible. Use a dull object, such as a fingernail or tweezers, to pull it straight out. If the stinger can't be removed quickly, stop trying. Go on to the next step.

Applying the tourniquet
● If you were stung on an arm or leg, apply a tourniquet between the sting site and your heart. Tighten the tourniquet by pulling the string.
● After 10 minutes, release the tourniquet by pulling on the metal ring.

Taking the antihistamine tablets
● Chew and swallow the antihistamine tablets. (Children age 12 and younger should follow the directions supplied by the practitioner or provided in the kit.)

Following up
● Apply ice packs, if available, to the sting site. Avoid exertion, keep warm, and see a physician or go to an emergency facility.
● *Important:* If you don't notice an improvement within 10 minutes, give yourself a second injection by following the directions in the kit. Proceed as before, following the injection instructions.

Special instructions
● Keep the kit handy at all times for emergency treatment.
● Ask the pharmacist for storage guidelines.
● Note the kit's expiration date, and replace the kit before that date.

DISCHARGE TEACHING

ANAPHYLAXIS TEACHING TOPICS

- After the acute anaphylactic event has been controlled, the patient must be told of the risk of delayed symptoms. Any recurrence of shortness of breath, chest tightness, sweating, angioedema, or other signs and symptoms must be reported immediately.
- Teach the patient to avoid exposure to known allergens. If he has a food or drug allergy, instruct him not to consume the offending food or drug in any of its combinations or forms. If he's allergic to insect stings, he should avoid open fields and wooded areas during the insect season.
- Tell the patient to wear a medical identification bracelet indicating his allergies and to carry a list of allergens and associated reactions in his wallet.

tivity. Closely monitor the patient during and after testing, making sure you have resuscitation equipment and epinephrine readily available.

- Monitor the patient undergoing diagnostic procedures that use radiographic contrast media, such as excretory urography, cardiac catheterization, and angiography. (See *Anaphylaxis teaching topics*.)

BRONCHOSPASM

Bronchospasm is an abnormal contraction of the smooth muscle of the bronchi, resulting in an acute narrowing and obstruction of the airway. The onset of bronchospasm may be sudden, usually resulting from anesthesia induction, or it may have a progressive onset over several minutes. The most common cause of bronchospasm is asthma; however, other causes include:

- allergic response to a drug or anesthesia
- history of pulmonary obstructive disease or allergies
- irritation of the airway from suctioning, airway insertion during an emergency, or endotracheal tube placement
- vigorous physical activity or exercise.

Pathophysiology

Bronchospasms result from the tightening of the muscles surrounding the bronchial tubes, resulting in narrowing of the air passages and an interruption in the normal flow of air into and out of the lungs. If bronchospasms aren't promptly diagnosed and treated, air exchange is hindered as air is trapped in the alveolar sacs of the lungs. Bronchospasms are commonly caused by a hyperreactive airway.

Exercise-induced bronchospasm generally occurs during exercise or within minutes of stopping. Hyperventilation of air that's cooler and dryer than the air in the respiratory tract results in the loss of heat and water from the lungs during episodes of physical exertion.

Bronchospasms can occur during the induction of anesthesia or at any time during the anesthetic or postoperative period. This occurs because the anesthetic agents can cause bronchoconstriction. The severity of this type of bronchospasm may be life-threatening, resulting in the inability to ventilate the patient. Patients at risk for bronchospasms related to anesthesia include those with a history of anesthesia-induced bronchospasm, history of reactive airway disease, significant smoking history, or recent history of an upper respiratory tract infection, making their airways irritable and possibly constricted.

Complications
- Hypoxia
- Respiratory arrest

Assessment findings
Signs and symptoms of bronchospasm may include:
- change in level of consciousness
- a slight cough with no further sound
- wheezing
- little or no movement of the chest
- inability to ventilate even with positive pressure
- change in oxygen saturation values (hypoxia)
- change in color due to lack of oxygen
- dyspnea
- respiratory distress at rest
- diminished breath sounds due to air trapping.

Diagnostic test results

- Pulmonary function tests reveal decreased vital capacity and increased total lung and residual capacities during an acute asthma attack. Peak and expiratory flow rate measurements are less than 60% of baseline.
- Pulse oximetry usually shows decreased oxygen saturation.
- Chest X-ray may show hyperinflation with areas of atelectasis and a flat diaphragm caused by increased intrathoracic volume.
- Arterial blood gas analysis reveals decreasing partial pressure of arterial oxygen and increasing partial pressure of arterial carbon dioxide ($PaCO_2$).
- An electrocardiogram may show sinus tachycardia.

Treatment

With bronchospasms, the patient is monitored closely for respiratory failure. Oxygen, bronchodilators, epinephrine, I.V. corticosteroids, and nebulizer therapy may be ordered. The patient may be intubated and placed on mechanical ventilation if $PaCO_2$ increases or if respiratory arrest occurs.

    If the patient has a history of asthma, the following treatment measures should be considered:

- prevention, by identifying and avoiding precipitating factors, such as environmental allergens or irritants or nonsteroidal anti-inflammatory drugs and aspirin, if appropriate
- desensitization to specific antigens, if the stimuli can't be removed entirely, which decreases the severity of asthma attacks with future exposure
- bronchodilators (epinephrine [Bronkaid Mist], albuterol [Proventil]), to decrease bronchoconstriction, reduce bronchial airway edema, and increase pulmonary ventilation
- anticholinergics, to increase the effects of bronchodilators
- corticosteroids (methylprednisolone [Depo-Medrol]), to decrease bronchoconstriction, reduce bronchial airway edema, and increase pulmonary ventilation
- montelukast (Singulair), to protect against bradykinin-induced bronchospasm
- I.M. epinephrine, to counteract the effects of mediators of an asthma attack

DISCHARGE TEACHING

BRONCHOSPASM TEACHING TOPICS

- Teach the patient and family to avoid allergens, irritants, smoke, and cold air.
- Teach the patient about his medications, including proper dosages, administration instructions, and possible adverse effects and when to notify the practitioner.
- Teach the patient how to use a metered-dose inhaler.

- mast cell stabilizers (cromolyn [Intal], nedocromil [Tilade]) in patients with atopic asthma who have seasonal disease; when given prophylactically, they block the acute obstructive effects of antigen exposure by inhibiting the degranulation of mast cells, thereby preventing the release of chemical mediators responsible for anaphylaxis
- humidified oxygen, to correct dyspnea, cyanosis, and hypoxemia and to maintain an oxygen saturation greater than 90%
- mechanical ventilation, to help the patient who doesn't respond to initial ventilatory support and drugs or who develops respiratory failure
- relaxation exercises, to increase circulation and aid recovery from an asthma attack. (See *Bronchospasm teaching topics*.)

Nursing interventions

Consider the following interventions when caring for a patient with bronchospasm:

- Conduct careful and frequent assessment of the patient's respiratory status, especially if he isn't intubated. Check his respiratory rate, auscultate breath sounds, and monitor oxygen saturation continually. Prepare the patient to be intubated, if necessary.
- Be alert with a patient who was wheezing but suddenly stops and continues to show signs of respiratory distress. This is a sign of imminent respiratory collapse, and the patient needs intubation and mechanical ventilation. Reassure the patient and stay with him. Help him to relax as much as possible.
- Assess the patient's mental status for confusion, agitation, or lethargy and early signs of respiratory compromise.

- Assess the patient's heart rate and rhythm. Be alert for cardiac arrhythmias related to bronchodilator therapy or hypoxemia.
- Obtain ordered tests and report results promptly.
- Give medications, as ordered (particularly bronchodilators).
- Give I.V. fluids to replace insensible fluid loss from hyperventilation.

RESPIRATORY ARREST

Effective pulmonary gas exchange involves several functions, including a clear airway, normal lungs and chest wall, and adequate pulmonary circulation. A compromise of any of these anatomical structures or functions can affect respiration. The three degrees of respiratory compromise are respiratory distress, respiratory failure, and respiratory arrest.

Respiratory distress may be mild or severe and results in changes in the respiratory rate, respiratory mechanism, or both.

Respiratory failure indicates that the respiratory system can no longer meet the oxygen requirements of the body, and if uncorrected, will cause the patient to progress to cardiac arrest. Respiratory arrest is the cessation of respiration, but may also be characterized by episodes of prolonged apnea.

Conditions that may lead to respiratory arrest include:
- stroke
- complete airway obstruction
- cardiac arrest
- shock
- heart disease
- cardiac arrhythmias
- seizures
- poisoning or inhalation of toxic substances
- injury to the lungs
- drowning or suffocation
- emphysema or asthma
- allergic reactions
- hyperventilation
- drugs
- prematurity
- head or brain stem injury.

Pathophysiology

Primary respiratory arrest results from airway obstruction, a decreased respiratory drive, or respiratory muscle weakness. Although airway obstruction can be partial or complete, the most common cause in an unconscious victim is tongue displacement into the oropharynx due to a loss of muscle tone. Other causes of upper airway obstruction include:

- accumulation of blood, mucus, or vomitus
- foreign body aspiration
- spasms or edema of the larynx
- edema of the pharynx
- inflammation of the upper airway
- neoplasm
- trauma.

Lower airway obstruction can be related to the aspiration of gastric contents, severe bronchospasm, or conditions that fill the alveoli with fluid such as heart failure or pulmonary hemorrhage or edema.

Secondary respiratory arrest results from insufficient circulation. Complete respiratory arrest is the absence of spontaneous ventilatory movement with cyanosis and may develop quickly in a conscious victim due to a foreign body obstruction. If respiratory arrest is prolonged, cardiac arrest follows from impairment of cardiac oxygenation and function related to hypoxemia.

Complications

- Coma
- Death

Assessment findings

Signs and symptoms of respiratory arrest include:

- depressed sensorium
- gasping for air
- irregular respiratory patterns
- tachycardia
- diaphoresis
- hypertension
- absence of spontaneous breathing
- no rise or fall of the chest

▨ inability to feel the movement of air from the mouth or nose
▨ cyanosis
▨ cool, clammy skin
▨ decreasing pulse oximetry and oxygen saturation level.

Diagnostic test results
Physical examination usually helps to diagnose respiratory arrest. For example, auscultating the chest determines the presence or absence of breath sounds. Placing a hand on the chest allows for assessment of chest movement with respirations or lack of movement. If tests are ordered, they may include:
▨ arterial blood gas (ABG) analysis
▨ chest X-ray
▨ electrocardiogram
▨ bronchoscopy and laryngoscopy for obstructed airway.

Treatment
Respiratory arrest is a medical emergency, and treatment focuses on correcting the cause, establishing an airway, and providing oxygenation. If respiratory arrest is related to an obstructed airway, treatment should focus on relieving the obstruction through a series of subdiaphragmatic, abdominal thrusts in the child or adult or five back blows followed by five chest thrusts in the infant. The pregnant woman requires chest thrusts. If the airway is patent and cardiac arrest occurs, cardiopulmonary resuscitation must be implemented.

Nursing interventions
Consider the following interventions when caring for a patient with respiratory arrest:
▨ Assess airway, breathing, and circulation.
▨ Start basic life support in the absence of circulation and respirations and in the presence of a patent airway.
▨ If the airway is obstructed, try to clear the obstruction.
▨ If a cervical spine injury is suspected after a fall, use the jaw-thrust maneuver to open the airway.
▨ Assess breath sounds.
▨ Monitor chest X-rays and ABG results after the obstruction is relieved.
▨ Watch for "seesaw" respirations.

- Apply pulse oximetry to assess the patient's oxygenation status.
- Continually assess for stridor, cyanosis, and changes in level of consciousness, and notify the practitioner immediately.
- Prepare for endotracheal intubation or a tracheostomy, within the hospital setting, if an airway can't be established.
- Anticipate cardiac arrest if the obstruction isn't cleared promptly.
- Give oxygen.
- Start or continue cardiac monitoring.
- Give I.V. fluids and medications, as ordered.

RESPIRATORY DEPRESSION

Respiratory depression is related to inadequate ventilation and, if not corrected, leads to acidemia.

Respiratory depression may be caused by:
- cerebral trauma from birth injuries
- intracranial tumors
- vascular lesions
- central nervous system (CNS) infections (meningitis, encephalitis, or sepsis)
- overdose of medications (see *Respiratory depression related to poisoning in children,* page 398)
- severe asphyxia
- aspiration
- strangulation
- pulmonary edema
- pneumothorax
- flail chest
- carbon monoxide or cyanide poisoning
- severe anemia
- tetanus
- anesthesia.

RESPIRATORY DEPRESSION RELATED TO POISONING IN CHILDREN

Because of their curiosity and ignorance, children are the most common group of poison victims. Accidental poisoning, usually from ingestion of salicylates (aspirin), acetaminophen (Tylenol), cleansers, insecticides, paints, cosmetics, or plants, is the fourth leading cause of death in children.

Assessment of the patient with a toxic ingestion includes a simultaneous history from parent or caregiver; assessment of the airway, breathing, and circulation; and initiation of life support, as indicated. The patient's history should reveal the source of poison, the form of exposure (ingestion, inhalation, injection, or skin contact), amount the child was exposed to, estimated time of poisoning, treatment provided, and whether the child vomited. Assessment findings vary with the poison.

Pathophysiology

Respiratory depression is a serious emergency that commonly occurs in patients sedated with anesthesia or medications, such as opioids, and can be sudden or gradual in onset.

Respiratory depression should be suspected with any change in respiratory function based on earlier assessments and data. If the condition goes uncorrected, progressive carbon dioxide retention and hypoxemia can result in systemic acidemia. Respiratory depression may result from impairment at various levels of the respiratory system, including the CNS, upper and lower airways, alveolar spaces, or chest wall. It may also result from impairment of normal mechanisms of ventilation or from blood and circulatory system impairment.

Complications

- Hypoxia
- Cardiac arrest

Assessment findings

Signs and symptoms of respiratory depression may include:

- respiratory rate below 10 breaths/minute (normal adult respiratory rate: 12 to 18 breaths/minute)
- shortness of breath

- tachycardia
- dyspnea
- change in the depth of respirations
- tidal volume below 10 ml/kg
- restlessness or agitation
- unresponsiveness
- decreased level of consciousness (LOC)
- air hunger
- low partial pressure of arterial oxygen and high partial pressure of arterial carbon dioxide ($PaCO_2$)
- decreased oxygen saturation level
- pale or cyanotic skin color
- hypoventilation, diaphoresis, dilated or constricted pupils, coma, tremors, or seizure activity or neurologic posturing (with an overdose of sedatives or opiates).

Diagnostic test results
- Arterial blood gas (ABG) analysis confirms the presence of hypoxemia and hypercapnia (hypercarbia).
- Pulse oximetry provides oxygen saturation level.
- Chest X-ray may reveal pulmonary pathology.
- ABG analysis provides information on carbon dioxide and $PaCO_2$ levels and acid-base balance.
- A blood glucose test result helps rule out hypoglycemia as the cause of the patient's altered LOC.
- Electrocardiogram readings reveal ischemia and arrhythmias.
- Toxicology studies (including drug screens) of drug levels in the mouth, vomitus, urine, stool, or blood or on the victim's hands or clothing help to confirm respiratory depression related to a drug overdose.

Treatment
Initial treatment includes support for the patient's airway, breathing, and circulation and administration of the antidote, if an overdose is diagnosed. (See *Common antidotes,* page 400.) Ventilation with a bag and mask, tracheal intubation, or reversal of the agent causing the respiratory depression is commonly warranted.

COMMON ANTIDOTES

This table lists drugs or toxins commonly involved in respiratory depression and their antidotes.

DRUG OR TOXIN	ANTIDOTE
Acetaminophen (Acephen)	Acetylcysteine (Mucomyst, Acetadote)
Anticholinergics, tricyclic antidepressants	Physostigmine (Antilirium)
Benzodiazepines	Flumazenil (Romazicon)
Calcium channel blockers	Calcium chloride
Cyanide	Amyl nitrite, sodium nitrite, and sodium thiosulfate; methylene blue
Digoxin (Lanoxin), cardiac glycosides	Digoxin immune fab (Digibind)
Ethylene glycol (Co-Lav) or methanol	Fomepizole (Antizol)
Heparin	Protamine sulfate
Insulin	Glucagon
Iron	Deferoxamine (Desferal)
Lead	Edetate calcium disodium (Calcium Disodium Versenate)
Opioids	Naloxone (Narcan), nalmefene (Revex), naltrexone (ReVia)
Organophosphates, anticholinesterases	Atropine, pralidoxime (Protopam)

Nursing interventions

Consider the following interventions when caring for a patient with respiratory depression:

■ Immediately assess the patient's airway, breathing, and circulation. Institute emergency resuscitative measures, as necessary.

- Monitor the patient's neurologic, cardiac, and respiratory status closely, at least every 15 minutes or more frequently, depending on his condition.
- Assess the patient's LOC for changes, such as increasing confusion, restlessness, or decreased responsiveness.
- Auscultate lung sounds for crackles, rhonchi, or stridor.
- Observe for signs of airway obstruction, including labored breathing, severe hoarseness, and dyspnea.
- If oxygen saturation worsens, obtain ABG levels and notify the practitioner of the results.
- Give supplemental humidified oxygen, as ordered.
- Monitor oxygen saturation via continuous pulse oximetry and serial ABG analysis for evidence of hypoxemia, and anticipate the need for endotracheal intubation and mechanical ventilation should the patient's respiratory status deteriorate.
- Initiate I.V. access and give I.V. fluids, as ordered.
- Obtain laboratory specimens to assess for drug, electrolyte, and glucose levels.
- Anticipate giving normal saline solution and vasopressors if the patient is hypotensive; give dextrose 5% in water if the patient is hypoglycemic.
- Place the patient in semi-Fowler's position to maximize chest expansion. Keep him as relaxed and comfortable as possible to minimize oxygen demands.
- Give bronchodilators, as ordered.
- Perform oropharyngeal or tracheal suctioning, as indicated by the patient's inability to clear the airway or by abnormal breath sounds.
- Monitor the patient's vital signs continuously for changes.
- Help with the insertion of a pulmonary artery catheter, if indicated, to evaluate the patient's hemodynamic status. Monitor such hemodynamic parameters as central venous pressure, pulmonary artery wedge pressure, and cardiac output (and cardiac index) frequently.
- Institute continuous cardiac monitoring to evaluate for possible arrhythmias. If the patient develops heart block, prepare for cardiac pacing. Give antiarrhythmics, as ordered.
- Assess intake and output every hour; insert an indwelling urinary catheter, as indicated, to ensure accurate urine measurement.

■ Give antidotes, as ordered and available. When giving flumazenil (Romazicon) and naloxone (Narcan), watch for signs of withdrawal. Flumazenil may precipitate seizures, especially in patients who have ingested antidepressants or who have been on long-term sedation with benzodiazepines.

■ Monitor the patient with respiratory distress from an overdose for the return of overdose symptoms because the drug may last longer in the patient's system than the dose of antidote.

■ Monitor laboratory test results.

COMPLICATIONS

RESPIRATORY ACIDOSIS

Respiratory acidosis is an acid-base disturbance characterized by reduced alveolar ventilation and manifested by hypercapnia (partial pressure of carbon dioxide [$PaCO_2$] greater than 45 mm Hg). Respiratory acidosis may be acute (resulting from sudden failure in ventilation) or chronic (resulting from long-term pulmonary disease). (See *What happens in respiratory acidosis.*)

The prognosis depends on the severity of the underlying disturbance and the patient's general clinical condition.

Factors that predispose a patient to respiratory acidosis include:

■ drugs (such as opioids, anesthetics, hypnotics, and sedatives), central sleep apnea, and obesity, which inhibit the respiratory drive center

■ central nervous system (CNS) trauma, such as medullary injury, which may impair ventilatory drive

■ chronic metabolic alkalosis, which may occur when respiratory compensatory mechanisms attempt to normalize pH by decreasing alveolar ventilation

■ neuromuscular diseases, such as Guillain-Barré syndrome, spinal cord injury, multiple sclerosis, myasthenia gravis, and poliomyelitis, in which respiratory muscles fail to respond properly to respiratory drive, thus reducing alveolar ventilation.

In addition, respiratory acidosis can result from an airway obstruction (such as aspiration) or a parenchymal lung disease

UP CLOSE

WHAT HAPPENS IN RESPIRATORY ACIDOSIS

These illustrations explain the basic pathophysiology of respiratory acidosis.

1. Pulmonary ventilation diminishes.

When pulmonary ventilation decreases, retained carbon dioxide (CO_2) in the red blood cells (RBCs) combines with water (H_2O) to form excess carbonic acid (H_2CO_3). The H_2CO_3 dissociates to release free hydrogen (H^+) and bicarbonate ions (HCO_3^-). In this condition, arterial blood gas (ABG) analysis shows increased partial pressure of arterial carbon dioxide ($PaCO_2$) (over 45 mm Hg) and reduced blood pH (below 7.35).

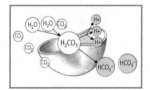

2. Oxygen saturation decreases.

As pH decreases and 2,3-diphosphoglycerate (2,3-DPG) increases in RBCs, 2,3-DPG alters hemoglobin (Hb) so it releases oxygen (O_2). This reduced Hb, which is strongly alkaline, picks up H^+ and CO_2, eliminating some free H^+ and excess CO_2. At this stage, arterial oxygen saturation levels decrease, and the Hb dissociation curve shifts to the right.

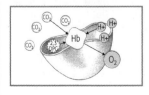

3. Respiratory rate rises.

Whenever $PaCO_2$ increases, CO_2 levels increase in all tissues and fluids. CO_2 reacts with H_2O to form H_2CO_3, which dissociates into H^+ and HCO_3^-. Elevated $PaCO_2$ and H^+ have a potent stimulatory effect on the medulla, increasing respirations to blow off CO_2. Look for rapid, shallow respirations and diminishing $PaCO_2$.

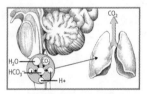

4. Blood flows to brain.

The free H^+ and excess CO_2 dilate cerebral vessels and increase blood flow to the brain, causing cerebral edema and depressed central nervous system activity. At this stage, the patient experiences headache, confusion, lethargy, nausea, and vomiting.

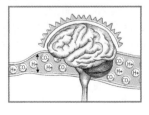

(continued)

WHAT HAPPENS IN RESPIRATORY ACIDOSIS
(continued)

5. Kidneys compensate.
As respiratory mechanisms fail, increasing $PaCO_2$ stimulates the kidneys to retain HCO_3^- and sodium ions (Na^+) and to excrete H^+. As a result, more sodium bicarbonate ($NaHCO_3$) is available to buffer free H^+. Ammonium ions (NH_4^+) are also excreted to remove H^+. A patient in this condition has increased urine acidity and ammonium levels, elevated serum pH and HCO_3^- levels, and shallow, depressed respirations.

6. Acid-base balance fails.
As H^+ concentration overwhelms compensatory mechanisms, H^+ move into the cells and potassium ions (K^+) move out. Without sufficient O_2, anaerobic metabolism produces lactic acid. Electrolyte imbalance and acidosis critically depress brain and cardiac function. ABG values in a patient in this condition show elevated $PaCO_2$ and decreased partial pressure of arterial oxygen and pH. The patient experiences hyperkalemia, arrhythmias, tremors, decreased level of consciousness and, possibly, coma.

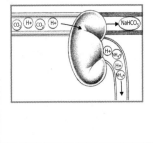

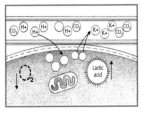

that interferes with alveolar ventilation, or from chronic obstructive pulmonary disease (COPD), asthma, severe acute respiratory distress syndrome, chronic bronchitis, large pneumothorax, extensive pneumonia, and pulmonary edema.

Pathophysiology

When pulmonary ventilation decreases, $PaCO_2$ is increased, and the level of carbon dioxide (CO_2) rises in all tissues and fluids, including the medulla and cerebrospinal fluid. Retained CO_2 combines with water to form carbonic acid, which then dissociates to release free hydrogen (H^+) and bicarbonate ions. Increased $PaCO_2$ and H^+ drive and expel CO_2.

As pH falls, 2,3-diphosphloglycerate accumulates in the red blood cells, where it alters hemoglobin so it releases oxygen.

This reduced hemoglobin, which is strongly alkaline, picks up H+ and CO_2 and removes them from the serum.

As respiratory mechanisms fall, rising $PaCO_2$ stimulates the kidneys to retain bicarbonate and sodium ions and excrete H+. As a result, more sodium bicarbonate is available to buffer free H+. Some hydrogen is excreted in the form of ammonium ions, neutralizing ammonia, which is an important CNS toxin.

As the H+ concentration overwhelms compensatory mechanisms, H+ move into the cells and potassium ions move out. Without enough oxygen, anaerobic metabolism produces lactic acid. Electrolyte imbalances and acidosis critically depress neurologic and cardiac functions.

Complications
■ Cardiac arrest
■ Shock

Assessment findings
Signs and symptoms of respiratory acidosis include:
■ headache
■ predisposing conditions for respiratory acidosis (drugs, CNS trauma, neuromuscular disease)
■ dyspnea
■ diaphoresis
■ nausea and vomiting
■ bounding pulses
■ rapid, shallow respirations
■ tachycardia
■ hypotension
■ papilledema
■ level of consciousness (LOC) ranging from restlessness, confusion, and apprehension to somnolence
■ fine or flapping tremor (asterixis)
■ depressed reflexes.

Diagnostic test results
■ Arterial blood gas (ABG) analysis confirms respiratory acidosis when the $PaCO_2$ is greater than the normal 45 mm Hg; pH is typically below the normal range of 7.35 to 7.45; and bi-

carbonate levels are normal in acute respiratory acidosis, but elevated in chronic respiratory acidosis.

Treatment

The goal of treatment is to correct the source of alveolar hypo-ventilation. If alveolar ventilation is significantly reduced, the patient may need the support of noninvasive positive pressure ventilation or mechanical ventilation until his underlying condition can be treated. In patients with COPD, noninvasive positive pressure ventilation lets the patient rest while it performs the work of breathing, to return the patient's acid-base balance to normal without requiring intubation and mechanical ventilation.

Other therapy includes administration of bronchodilators, oxygen, and antibiotics for patients with COPD; drug therapy for conditions such as myasthenia gravis; removal of foreign bodies from the airway in cases of obstruction; antibiotics for pneumonia; dialysis to eliminate toxic drugs; and correction of metabolic alkalosis.

Dangerously low pH levels (less than 7.15) can produce profound CNS and cardiovascular deterioration and may require the administration of I.V. sodium bicarbonate. However, in chronic lung disease, elevated CO_2 levels may persist despite treatment.

Nursing interventions

- Assess changes in level of consciousness, behavior, and mood, and watch for increased fatigue, sleep, and irritability.
- Be prepared to treat or remove the underlying cause such as an airway obstruction.
- Be alert for critical changes in the patient's respiratory, CNS, and cardiovascular functions. Report these changes immediately. Also report variations in ABG levels and electrolyte status.
- Maintain adequate hydration by giving I.V. fluids.
- Maintain continuous cardiac monitoring, and be prepared to treat arrhythmias related to electrolyte imbalances.
- Give oxygen (only at low concentrations in the patient with COPD) if the $Paco_2$ drops.

■ Give aerosolized or I.V bronchodilators. Monitor and record the patient's response to these medications.

■ Start noninvasive or mechanical ventilation, as ordered, if hypoventilation can't be corrected immediately. Continuously monitor the ventilator's settings.

■ Maintain a patent airway, and provide adequate humidification if acidosis requires mechanical ventilation.

■ Perform tracheal suctioning regularly and chest physiotherapy, if ordered.

■ To detect developing respiratory acidosis, closely monitor patients with COPD and chronic CO_2 retention for signs of acidosis. Give oxygen at low flow rates and closely monitor all patients who receive opioids and sedatives.

■ Reassure the patient as much as possible, depending on his LOC. Ease the fears and concerns of family members by keeping them informed of the patient's status. (See *Respiratory acidosis teaching topics*.)

RESPIRATORY ALKALOSIS

Respiratory alkalosis results from alveolar hyperventilation. It's marked by a decrease in partial pressure of arterial carbon dioxide ($PaCO_2$) (less than 35 mm Hg) and an increase in blood pH over 7.45. Uncomplicated respiratory alkalosis leads to a decrease in hydrogen ion concentration, which raises the blood pH. Hypocapnia occurs when the lungs eliminate more carbon dioxide (CO_2) than the body produces at the cellular level. In the acute stage, respiratory alkalosis is also called *hyperventilation syndrome*.

Predisposing conditions to respiratory alkalosis include:

- heart failure
- central nervous system (CNS) injury to the respiratory control center
- extreme anxiety
- fever
- pregnancy
- hypoxemia
- overventilation during mechanical ventilation
- pulmonary embolism
- salicylate intoxication (early).

Pathophysiology

When pulmonary ventilation increases to more than is needed to maintain normal CO_2 levels, excessive amounts of CO_2 are exhaled. The resulting hypocapnia leads to a chemical reduction of carbonic acid, excretion of hydrogen and bicarbonate ions, and a rising pH.

In defense against the increasing serum pH, the hydrogen-potassium buffer system pulls hydrogen ions out of the cells and into the blood in exchange for potassium ions. The hydrogen ions entering the blood combine with available bicarbonate ions to form carbonic acid, resulting in falling pH.

Hypocapnia stimulates the carotid and aortic bodies as well as the medulla; it also increases the heart rate (which hypokalemia can further aggravate), but not blood pressure. At the same time, hypocapnia causes cerebral vasoconstriction and decreased cerebral blood flow. It also overexcites the medulla, pons, and other parts of the autonomic nervous system. When hypocapnia lasts more than 6 hours, the kidneys secrete more bicarbonate and less hydrogen. Full renal adaptation to respiratory alkalosis requires normal volume status and renal function and may take several days to be noticed.

Continued low $PaCO_2$ and the vasoconstriction it causes increases cerebral and peripheral hypoxia. Severe alkalosis inhibits calcium ionization; as calcium ions become unavailable, nerves and muscles become progressively more excitable. Eventually, alkalosis overwhelms the CNS and the heart. (See *What happens in respiratory alkalosis,* pages 410 and 411.)

Complications
- Cardiac arrhythmias
- Seizures

Assessment findings
Signs and symptoms of respiratory alkalosis include:
- predisposing factors associated with respiratory alkalosis (heart failure, CNS injury, pulmonary embolism, anxiety, fever, overventilation during mechanical ventilation)
- light-headedness
- paresthesia
- cramping
- carpopedal spasms
- anxiety
- tetany
- tachycardia
- deep, rapid breathing.

Diagnostic test results
- Arterial blood gas (ABG) analysis confirms respiratory alkalosis and rules out compensation for metabolic acidosis. The $PaCO_2$ falls below 35 mm Hg; blood pH increases in proportion to a decrease in the $PaCO_2$ in the acute stage but drops toward normal in the chronic stage. The bicarbonate level is normal in the acute stage but below normal in the chronic stage.
- Serum electrolyte studies detect metabolic acid-base disorders.

Treatment
In respiratory alkalosis, the goal of treatment is to eradicate the underlying condition—for example, by removing ingested toxins or by treating fever, sepsis, or CNS disease. In severe respiratory alkalosis, the patient may need to breathe into a paper bag,

WHAT HAPPENS IN RESPIRATORY ALKALOSIS

This series of illustrations shows how respiratory alkalosis develops at the cellular level.

When pulmonary ventilation increases above the amount needed to maintain normal carbon dioxide (CO_2) levels, excessive amounts of CO_2 are exhaled. This causes hypocapnia (a fall in partial pressure of arterial carbon dioxide [$PaCO_2$]), which leads to reduced carbonic acid (H_2CO_3) production, a loss of hydrogen (H^+) and bicarbonate ions (HCO_3^-), and a subsequent rise in pH. Look for pH above 7.45, $PaCO_2$ below 35 mm Hg, and a bicarbonate level below 22 mEq/L.

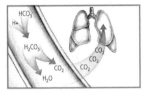

In defense against the rising pH, H^+ are pulled out of the cells and into the blood in exchange for potassium ions (K^+). The H^+ entering the blood combine with HCO_3^- to form H_2CO_3, which lowers pH. Look for a further decrease in HCO_3^- levels, a fall in pH, and a fall in serum potassium levels (hypokalemia).

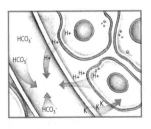

Hypocapnia stimulates the carotid and aortic bodies and the medulla, which causes an increase in heart rate without an increase in blood pressure. Look for angina, electrocardiogram changes, restlessness, and anxiety.

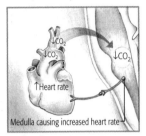

Medulla causing increased heart rate

Simultaneously, hypocapnia produces cerebral vasoconstriction, which prompts reduced cerebral blood flow. Hypocapnia also overexcites the medulla, pons, and other parts of the autonomic nervous system. Look for increasing anxiety, diaphoresis, dyspnea, alternating periods of apnea and hyperventilation, dizziness, and tingling in the fingers or toes.

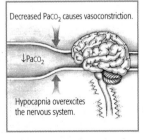

Decreased $PaCO_2$ causes vasoconstriction.

$\downarrow PaCO_2$

Hypocapnia overexcites the nervous system.

WHAT HAPPENS IN RESPIRATORY ALKALOSIS
(continued)

When hypocapnia lasts more than 6 hours, the kidneys increase bicarbonate secretion and reduce hydrogen excretion. Periods of apnea may result if the pH remains high and the $PaCO_2$ remains low. Look for a slowed respiratory rate, hypoventilation, and Cheyne-Stokes respirations.

striction. Severe alkalosis inhibits calcium (Ca) ionization, which in turn causes increased nerve excitability and muscle contractions. Eventually, the alkalosis overwhelms the central nervous system and the heart. Look for a decreasing level of consciousness, hyperreflexia, carpopedal spasm, tetany, arrhythmias, seizures, and coma.

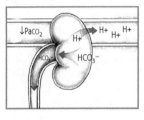

Continued low $PaCO_2$ increases cerebral and peripheral hypoxia from vasocon-

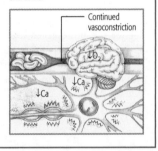

which helps relieve acute anxiety and lower CO_2 levels. If respiratory alkalosis results from anxiety, sedatives and tranquilizers may be necessary.

To prevent hyperventilation in patients receiving mechanical ventilation, ABG levels are monitored and dead-space or minute ventilation volume is adjusted.

Nursing interventions
- Watch for and report changes in the patient's neurologic, neuromuscular, and cardiovascular functioning.
- Remember that twitching and cardiac arrhythmias may be associated with alkalemia and electrolyte imbalances. Monitor ABG and serum electrolyte levels closely. Report any variations immediately.

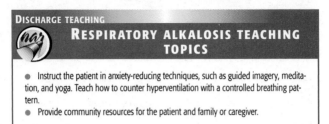

RESPIRATORY ALKALOSIS TEACHING TOPICS

● Instruct the patient in anxiety-reducing techniques, such as guided imagery, meditation, and yoga. Teach how to counter hyperventilation with a controlled breathing pattern.
● Provide community resources for the patient and family or caregiver.

■ Stay with the patient during periods of extreme stress and anxiety. Offer reassurance and maintain a calm, quiet environment. Monitor the effects of any sedation given.
■ Institute I.V. access and administer medications, as ordered.
■ Maintain continuous cardiac monitoring.
■ If the patient is coping with anxiety-induced respiratory alkalosis, help him identify factors that precipitate anxiety. Also help him find coping mechanisms and activities that promote relaxation. (See *Respiratory alkalosis teaching topics*.)

Appendices
Selected references
Index

English-Spanish respiratory assessment

―――――――――○―――――――――

When examining the respiratory system, be sure to ask about chest pain, coughing, weight gain, and medication use.

Aches and pains

Do you have chest pain?
¿Tiene Ud. dolor de pecho?

–Is it intermittent?
–¿Es intermitente?

–Is it constant?
–¿Es constante?

–Where is it located?
–¿Dónde se localiza el dolor?

–Do any activities produce the pain?
–¿Qué actividad o actividades producen el dolor?

Does it hurt when you breathe normally or when you breathe deeply?
¿Tiene Ud. el dolor cuando respira normalmente o cuando respira profundamente?

Does it hurt when you cough?
¿Le duele cuando tose?

Confusion, restlessness, and faintness

Do you ever feel confused, restless, or faint?
¿Alguna vez siente Ud. confusión, desasosiego o desmayo?

–When does the feeling occur?
–¿Cuándo ocurre esto?

–How long does it last?
–¿Cuánto tiempo dura?

Types of cough

Do you have a cough?
¿Tiene Ud. tos?

–What does it sound like?
–¿Qué sonido tiene?

   Hacking?
   ¿Tos seca?

   Barking?
   ¿Tos perruna?

   Congested?
   ¿Congestionada?

–Does it usually occur at a certain time of day?

When?

Do you cough up sputum?

–How much do you cough up each day?

–What color is it?

Red?

Pink?

With streaks of blood?

Yellow?

Green?

White?

Clear?

–How does it smell?

–Is it thick?

–Is it thin?

–What time of day do you cough up the most sputum?

Morning?

Night?

After meals?

–¿Por lo general, ocurre a cierta hora del día?

¿Cuándo?

¿Expectora Ud.?

–¿Cuánto expectora Ud. al día?

–¿De qué color es?

¿Rojo?

¿Rosado?

¿Sanguino lento?

¿Amarillo?

¿Verde?

¿Blanco?

¿Transparente o claro?

–¿Qué olor tiene?

–¿Es el esputo denso?

–¿Es el esputo claro?

–¿A qué hora del día expectora Ud. más?

¿Por la mañana?

¿Por la noche?

¿Después de las comidas?

Weight gain

Do you suffer from foot or ankle swelling?

Have you noticed any weight gain recently?

–How much weight have you gained?

–In what time frame?

¿Sufre Ud. de inflamación (hinchazón) del tobillo?

¿Ha notado Ud. algún aumento de peso recientemente?

–¿Cuánto peso ha aumentado?

–¿En qué tiempo?

Shortness of breath

Do you have shortness of breath?

–Is it constant?

–Is it intermittent?

¿Sufre Ud. de falta de respiración?

–¿Es constante?

–¿Es intermitente?

–Does position, medication, or relaxation relieve it?

–¿Se alivia Ud. con el descanso, algún medicamento, o cambio de postura?

Do your lips or nail beds ever turn blue?

¿Alguna vez se le ponen azules los labios o el lecho de la uña?

Does body position affect your breathing?

¿Le afecta la respiración la postura del cuerpo?

–How?

–¿Cómo?

Does time of day affect your breathing?

¿Le afecta la respiración la hora del día?

–What time of day?

–¿A qué hora del día se siente peor?

Specific activities

Does a particular activity affect your breathing?

¿Alguna actividad en particular afecta su respiración?

–Which activity?

–¿Qué actividad?

  Bathing?

  ¿Bañarse?

  Walking?

  ¿Caminar?

  Running?

  ¿Correr?

  Climbing stairs?

  ¿Subir escaleras?

  Other?

  ¿Otra?

How many stairs can you climb before you feel short of breath?

¿Cuántos escalones puede Ud. subir antes de sentir falta de respiración?

How many blocks can you walk before you feel short of breath?

¿Cuántas calles puede caminar antes de sentir falta de respiración?

Inhalers and nebulizers

Do you ever use over-the-counter nasal sprays or inhalers?

¿Usa Ud. alguna vez rociadores nasales o inhaladores?

–What kind do you use?

–¿Qué clase usa Ud.?

–How frequently do you use them?

–¿Con qué frecuencia lo usa Ud.?

Do you take any over-the-counter or prescription drugs for your respiratory difficulties?

¿Toma Ud. medicamentos con receta o sin receta médica para sus dificultades respiratorias?

–Which drugs? / –¿Qué medicamentos?

–Any steroids? / –¿Esteroides?

–How often do you take them? / –¿Con qué frecuencia los toma Ud.?

–When did you last take these drugs? / –¿Cuándo fue la última vez que tomó estos medicamentos?

Do you use a nebulizer or other breathing treatment? / ¿Usa Ud. un nebulizador u otro tratamiento para respirar?

–What condition does it treat? / –¿Para qué enfermedad usa Ud. el tratamiento?

–What dose do you use? / –¿Qué dosis se le dió?

–How often do you have a treatment? / –¿Con qué frecuencia sigue Ud. un tratamiento?

–Do you ever experience any adverse effects from the treatment? / –¿Alguna vez tiene Ud. efectos adversos a causa del tratamiento?

–Do you follow special instructions for using the treatment? / –¿Sigue Ud. instrucciones especiales para el uso del tratamiento?

–When did you last do a treatment? / –¿Cuándo recibió el último tratamiento?

Using oxygen

Do you use oxygen at home? / ¿Usa Ud. oxígeno en casa?

–Do you use a cannula or a mask? / –¿Usa Ud. una cánula o máscara?

–How often do you use it? Continuously? Intermittently? / –¿Con qué frecuencia la usa? ¿Continuamente? ¿Intermitentemente?

–How long have you been using oxygen at home? / –¿Hace cuánto tiempo que Ud. usa oxígeno en casa?

Medical history

In the medical history, determine if the patient has a history of respiratory problems or has had tuberculosis, a chest X-ray, a flu vaccination, or a sinus infection.

Past problems

Have you had any lung problems?	¿Ha tenido Ud. problemas de los pulmones?
–Asthma?	–¿Asma?
–Tuberculosis?	–¿Tuberculosis?
–Pneumonia?	–¿Pulmonía?
–Influenza?	–¿Gripe?
–Sinus problems?	–¿Sinusitis?
–Emphysema?	–¿Enfisema?
–Allergies?	–¿Alergias?
–Other?	–¿Otros?
How long did the problem last?	¿Cuánto tiempo le duró el problema?
How was the problem treated?	¿Qué tratamiento recibió?

Previous exposure

Have you been exposed to anyone with a respiratory disease?	¿Ha estado Ud. expuesto(a) a alguna persona que tenga una enfermedad respiratoria?
–What type of disease?	–¿Qué clase de enfermedad?
–When were you exposed?	–¿Cuándo estuvo Ud. expuesto(a)?

Previous tests

Have you had chest surgery?	¿Lo han operado del pecho?
Have you had surgery on your___?	¿Fue operado_____?
–lungs	–de los pulmones
–sinuses	–de los senos nasales
–mouth, nose, or throat?	–de la boca, nariz, o garganta
Have you had a diagnostic study of the lungs?	¿Le han hecho una revisión de los pulmones?
–What type?	–¿De qué tipo?

–Why did you have it?

–¿Por qué tuvo la cirugía o por qué se le hizo el estudio?

When was your last chest X-ray?

¿Cuándo se le tomó la última radiografía de los pulmones?

When was your last tuberculosis test?

¿Cuándo se le hizo el último análisis para la tuberculosis?

–What was the result?

–¿Cuál fue el resultado?

Do you use home remedies for respiratory problems?

¿Usa Ud. remedios caseros para sus problemas respiratorios?

–What do you use?

–¿Qué usa Ud.?

Known allergies

Do you have allergies that flare up in different seasons?

¿Tiene Ud. alergias que se agravan durante diferentes temporadas del año?

–What causes them?

–¿Qué es lo que las causa?

–Do they cause any of these symptoms:

–¿Le causan alguno de los siguientes síntomas:

runny nose?

¿le gotea la nariz?

itching eyes?

¿picazón en los ojos?

congestion?

¿congestión?

other symptoms?

¿otros síntomas?

–What do you do to relieve these symptoms?

–¿Qué hace Ud. para aliviar estos síntomas?

Previous reactions

In the last 2 months, have you had:

¿En los últimos dos meses ha tenido:

–fever?

–fiebre?

–chills?

–escalofríos?

–fatigue?

–fatiga?

–night sweats?

–sudores nocturnos?

Have you ever had a blood test that showed you had anemia?

¿Alguno de sus análisis de sangre ha indicado que tenía anemia?

–When?

–¿Cuándo?

Do you ever have sinus pain?	¿Le han dolido alguna vez los senos nasales?
Do you ever have nasal discharge or postnasal drip?	¿Ha tenido alguna vez secreción nasal o goteo posnasal?
Do you ever have a bad taste in your mouth or bad breath?	¿Tiene alguna vez mal sabor en la boca o mal aliento?

Family history

Ask the patient about a family history of emphysema, asthma, respiratory allergies, and tuberculosis.

Has any member of your family had:	¿Algún miembro de su familia tuvo alguna de las siguientes enfermedades:
–emphysema?	–enfisema?
–asthma?	–asma?
–respiratory allergies?	–alergias del sistema respiratorio?
–tuberculosis?	–tuberculosis?
–sarcoidosis?	–sarcoidosis?
Did you have contact with the family member who had tuberculosis?	¿Estuvo Ud. en contacto con el miembro de la familia que tuvo tuberculosis?
–When?	–¿Cuándo?
–Do they live with you?	–¿Vive con Ud.?

Lifestyle

Ask the patient about lifestyle issues, such as smoking and sleep patterns. Also ask about factors at home or work that might cause respiratory problems, such as pets, excessive stress, and workplace irritants.

Use of tobacco

Do you smoke or chew tobacco?	¿Fuma Ud. o masca tabaco?
–What do you smoke?	–¿Qué fuma Ud.?
Cigarettes?	¿Cigarrillos?
Cigars?	¿Cigarros (puros)?

Pipes?

¿Pipas?

–How long have you smoked or chewed tobacco?

–¿Hace cuánto tiempo que Ud. fuma o masca tabaco?

–How many cigarettes, cigars, or pipes of tobacco do you smoke each day?

–¿Cuántos cigarrillos, cigarros (puros) o pipas de tabaco fuma Ud. al día?

–How much tobacco do you chew each day?

–¿Cuánto tabaco masca Ud. diariamente?

–Did you ever stop?

–¿Dejó Ud. alguna vez de fumar o mascar tabaco?

How long did it last?

¿Cuánto tiempo duró?

What method did you use to stop?

¿Qué método usó Ud. para dejar de fumar o mascar?

Do you remember why you started again?

¿Recuerda Ud. por qué volvió a comenzar a fumar o mascar tabaco otra vez?

–Have you smoked or chewed tobacco in the past?

–¿Ha Ud. fumado o mascado tabaco en el pasado?

What influenced you to stop?

¿Qué influenció sobre Ud. para parar?

Sleep patterns

How many pillows do you use when you sleep?

¿Cuántas almohadas usa Ud. para dormir?

–Are you using more or fewer pillows than you used to?

–¿Usa Ud. más o menos almohadas de las que usaba antes?

Have your sleep patterns changed because of breathing problems?

¿Han cambiado sus hábitos de dormir a causa de sus problemas respiratorios?

How many hours of sleep do you get each night?

¿Cuántas horas duerme por noche?

Living situation

How many people live with you?

¿Cuántas personas viven con Ud.?

Do you have pets?

¿Tiene Ud. animales en la casa?

–What type of pets do you have?

–¿Qué tipo de mascotas tiene Ud.?

–Does the animal's fur or feathers bother you?

–¿Le molestan a Ud. el pelaje o las plumas del animal?

–How does it bother you?

–¿Cómo le molestan?

  Runny nose?

  ¿Le gotea a Ud. la nariz?

  Cough?

  ¿Tose?

  Wheezing?

  ¿Respira con dificultad?

  Other?

  ¿Otro síntoma?

What type of home heating do you have?

¿Qué tipo de calefacción tiene Ud. en casa?

Are there any respiratory irritants in your home, such as fresh paint, cleaning sprays, or heavy cigarette smoke?

¿Hay en su casa agentes irritantes que le afectan la respiración, tales como pintura fresca, nebulización de productos de limpieza o humo de cigarrillos?

Do you have steps leading to or in your home?

¿Tiene escalones para entror en su casa o escaleras en su casa?

Do you have to walk up and down them often?

¿Tiene que subirlos o bajarlos con frecuencia?

Stress

Does stress at home or work affect your breathing?

¿Le afecta la respiración el estrés en casa o en el trabajo?

Do you have any special measures for stress management?

¿Toma Ud. algunas medidas especiales para controlar el estrés?

–What are they?

–¿Cuáles son?

Occupational concerns

What's your current occupation?

¿Cuál es su ocupación o empleo actual?

What were your previous occupations?

¿Qué otros empleos ha tenido anteriormente?

Are you exposed to any known respiratory irritants at work?

¿Sabe Ud. si está expuesto en su trabajo a agentes irritantes que afecten su respiración?

–Do you use safety measures during exposure?

–¿Usa Ud. medidas de seguridad mientras está expuesto(a)?

Selected references

———————————————○———————————————

American Association for Respiratory Care. "AARC Clinical Practice Guideline: Nasotracheal Suctioning," *Respiratory Care* 49(9):1080-84, September 2004.

American Association for Respiratory Care. "AARC Clinical Practice Guideline: Resuscitation and Defibrillation in the Health Care Setting," *Respiratory Care* 49(9):1085-99, September 2004.

American Heart Association. "2005 AHA Guidelines for Cardiopulmonary Resuscitation and Emergency Cardiovascular Care: International Consensus on Science," *Circulation* 112(22 Suppl):IV-1-IV-211, November 2005.

Buemi, M., et al. "From the Oxygen to the Organ Protection: Erythro-poietin as Protagonist in Internal Medicine," *Cardiovascular & Hematological Agents in Medicinal Chemistry* 4(4):299-311, October 2006.

Cecconi, M., et al. "What Role Does the Right Side of the Heart Play in Circulation?" *Critical Care* 10(Suppl 3):S5, 2006.

Hansel, N.N., and Diette, G.B. "Gene Expression Profiling in Human Asthma," *Proceedings of the American Thoracic Society* 4(1):32-36, January 2007.

Henke, M.O., et al. "The Role of Airway Secretions in COPD—Clinical Applications," *COPD* 2(3):377-90, September 2005.

Hoshi, S., et al. "Silico-Asbestosis that Responded to Steroid Therapy," *Internal Medicine* 45(15):917-21, 2006.

Ignatavicius, D.D., and Workman, M.L. *Medical-Surgical Nursing*, 5th ed. Philadelphia: W.B. Saunders Co., 2006.

Ijaz, K., et al. "Safety of the Rifampin and Pyrazinamide Short-Course Regimen for Treating Latent Tuberculosis Infection," *Clinical Infectious Diseases* 44(3):464-65, February 2007.

Lumb, A.B. *Nunn's Applied Respiratory Physiology*, 6th ed. Philadelphia: Butterworth-Heinemann, 2005.

Mistry, R, et al. "Gene-Expression Patterns in Whole Blood Identify Subjects at Risk for Recurrent Tuberculosis," *Journal of Infectious Disease* 195(3):357-65, February 2007.

Ng, T.P., et al. "Factors Associated with Acute Health Care Use in a National Adult Asthma Management Program," *Annals of Allergy, Asthma, and Immunology* 97(6):784-93, December 2006.

Paje, D.T., and Kremer, M.J. "The Perioperative Implications of Obstructive Sleep Apnea," *Orthopedic Nurse* 25(5):291-97, September-October 2006.

Phillips, B.A. *Year Book of Pulmonary Disease*. St. Louis: Mosby–Year Book, Inc., 2007.

Randhawa, K., et al. "Acute Effect of Cigarette Smoke and Nicotine on Airway Blood Flow and Airflow in Healthy Smokers," *Lung* 184(6):363-68, November-December 2006.

Razi, C., et al. "Effect of Montelukast on Symptoms and Exhaled Nitric Oxide Levels in 7- to 14-year-old Children with Seasonal Allergic Rhinitis," *Annals of Allergy, Asthma, and Immunology* 97(6):767-74, December 2006.

Schwartzstein, R.M., and Parker, M.J. *Respiratory Physiology: A Clinical Approach*. Philadelphia: Lippincott Williams & Wilkins, 2005.

Voelkel, N.F., et al. "Right Ventricular Function and Failure: Report of a National Heart, Lung, and Blood Institute Working Group on Cellular and Molecular Mechanisms of Right Heart Failure," *Circulation* 114(17):1883-91, October 2006.

Zervos, M., et al. "Efficacy and Safety of 3-day Azithromycin Versus 5-day Moxifloxacin for the Treatment of Acute Bacterial Exacerbations of Chronic Bronchitis," *International Journal of Antimicrobial Agents* 29(1):56-61, January 2007.

Zhanel, G.G., et al. "A Review of New Fluoroquinolones: Focus on their Use in Respiratory Tract Infections," *Treatments in Respiratory Medicine* 5(6):437-65, 2006.

Index

---

i refers to an illustration; t refers to a table.

i refers to an illustration; t refers to a table.

---

i refers to an illustration; t refers to a table.

i refers to an illustration; t refers to a table.

---

i refers to an illustration; t refers to a table.

i refers to an illustration; t refers to a table.

---

i refers to an illustration; t refers to a table.

i refers to an illustration; t refers to a table.

---

i refers to an illustration; t refers to a table.

i refers to an illustration; t refers to a table.

---

i refers to an illustration; t refers to a table.